Imperial Contagions

Centre for the Humanities and Medicine
The University of Hong Kong

Since its inauguration in 2009, the Centre for the Humanities and Medicine has fostered cross-disciplinary research on the interrelationship between disease, health, culture, and society. In collaboration with Hong Kong University Press, the Centre publishes work that promotes exchanges between the humanities and medicine.

Imperial Contagions

Medicine, Hygiene, and Cultures of Planning in Asia

Edited by Robert Peckham and David M. Pomfret

香港大學出版社
HONG KONG UNIVERSITY PRESS

Hong Kong University Press
The University of Hong Kong
Pokfulam Road
Hong Kong
www.hkupress.org

ISBN 978-988-8139-12-5 *(Hardback)*
ISBN 978-988-8139-52-1 *(Paperback)*

British Library Cataloguing-in-Publication Data
A catalogue record for this book is available from the British Library.

Cover image: "Drs. Young and Chai in Vaccine Laboratory, Changchun," lantern slide, 1911. Courtesy of the Harvard Medical Library in the Francis A. Countway Library of Medicine.

10   9   8   7   6   5   4   3   2   1

Printed and bound by Goodrich Int'l Printing Co., Ltd. in Hong Kong, China

Contents

Part III Circulations

Acknowledgments

The preparation of *Imperial Contagions* was made possible with generous support from the University of Hong Kong's Faculty of Arts in the form of a grant from the Louis Cha Fund under the China-West Studies Research Theme Initiative. We are also grateful to our colleagues in the Department of History who supported the project through the History Endowment Fund. The Centre for the Humanities and Medicine offered invaluable assistance throughout and we would like to thank, in particular, Maria Sin, for all her help in the preparation of the manuscript. We benefited greatly from the input of two anonymous reviewers and would like to take this opportunity to thank them for their comments on the original manuscript. We would also like to thank Clara Ho and Serina Poon from Hong Kong University Press for their help in the production of this book. Finally, many thanks to Christopher Cowell, and to the following for their encouragement and advice: Daniel Chua, Michael Duckworth, James Duncan, Kam Louie, Christopher Munn, Maureen Sabine, and Helen Meller.

Contributors

Sunil S. Amrith is Reader in the Department of History, Classics and Archaeology at Birkbeck College, University of London. His research is on the Bay of Bengal as a space of economic and cultural interaction, with a particular focus on the history of migration between South India and Southeast Asia in the nineteenth and twentieth centuries. He is the author of *Decolonizing International Health: India and Southeast Asia, 1930–65* (2006), *Migration and Diaspora in Modern Asia* (2011), and he is working on a volume entitled *Crossing the Bay of Bengal*.

Jiat-Hwee Chang is Assistant Professor in the Department of Architecture, School of Design and Environment at the National University of Singapore. His research focuses on the history of 'tropical architecture' in nineteenth-and twentieth-century British colonial and postcolonial networks, counter-histories and theories of sustainable architecture and urbanism in Asia.

Cecilia Chu is currently completing her Ph.D. thesis, entitled "Speculative Modern: Housing and the Politics of Representation in Colonial Hong Kong, 1900–1950," in the Department of Architecture at UC Berkeley.

Sander L. Gilman is Distinguished Professor of the Liberal Arts and Sciences at Emory University. A cultural and literary historian, his many works include *Smart Jews: The Construction of the Image of Jewish Superior Intelligence* (1996), *Making the Body Beautiful: A Cultural History of Aesthetic Surgery* (2000), and *Fat: A Cultural History of Obesity* (2008).

Richard Harris is Professor in the School of Geography and Earth Sciences at McMaster University. His research focuses on urban social and historical geography, including urban development in the British colonies, primarily between the 1920s and 1960s. He is the author of *Unplanned Suburbs: Toronto's*

American Tragedy, 1900–1950 (1996), *Creeping Conformity: How Canada Became Suburban, 1900–1960* (2004), and co-editor of *Changing Suburbs: Foundation, Form and Function* (1999).

Stephen Legg is Associate Professor in Cultural and Historical Geography at the University of Nottingham. He is the author of *Spaces of Colonialism: Delhi's Urban Governmentalities* (2007), a study of residential, policing, and infrastructural landscapes in India's new capital. He is currently completing a monograph, entitled *Scales of Prostitution: International Governmentalities and Interwar India*, which explores the politics of regulating prostitution in Delhi at the scale of national legislation, imperial campaigning, and the international covenant of the League of Nations.

Robert Lewis is Professor of Geography in the Department of Geography and Planning at the University of Toronto. His research focuses on the historical geographies of metropolitan economic and social processes in the United States and Canada between 1850 and 1960. He is the author of *Manufacturing Montreal: The Making of an Industrial Landscape, 1850 to 1930* (2000) and *Chicago Made: Factory Networks in the Industrial Metropolis, 1865–1940* (2008), and editor of *The Manufacturing Suburb: Building Work and Home on the Metropolitan Fringe* (2004).

Laurence Monnais is Associate Professor in the Department of History and the Centre for East Asian Studies (CETASE) at the Université de Montréal. She is a specialist in the history of medicine in colonial Vietnam; she also works on topics such as the healthcare practices of the Vietnamese diaspora in Canada and on the modern history of alternative medicines. She is the author of *Médecine et colonisation. L'aventure Indochinoise, 1860–1939* (1999) and is currently co-editing two further volumes, *Histories of Medicine in Southeast Asia* and *Vietnamese Medicine in the Making: Southern Medicine for Southern People*.

Robert Peckham is Co-Director of the Centre for the Humanities and Medicine at the University of Hong Kong, where he is also Assistant Professor in the Department of History. His current research focuses on histories of infectious disease and epidemic control, technologies of biopower, and the modern state's role in the supervision of public health. He is the editor of the volume *Disease and Crime: A History of Social Pathologies and the New Politics of Health* (forthcoming), and is currently completing a monograph entitled *Infective Economies: Plague and the Crisis of Empire*.

David M. Pomfret is Associate Professor in Modern European History at the University of Hong Kong. He is the author of *Young People and the European City: Age Relations in Nottingham and Saint-Etienne, 1890–1940* (2004).

Ruth Richardson is Visiting Professor in the School of Humanities at the University of Hong Kong. She is Affiliated Scholar in the History and Philosophy of Science at the University of Cambridge and Senior Visiting Research Fellow in the Centre for Life-Writing Research at King's College London. She is the author of numerous books, including *Death, Dissection and the Destitute* (2001), *The Making of Gray's Anatomy: Bodies, Books, Fortune, Fame* (2008), and *Dickens and the Workhouse: Oliver Twist and the London Poor* (2012).

Priscilla Wald is Professor of English at Duke University. She is the author of *Constituting Americans: Cultural Anxiety and Narrative Form* (1995). Her recent book-length study, *Contagious: Cultures, Carriers, and the Outbreak Narrative* (2008), considers the intersection of medicine and myth in the idea of contagion and the evolution of the contemporary stories we tell about the global health problem of 'emerging infections.' She is currently at work on a book-length study entitled *Human Being After Genocide*.

Introduction: Medicine, Hygiene, and the Re-ordering of Empire

Robert Peckham and David M. Pomfret

Fears of contagion played a critical role in the re-ordering of British and French colonial societies in Asia from the mid-nineteenth to the twentieth centuries. *Imperial Contagions* explores this key theme in the history of empire, investigating connections between the reconceptualization of disease and the construction of colonial cities in Europe's expanding empires. It shows how new, laboratory-based understandings of infection challenged and informed sanitary and environmental approaches to disease and health, and provided often contradictory rationales for the re-creation of colonial space. How were locales such as schools, clinics, and bacteriological laboratories—as well as apparatuses of governance such as censuses, sanitary interventions, and migration controls—implicated in this process? How did they connect with new meanings of disease? And to what extent was disease management intertwined with forms of social ordering, cultures of colonialism, and the disciplinary organization of new medico-scientific knowledge?

This book elaborates on the mutual idioms of medical science and empire, with their common focus on 'cultures' and 'colonies,' and examines the entanglement of medicine, public health, European overseas expansion, and entrenchment in the nineteenth and twentieth centuries. It explores this entanglement as a spatial predicament in Asia through a number of case studies that address intersecting themes in different settings and, in so doing, contribute to the "spatial turn" in the history of science and medicine.[1] The emphasis is on the emplacement of scientific and medical practices, the pathologization of colonized places, and spatial responses to colonial anxieties about contagion. Against this background, many of the chapters collected here demonstrate how colonial medicine and regimes of hygiene in Asia were constituted, not only to deal with infectious diseases, but to manage apprehensions that these 'tropical' afflictions induced in colonial communities.

1

To be sure, notions of empire had very different meanings in British, French, German, Spanish, and Portuguese contexts, as Nancy Leys Stepan has shown in her discussion of tropical nature, disease, and race.[2] The focus in this volume is predominantly on British and French colonial settings in Asia, ranging from the Indian Subcontinent to Indochina and Hong Kong. At the same time, *Imperial Contagions* contributes to current discussions about the extent to which, as Charlotte Furth has recently observed in the context of Chinese East Asia, "different regimes of empire […] do not produce an overarching narrative of imperialism."[3] Although medicine and public health tend to be understood as state-and nation-building projects, there is good reason, as Furth suggests, to "trace global genealogies of scientific practices in interaction with highly local situations."[4] Consequently, *Imperial Contagions* seeks to explore the dynamics between local situations and transcolonial and metropolitan networks, thereby problematizing neat divisions between colonizer and colonized and challenging the idea of colonialism as "a coherent symbolic order." As Nicholas Thomas has remarked, if colonizing projects were "frequently split between assimilationist and segregationist ways of dealing with indigenous populations," so "colonizing constantly generated obstacles to neat boundaries and hierarchies between populations."[5]

The book examines the contradictory impulses that informed colonial planning policies between approximately 1880 and 1949. Colonial administrators strove, on the one hand, to protect the integrity of colonial spaces from external and internal threats of contamination, while, on the other hand, facilitating mobility across and between colonial states with a view to safeguarding the economic vitality upon which empire was predicated. Each of the essays in the volume investigates the "frictions" and contradictions of empire through these themes, but from different vantage points.[6]

In the 1880s, the word 'pathogen' gained currency, reflecting a new understanding of disease and its etiology. The rise of germ theory and laboratory science informed the implementation of state-sponsored measures designed not only to protect public health, but to manage and make legible governed populations. The term 'medicine,' however, with its suggestion of internal coherence, continued to obscure the complex and often conflicting interpretations of disease that persisted well into the twentieth century, and the tendency for overlap between the new laboratory science, medical practice, and hygienic and sanitary approaches to health. Thus, in 1931, when the bacteriologist Aldo Castellani published *Climate and Acclimatization*, he felt able to condemn what he saw as the "fashion" for denying that "climate has any injurious influence on the health of Europeans living in the tropics."[7] Castellani—noted for his work on the cause and transmission of sleeping sickness—did not deny the role played by parasites and hygienic conditions in the dissemination of disease, but he reasserted the influence of telluric agents in contagion, arguing that "there have been signs in various quarters tending to show that the importance of climatic factors is again going to be generally recognised."[8] This example is suggestive of the way in which older ideas and technologies continued to influence newer scientific particularities, even as they were being extrapolated into colonial policy. Beyond the new disciplinary and spatial infrastructures through which public health was advanced, this book considers the enduring significance, after the "bacteriological turn," of older models of disease transmission and the hygienic enclaves they produced.[9]

An important focus in *Imperial Contagions* is on the contestation of colonial medical knowledge and on challenging assumptions that remain prevalent about medicine's appropriation by colonial government as a critical "tool of empire."[10] The book draws attention to the complex outcomes of the situated encounters between 'Western' medicine and non-Western contexts. It does so by showing how imperialist exploitation took a variety of forms, extending from coercive interventionism to outright neglect. Medicine and public health were never simply diffused from 'center' to 'periphery' or imposed upon colonies in any straightforward way. At the same time, as several chapters in the volume make clear, colonial authorities were acutely aware of the shortcomings of public health initiatives launched from within colonial states. Indigenous agents sometimes appropriated—but could also act as a brake upon—the professional practices being imported into their midst. Discourses and technologies of health used to delimit and define subject peoples' identities and to manage urban populations also produced indigenous engagements with such framings.[11] This book thus moves beyond the dichotomies of dominance and resistance to illustrate how medicine and health, as key dimensions of European colonial culture, were transformed, re-oriented, and reproduced through contact with local agency and indigenous practice.

Laboratory science, as Bruno Latour has noted, provides a suggestive way for rethinking agency in a colonial setting. Bacteria, as agents of identifiable diseases, were never simply natural 'objects' to be studied; they were also in some sense 'subjects,' since they were construed as being equipped with a capacity and volition to infect. As such, following Latour, bacteria might be deemed "quasi-objects."[12] The ambiguous status of microbiological life, which underpinned scientific medicine, mirrored, it might be argued, the similarly equivocal status of the colonial subject within imperial planning policy, remaining at once a pliable object of government and a recalcitrant agent of disruption: in short, a "quasi-object" and "quasi-subject." In developing this theme, which links colonial cultures of planning with notions of agency, the essays in the volume explore colonial economies of scale, which ranged from the microscopic bacterium to macroscopic realms of empire. In different ways, each contributor engages with such questions as: How did these different levels connect with one another? How were they studied, mapped, represented, and responded to? How were scientific particularities, from there, extrapolated into colonial policy—or, indeed, were they?

In existing scholarship on colonial medicine and public health, discussions of the shift away from enclavism have tended to be framed in teleological and exclusivist terms, but the essays collected here suggest that it was precisely as colonial authorities began to extend the scope of their policies outwards that enclavist ideals became most clearly articulated, in carefully controlled and purportedly 'pure' or 'hygienic' spaces: schools, clubs, hospitals, botanical gardens, hill stations, and laboratories. In other words, *Imperial Contagions* argues that no straightforward shift from enclavism to public health occurred. On the contrary, the institutionalization of health and the refashioning of the urban environment were coterminous with the creation of circumscribed spaces, exemplified by the laboratory, wherein privileged bodies—those of children, scientists, and administrators—were protected from the threat of contamination. From this perspective, *Imperial Contagions* maintains that the era of colonial public health should perhaps be understood, not in terms of the demise of enclavism, but rather as its radical reaffirmation.

The debates surrounding the establishment of public gardens in Hong Kong, first mooted in the 1840s, and the subsequent drive to extend the plantation with a comprehensive program of afforestation, illustrate the impetus to push the 'enclave' outwards into the colony at large. As the British Empire expanded, so satellite Kew Gardens were set up across its dispersed dominions, forming "a network that circulated living plants, specimens, and information across the globe."[13] These botanical gardens were sites of scientific research, economic return (with the planting of valuable crops such as tea, sisal, and cinchona), as well as leisure.[14] They were also models of a 'healthy' environment and a reminder of the need for cultivation. As the colony's governor, Hercules

Robinson, noted in 1861, the formation of "Public Gardens" would "contribute to the embellishment of the City of Victoria and the health and enjoyment of its inhabitants."[15]

High rates of mortality in Hong Kong were attributed to the insalubrious tropical weather, particularly in the early colonial years, leading the government to afforest the island in the hope that this would reduce disease and improve health.[16] Charles Ford was appointed superintendent of gardens in 1871 and oversaw the afforestation of the colony.[17] Although the focus of *Imperial Contagions* is principally on the built environment, nonetheless the engineering of a hygienic 'nature' by colonial agencies and, more particularly, the extension of the 'garden' into the pathologized places of the colony, are reminders that the colonial 'cultures of planning,' evoked in the subtitle to this volume, involved the co-production of nature and society, and a complex interweaving of political, economic, and hygienic interests.

Empire was sustained, of course, by a fundamental mobility of people, commodities, capital, and information,[18] and by novel technologies of global communication.[19] Much has been written on the "web of empire,"[20] and the transnational or diasporic networks that formed within and between colonial cities.[21] Although the emphasis is often on the competitive nature of medical science, recent research has emphasized the collaborative, transnational network of researchers and clinicians who carried out drug therapy trials, for example, on sleeping sickness patients in African colonies at the turn of the century.[22] The theme of technological transference between colonial states and the metropole underlies many of the chapters in this volume. While the Contagious Diseases Acts (1864–69) were exported from Britain to its imperial dominions, the legislation to curb venereal disease had itself been profoundly shaped by Britain's colonial experience. Similarly, Charles Booth's survey of life and labor in London (1886–1903), which charted the 'black' areas of the metropole, was an important influence on the mapping of colonial cities.

A key focus of the chapters is on the ways in which colonial authorities sought to promote certain forms of 'healthy' circulations, even as they endeavored to restrict other forms of potentially 'unhealthy' trafficking, including the spread of infectious disease. Writing on the antecedents of contemporary globalization, Michael Hardt and Antonio Negri observe:

> The horror released by European conquest and colonialism is a horror of unlimited contact, flow, and exchange—or really the horror of contagion, miscegenation, and unbounded life. Hygiene requires protective barriers.

> European colonialism was continually plagued by contradictions between virtuous exchange and the danger of contagion, and hence it was characterized by a complex play of flows and hygienic boundaries between metropole and colony and among colonial territories.[23]

The Asian plague pandemic in the 1890s brought these issues of flow and counter-flow to the fore, as colonial authorities in Hong Kong and India sought to curb the movement of people, even as they strove to bolster trade. The report of the plague in Hong Kong published in *The Times* of London on June 13, 1894, is suggestive in this context:

> Half native population [of] Hongkong left, numbering 100,000. Leaving by thousands daily; 1,500 deaths; several Europeans seized, one died. Labour market paralyzed. Deaths nearly hundred daily. Government anticipates failure of opium revenue; proposes taking over and destroying all unhealthy native quarters.[24]

Here, the colonial imperative to keep trade routes open at all costs ran up against colonial fears of microbial invasion. Economics—the "labour market"—was conceptualized in pathological terms ("paralyzed"), while disease was equated with economic deterioration and dislocation: the failure of the opium revenue. In short, the passage attests to a complex conflation wherein movements of the "native" population, the spread of disease, and the destruction of "unhealthy native quarters," inscribe the connective and disruptive processes seen to lie at the core of empire.

Imperial Contagions is organized into three parts. In Part I, "Building for Health," the focus is on colonial governmentality and planning. Contributors explore the extent to which the priorities of colonial medicine and planning began to shift during the final decades of the nineteenth and beginning of the twentieth centuries, away from an 'enclavist' approach—servicing colonial officials and the military—towards a more all-encompassing 'public health' approach that integrated indigenous populations and their spaces into a more centralized colonial regime. Cecilia Chu demonstrates the extent to which colonial sanitary measures and housing reforms were contested by the local Chinese population in Hong Kong in the aftermath of the 1894 plague. More specifically, she considers debates about property rights and argues that an analysis of "the convergence of interests between the Chinese and European property owners and their shifting allegiance to the colonial state also reveals the complex power relations between these agencies." In his chapter on housing and sanitation in Singapore between 1907 and 1942, Jiat-Hwee Chang argues that the colonial state, despite gestural efforts at housing improvement, left the native population alone, reinforcing forms of segregation. Finally, Richard Harris and Robert Lewis in their chapter on the 1901 census in Bombay and Calcutta suggest that "the plague called into question [European] strategies for separating themselves from the native population and from disease, both contagious and otherwise."

The chapters in Part II, "Hygienic Enclaves," consider the expansion of the colonial 'enclave' from the 1880s. David Pomfret adopts a comparative perspective to focus on the Victoria Peak Hill Reservation in Hong Kong and the hill station of Dalat in the French 'protectorate' of Annam (modern Vietnam). He shows how the histories of these hygienic spaces were interwoven with a moral imperative to safeguard foreign children in 'tropical' contexts and to (re)produce governing elites. The production of the 'child' in empire informed efforts to carve out hygienic spaces and to support their expansion into the pathologized field. These moves drew heavily upon nascent laboratory science and gave expression to latent "anxieties about racial and cultural reproduction in the tropics."

Stephen Legg charts the "shift in the scientific episteme from that of contamination to that of contagion" as a conceptual underpinning for everything from medical practices to urban planning. Focusing on urban health and venereal diseases in interwar India, he demonstrates how new regulations concerning public health manifest "a contagionist but individualist concern with infection, as well as a newly internationalist concern both with imperial race and the potential of a postcolonial scientific modernity."

Finally, Robert Peckham explores the history of Alexandre Yersin's makeshift 'matshed' laboratory, constructed in Hong Kong in 1894 during the plague epidemic. Peckham investigates the properties of the improvised colonial laboratory and argues that they reveal a fundamental ambivalence about the constitution of 'healthy' and 'unhealthy' dwellings, throwing into relief the equivocal boundaries between colonial and indigenous spaces, as well as underscoring a colonial discourse that construed scientific research as a form of 'exploration.'

Part III of the volume, "Circulations," examines different forms of colonial mobility across and between colonies and the metropole. It considers public health and colonial medicine as a multicentered process connecting actors and forming bridges across borders. Sunil Amrith explores how the "mobile bodies" of Indian migrants to Southeast Asia gave rise to deep-rooted colonial anxieties about the threat of 'contagion.' He argues that new economic systems emerged between the mid-nineteenth and mid-twentieth centuries requiring new forms of labor, which created new social networks as migrant labor moved "from the heartlands of India and China" into "Asia's frontier zones."

Professional 'experts' and the working and personal relationships that they developed were critical to the circulation of knowledge and the technologies it produced between colonies and metropole. Adopting a transnational approach to the history of contagion can shed new light upon the entanglements of these actors within the structures of colonial states.[25] In her account of Henry Vandyke Carter's work on leprosy in India, Ruth Richardson explores how circulation was integral to the tensions and contradictions of colonial science and medicine on the ground. Carter was an imperial agent working across and between Europe and India. On the one hand, his efforts to map the distribution of leprosy—and thereby to make contagious native populations legible—helped to sustain the colonial state. At the same time, however, Carter was at pains to assert leprosy as a transnational phenomenon. Indeed, in many respects Carter's contribution to the state was premised upon his ability to transcend its boundaries in what Richardson calls a new "humanitarianism."

Sander Gilman considers the contemporary "obesity epidemic" in China within the context of nineteenth-and twentieth-century histories of China–West interactions, and particularly the ways in which circulations of Western medical and health discourses have helped to shape Chinese identity. Elsewhere, Larissa N. Heinrich has demonstrated the naturalizing powers of medical representations and argued for the role of Western medicine in the formation of Chinese ideas about the body and the nation.[26] Gilman here develops these ideas to consider obesity as both a 'real' condition and a construction produced by the circulation of medical and health discourses, as well as fears about the contaminating 'invasion' of Western products, such as tinned milk, into China.

Finally, Laurence Monnais considers the distribution of quinine as a cornerstone of the colonial state's preventive public health policy against malaria in Indochina. Examining the history of the State Quinine Service, an institution invested with the task of distributing subsidized quinine, Monnais points to the failure of the program and argues that quinine cannot be considered an effective "tool of empire." Her study reveals the fundamental disjuncture between the system of quinine distribution and the geographical diffusion of the disease. French colonials not only failed to curtail contagion but, through the development of an infrastructure intended to support the *mise en valeur*, were complicit in spreading disease from the "modernizing front" into the native village. Concluding that under French rule "the development of natural resources was prioritised over the development of human resources," Monnais offers an insight into a key theme: the devastating demographic impact of public health systems and colonial medicine.[27]

Notwithstanding the book's thematic organization, the chapters intersect in terms of theoretical approach and focus. Chang and Peckham, for example, both deal with the historical evolution of architectural forms and their mobility between metropole and colonies and across empire. Many of the chapters explore the interrelationship between individuals—as agents of colonial scientific, medical, health and planning policy—and broader social, political, and economic processes. In so doing, they engage with recent scholarship on urban modernity, which has stressed the role of technologically savvy cadres of professionals in the construction of modern cities from Chicago to Tokyo.[28]

Moreover, this collection of essays engages with the racial segregation of colonial communities, a theme in the history of colonial urban planning currently being re-examined in relation to the transnational movements of professional experts and modern planning ideas.[29] Professional planners reveled in the relative freedom that colonial contexts seemed to afford for the realization of modern, hygienically informed city planning. Although 'on the ground' these freedoms proved to be chimeric, scores of experts drew inspiration from the notion of the colony as laboratory and compared and constrasted ameliorative interventions across empires. Professor W. J. R. Simpson, for example, as Chang shows in this volume, assessed sanitary conditions and advised British colonial administrations from East Africa to Singapore.[30] Similarly, Ernest Hébrard drew upon his knowledge of the hill station of Baguio (in the Philippines), the garden city in Welwyn, London, and his own earlier work in Thessaloniki, Greece, when formulating a master plan for Dalat in 1923.[31]

As Ilana Löwy has recently observed in the context of biomedical research in ex-colonial countries, "the visualization of plagues was at the same time antithetical to modernity and a symbol of modernization."[32] Scientific technologies made visible 'backwardness,' even as scientists and colonial agents sought to represent themselves as embodiments of progress. Chapters in this collection expose the contradictions of empire in many places, particularly the ways in which colonial authorities created the very conditions that promoted the diseases they were seeking to eradicate. Thus, Legg shows how the British in India attributed the spread of venereal disease to the behavior of local populations, even though it is generally recognized that the British colonial economy sponsored the cities and mobile labor that created modern prostitution in India. And Monnais suggests that French efforts to counter the spread of malaria in Indochina by promoting new technologies, notably the railway, were partially self-defeating, since the railways arguably facilitated the dissemination of infection.

These forms of colonial contradiction and their capacity to destabilize are highlighted within several studies in this volume, both with reference to actual epidemic and disease episodes and metaphorical representations of disease threats. For example, the impetus to control contagion prompted colonial authorities to devise strategies for managing colonized people in certain spaces and across certain boundaries—as Harris and Lewis argue in relation to the census of 1901—thus inadvertently producing the conditions within which colonized peoples acceded to a form of subjecthood (albeit one defined in terms of physical health rather than political rights) that was to herald proliferating and ultimately uncontrollable demands for political representation.

'Colony,' 'culture,' and 'immunity' have been loaded terms, particularly from the 1880s. The shifting meaning of this 'colonial' terminology points to the entanglement of imperialism, governmentality, public health, and laboratory-based science, as many of the contributors to this volume demonstrate. It also suggests a complex interrelationship between microcultures and macrocultures, microparasites and macroparasites. Thus, European colonies, 'colonies' of bacteria on petri dishes and leper 'colonies'; immunity from the invasion of disease and diplomatic immunity;[33] resistance to disease and native resistance to colonial authority; the acculturation of the 'child peoples' of empire, and the inoculation of children of colonial subjects with vaccine cultures.

As one commentator has observed on the development of Kochian bacteriology in the Japanese colonial context:

> It is possible to take this process as an analogy for the production of Japanese cultures in colonies such as Korea and Taiwan. There, analogous attempts were made to construct a transparent medium for cultivation with the establishment of Japanese education and standardized language. It was a process of selection and purification.[34]

In the Philippines, a Bureau of Government Laboratories was established in 1901 with the aim of finding scientific solutions that would, as Warwick

Anderson has noted, "transcend" the tropical environment and enable white colonizers to survive the tropics. At the same time, the laboratory was extended outwards so that the Philippine archipelago was itself increasingly conceived as an "incipient colonial laboratory."[35]

At least from the 1870s, as scientist-investigators began to focus on the causal, bacteriological agents of disease, medicine began to move into the new sphere of public health. The resistance of British military and government elites to the laboratory on the grounds that it constituted a rarefied space for 'bacteriological speculation'—one that was fundamentally cut off from the practical issues of managing society—sits at odds with the ambiguities in the very idiom of colonial governmentality, which suggest, on the contrary, a profound intertwining of biomedical research and urban management from at least the 1870s. How should we explain these apparently contradictory trajectories, particularly in the colonies—the contiguous move into the laboratorial 'sanctuary' and out into the teeming 'pathogenic' colonial city? The issue at stake is the extent to which laboratories—particularly colonial laboratories from the 1890s, and in the wake of the plague pandemic—contributed to the transformation of an enclavist approach to health into a more interventionist and expansionist public health. Or indeed, whether such a transformation ever took place. Certainly in Taiwan, Korea, and to a lesser extent in Japan's 'informal empire' in China, epidemic episodes, notably the Manchurian plague outbreak of 1910–11, served as a spur to the development of sanitary infrastructures and a new focus on the "hygienic 'uplift' of the indigenous population."[36] Public health measures were extended in the Dutch East Indies and British Malaya following World War I.[37] Within the French empire, in the specific case of Indochina, the scope and ambition of the colonial government's efforts from 1905 to effect such improvements and to extend recognition of individual behaviors as part of a wider 'public health' was far greater, though the effectiveness of this drive (which was intimately informed by the Pastorian laboratory infrastructure) must remain in question.[38]

Whatever the extent of the expansion of public health, the laboratory represented an ideal of hygienic modernity and a locus of somatic regulation, as Pomfret and Peckham both argue in this volume. As such, the laboratory furnished a model for the colony writ large. Yet, the laboratory was only ever that: a model. The notion of the colony as a "laboratory of modernity," the chapters in this volume suggest, is fundamentally flawed in that it presupposes a standardization of practice and a uniformity of disciplinary power within empire that was often absent. As Peter Zinoman has argued in his account of the Indochinese prison system, regimes of colonial power were complex, heterogenous, and often "ill-disciplined."[39] Colonial space was fraught with tensions and contradictions between ideology and practical exigencies, between local and central government, indigenous resistance and colonial indigenization. Though administrators and planners referred to their work in colonial contexts as a kind of 'experiment' conducted upon supposedly neutral 'testing grounds,' these tensions and conflicts ensured that the implementation of plans (in which segregation remained a guiding principle) tended to be messy and, at best, partial.[40] As several chapters contend in this volume, exploring the shifting relationship between institutional spaces and the 'field' becomes a way of highlighting the unstable frameworks of colonial segregation.

Ironically, the conceptualization of the colony as a 'laboratory' for the production of new knowledges has been re-inscribed in much postcolonial theorizing of empire. On the one hand, it has been argued that, from the mid-nineteenth century, India was perceived as a laboratory for the creation of the liberal administrative state.[41] On the other hand, colonies have been construed as "laboratories of modernity": places "where missionaries, educators, and doctors could carry out experiments in social engineering without confronting the popular resistances and bourgeois rigidness of European society at home."[42]

In particular, the colonial city, whether French or British, has been viewed as a laboratory where Western rationalism could be imposed upon "rampant sensuality, irrationality, and decadence."[43] Hanoi, for example, has been described as "an experimental laboratory for the demonstration of the latest planning ideas and regulations introduced in France . . . Hanoi was seen as an experimental laboratory for achieving the perfect colonial society."[44] There has thus been an unconscious re-inscription of the term so that nineteenth-century notions of the colonial laboratory continue to be evoked as justifications for the study of the colonial and postcolonial city. Thus, Anthony D. King:

> What insights or data can we derive from studying colonial cities? … It is a laboratory for testing hypotheses: for geographers, on the cultural variable in environments; for anthropologists, on the dynamics of social change and the 'Westernisation' of material culture; . . . for architects and planners, it demonstrates the distinction between 'ethnic planning' and the 'rational professionalism' of the Western capitalist city . . .[45]

Or Gwendolyn Wright:

> The colonies provided more than the ideal laboratory so often evoked, and more than the mirror we might refer to today. They functioned like a magnifying glass, revealing with startling clarity the ambitions and fears, the techniques and policies that pertained at home, here carried out almost without restraints.[46]

The notion of empires, or individual colonies, as "laboratories of modernity" continues to be reiterated within postcolonial studies, even though such allusions inadvertently reaffirm a colonial discourse that sought to legitimate colonial rule in pseudo-scientific terms as 'experiment.' The essays in *Imperial Contagions* seek, in different ways, to dismantle the rhetorical construction of the "laboratory of modernity" in postcolonial theory by exploring how medico-scientific ideas of contagion were materialized in a variety of colonial settings. What has sometimes been understated in studies of transnational mobility, of course, is immobility and, particularly, the local.[47] The aim here is to demonstrate the ways in which, on a material level, medical knowledge was extended outwards to shape colonial cities and the governance of their populations, even as empire and its planning cultures migrated inwards to determine the spaces of medical research where the microscopic agents of disease were contemporaneously coming to be identified.

Imperial Contagions provides a comparative, transnational framework for rethinking colonial medicine, hygiene, and cultures of planning in Asia, thereby extending the scope of previous scholarship, which has tended to focus on discrete regions or single empires.[48] The geographical scope of the book encompasses a variety of colonial contexts, from South Asia through Southeast Asia, and along the China coast. By extending its focus within and across empires in Asia, the book provides comparative breadth, allowing it to shed new light upon the ways in which health and colonial medicine were implemented across borders and transregionally.[49]

The volume brings together scholars from the history of medicine and science, comparative urban planning, cultural geography, literary studies, and cultural history to re-orient debate about the ways in which medicine, public health, and planning were created by and helped to produce empire. At a time when the origins and meaning of pandemic disease are being hotly debated, the book will broaden understandings of contagion as a biological, cultural, and political phenomenon.[50] It provides new theoretical insights into the ways in which contagion worked as metaphor and practice through the development, planning, and segregation of colonial-era East and South Asian cities.[51] It also

complements and nuances recent studies of the tensions and ambiguities that
have characterized colonial responses towards the problem of public health,
and explores the gulf between discourses of power and the spatial practices that
actually resulted.[52] By the same token, as Priscilla Wald observes in the after-
word to this volume, each of the contributors illuminates, from a different perspective, the ways in which the re-ordering of colonial space in the nineteenth
and twentieth centuries continues to have consequences for the ways in which
we imagine and manage communicable disease today.

I

Building for Health

1
Combating Nuisance: Sanitation, Regulation, and the Politics of Property in Colonial Hong Kong

Cecilia Chu

Introduction

Despite important breakthroughs in medical science, in the nineteenth century infectious diseases ravaged crowded cities and towns across the globe with growing intensity. In the absence of reliable explanations for the causes of many deadly diseases, anxiety over epidemic outbreaks was often manifested in a powerful mixture of moral and cultural prejudice that saw the destitute and the impoverished designated as the likely carriers of diseases due to their "uncleanly habits."[1] In colonial territories, this prejudice was mapped onto native populations, perceived by many Europeans to belong to inferior races that had yet to acquire the basic concepts of hygiene and 'civilized' habits of living. The drawing of racial boundaries along the lines of health and cultural practices also allowed colonial authorities to implement racial segregation and other discriminatory legislations through which different rules were applied.[2]

Recent research on colonial urbanism has shown that the regulation of the colonial built environment was far more contested than has been previously assumed. As a major site of ongoing resistance and control, efforts to improve sanitation and public health in colonial cities have attracted interest from a growing number of scholars.[3] By examining the ways in which rules and regulations were resisted and appropriated in everyday practices, their studies have helped challenge the long-accepted dominance of the colonial state. Comparisons between housing and sanitary reforms in the metropole and the colonies, as well as indigenous responses to modernization efforts, have also enabled the articulation of the term "indigenous modernities,"[4] which seeks to acknowledge the multiple forms of colonial development and the roles of native peoples in transforming the built environment according to their own motivations.

The emphasis on the opposition between 'indigenous agency' and the 'colonial order' can sometimes be misleading, however. The tendency of historical accounts to focus on selected moments of conflict may leave out the more nuanced but arguably influential perspectives, such as those of colonial officials sympathetic to the natives or indigenous elites who aligned themselves with the colonial regimes. By slipping too easily from identifying the unequal power relations between the 'colonizers' and the 'colonized' to making broad assertions about collective ideologies, there is risk of overlooking the more complex political and economic processes that shaped historical change.[5]

Although much has been written about the role of colonial medicine as a tool of imperialism, the history of public health is still largely understood as an uncomplicated story of scientific progress. As Christopher Hamlin contends, the fact that so many of the technological achievements, such as underground drainage and water supplies, that came to define the modern built environment were no longer seen as questionable only proves the extent to which they have been "blackboxed."[6] But although a world in which modern sanitation is rejected might seem inconceivable in the present, it was not so in the nineteenth century. The now widely praised Chadwickean public health reforms, which involved heavy expenditure and state intervention, were constantly challenged in respect to their rationality, practicality, and cultural appropriateness when they were first introduced. Widespread resistance against regulations to improve housing and sanitation can be found in cities across the British Empire, where concepts of health and culture and the meanings of rights and obligations were being debated and constructed anew by different groups. While competing theories of medicine coexisted in many places, they were selectively endorsed by local administrators who used them to legitimize policies that suited their political agendas.[7] Meanwhile, colonial doctors, engineers, European and native landlords, and many others with stakes in housing and sanitary reform all sought to rationalize their priorities as those that served society's best interests.

To excavate some of the ways in which ideas and knowledge of health and sanitation were constructed and made useful for specific purposes, this chapter examines a number of controversies over British efforts to eliminate nuisance and improve sanitary conditions in Hong Kong in the last quarter of the nineteenth century. In keeping with the theme of this volume, which explores the complex entanglement between medicine, public health, and colonial planning in Asia, this chapter demonstrates the extent to which colonial sanitary measures were contested and appropriated by the local Chinese population. The first of these controversies involves a challenge launched by Chinese property owners against a set of building regulations that aimed to make the Chinese tenements more 'healthy'. The second concerns the provision of a universal water supply for the native population—an initiative that colonial sanitary engineers argued was essential for inducing personal cleanliness and preventing epidemic outbreaks. Finally, the chapter considers the debate over the demolition of a large number of 'unsanitary' Chinese houses after the 1894 bubonic plague outbreak, which incited a flurry of debate over the colonial state's simultaneous obligation to protect private property rights and the health and wellbeing of its subjects.

While all the cases concern specific issues and policy actions (and inaction), taken together they indicate how certain rationalities about development, public health, property rights, and Hong Kong as a colonial 'laissez-faire' polity itself came to be accepted and consolidated over time despite the apparent disputes over many initiatives when they were first introduced. It is argued that what needs to be examined is not so much the extent to which native populations were being discriminated against in specific policies or projects, but the emergence of new modes of governance wherein the 'colonizers' and the 'colonized' both adapted themselves to a changing political and economic order.[8] This is certainly not to downplay the inequalities and coercion existing in a colonial situation. But more attention to co-options and dialogues—not just outright contestation and conflicts—is needed because all are essential elements in the construction of discourse. As Robert Peckham and David Pomfret point out in the introduction to this volume, the discourses and technologies of health used to construct subject peoples' identities formed an essential part of indigenous agents' interactions with such framings. Attending to the shifting allegiances between Chinese property owners and the colonial state in three cases, this chapter seeks to bring to light the contradictions within the colonial planning culture of Hong Kong and the market system which underpinned it. A further aim, is to explore the formation of "epistemic communities," investigating the ways in which these communities both challenged and helped to shape Hong Kong's colonial culture.[9]

Speculation, Regulation, and the Colonial Conundrum

The urban condition of early Hong Kong exemplifies the laissez-faire development characteristic of so many of the colonial entrepôts that emerged in the nineteenth century. Constrained by an imperial fiscal policy that required it to pay for its own public works and administrative expenses, the colonial administration had been reluctant to commit to long-term planning and urban investment.[10] Because Hong Kong was designated as a free port and thus could not impose taxes on imported goods, its options for raising public funds were limited mainly to the collection of land rent, property rate, and licensing fees for local trades and services. To maximize revenue, the government adopted a 'high land price policy' within a leasehold system. By keeping a strict limit on land supply while not imposing too many regulations on development, it was able to ensure a good return from land auctions and property taxes.[11] While this system was lauded for its success in boosting fiscal revenue and creating a competitive 'free' land market, it also led to a chronic housing shortage and rampant property speculation that drove up rental costs to an exorbitant level. The problem was worst in the Chinese districts, where many low-income laborers had little choice but to share bed spaces in crowded and often poorly constructed tenements.[12] Ironically, the high rental return offered by these tenements through subdivision also made them an extremely profitable property holding. Moreover, many European and Chinese landowners preferred to invest in this type of building rather than the better-built European houses designed for single families.

From the very beginning of colonial rule, the government was keen to encourage Chinese property ownership (even though the most valuable properties were always reserved for lease to Europeans).[13] This was because the British understood that, as a non-settler colony with a small European population, Hong Kong's economic viability would depend on attracting native capital to help foster development and trade. By allowing the Chinese to buy and sell properties, the government also hoped to create new legal obligations between the colonial state and its subjects, thus achieving lasting stability through the rule of law. From early on, the highly lucrative housing market attracted many Chinese to invest in the colony. Like their European counterparts, many were able to amass substantial fortunes from their investments and came to assume control over a large number of property holdings. By the 1870s, the Chinese outnumbered Europeans as the largest taxpayers, with their assets concentrated in rental properties in Taipingshan and Kennedy Town—the two largest Chinese settlements in Hong Kong.

The shortage of housing was exacerbated after the mid-1850s, when continual political unrest in China drove multiple waves of refugees to the colony, seeking shelter and jobs.[14] Although the number of houses had increased more than threefold by the 1870s, the housing crisis continued unabated, fueling even more speculation that further pushed up property prices. The situation made some European property owners grow uneasy, as they feared the rapid growth and rising prices of the tenements would depreciate the value of European buildings. Meanwhile, articles in the local English press began to warn of the danger of potential epidemic outbreaks in the Chinese districts, where overcrowding and the unsanitary conditions of tenement houses made perfect breeding grounds for diseases. These concerns were further intensified during the property boom in the late 1870s, when a number of European buildings in the central business district were torn down to make way for the construction of Chinese tenements.[15] These incidents raised widespread criticism in the press against the property speculators' greed and the government's failure to protect the security and wellbeing of the (European) community.

The colonial administration was certainly not unaware of the poor state of the tenements. Successive colonial surgeons and surveyors general, for example, had for years been calling for more stringent construction standards for Chinese houses and better provision of infrastructure services. These recommendations were repeatedly made in the annual medical and sanitary reports, which also provided detailed documentation of the existing housing conditions and 'habits' of the native inhabitants. Written in a language that reflects the emerging discourse of public health, these reports were vehement in their criticism of the Chinese tenements, which were deemed to be "against every rule of sanitation in regards to drainage, ventilation, and cleanliness."[16] While the Chinese were condemned for their "dirty habits," which were said to further worsen the conditions of their dwellings, it was the property speculators and the colonial administration who were blamed for creating the high-rent situation that was the root of the problem.

Despite their vivid depictions of squalor and grave warnings of disease outbreaks in these spaces, the reports failed to usher in any significant policy changes (at least not until the outbreak of the bubonic plague in 1894). Although government officials frequently denigrated the Chinese houses as slum dwellings, the worry that excessive building regulations would drive away property investment and lower tax revenue had created a long-standing impediment to sanitary reform. Within the colonial administration, opinions were divided between those who believed that some control was needed to cool down speculation, and others who adhered to the laissez-faire principle that opposed any intervention in the market or tightening of building regulations. A salient representative of the latter was Governor John Pope-Hennessy, whose tenure coincided with the colony's economic boom at the end of the 1870s. In his attempt to convince other officials that sanitary reform was unnecessary, the governor argued that the 'Western' concept of public health was not appropriate to apply to the native Chinese, who, he claimed, possessed different customs and health practices from those of the Europeans.[17] Referring to the overall decline in death rates in the population, Hennessy insisted that Hong Kong was in fact becoming a more 'healthy' city—a development that paralleled the colony's unprecedented economic growth that was primarily due to increased investment by the Chinese.

Although Hennessy's 'pro-Chinese' position proved controversial among his contemporaries,[18] the support that he won from the Chinese suggests that this strategy was successful. Hennessy's invocation of 'cultural difference' between the natives and Europeans illustrates how the discourse of culture was used to legitimize particular political priorities, and in the process opened up new channels for the application of colonial power. Contrary to the opinions of the colonial doctors and sanitary engineers who believed that the natives could become more hygienic and 'civilized' like the Europeans through positive environments and proper education, the notion of 'difference' was presented by Hennessy as a reason for maintaining the status quo. At the same time, by asserting that the uniqueness of Chinese customs should be respected, Hennessy also set his claim against that of many Europeans who saw the difference between China and the 'West' to be about different stages of human development. As will be discussed in the following section, this rationality of cultural distinctions was also deployed by the Chinese in a different way in their attempt to contest legislation that would impinge upon their economic interests.

Re-appropriating Chineseness: The Petition against the Improved Tenements

In short, the 1860s and 1870s were boom decades marked by a rapid rise of property ownership by the Chinese, who continued to buy up existing properties from the Europeans while acquiring new land for development. Although these native landlords were subjected to colonial overlordship, they were highly aware of the political bargaining power enabled by their growing capital. One of the ways in which the Chinese property owners tried to use their leverage was through petitioning the governor and the Colonial Office on matters affecting their interests, particularly on taxation, land rent, and the regulation of housing properties. Depending on the issues, these petitions sometimes drew upon the support of other European landholders, and at other times claimed to speak on behalf of the 'Chinese community.'

One telling example that illustrates the contest against sanitary reform is a development proposal initiated by one Chinese landholder, Li Tak-cheong. In 1879, Li sent an application to Surveyor General J. M. Price for the construction of a total of 79 houses at the new Praya recently reclaimed by the government.[19] Upon seeing these plans, which showed that most of the houses would be constructed back-to-back, Price decided not to grant his approval unless the design was significantly modified to take on board his sanitary concerns. Specifically, Price requested that additional alleyways, windows, and backyards be included to allow more light and ventilation. He also remarked that the plans did not show any privy or sinks, which were deemed necessary according to the "European point of view." Calling the proposed houses "the most aggravated type of fever-den," Price lamented that part of the problem lay with the Chinese tenants' ignorance about sanitation, which allowed speculative landlords such as Li to extract high rent for such poorly designed dwellings.[20]

The proposed houses were in fact not very different from the colony's existing Chinese tenements, which were typically built to accommodate a large number of laborers by subdividing the upper floors into cubicles—conditions that had long been condemned by successive colonial surgeons and surveyors general. What made this case particularly alarming to Price was the development's unprecedented scale, which involved not only house-building but also the creation of many privately constructed streets and alleyways on newly reclaimed land. In his letter to the colonial secretary, Price pointed out that Li had become by far the largest builder in the colony and had been carrying out his operations on a large scale.[21] As Li's only concern was to maximize his rental income with no regard whatsoever for sanitation and the wellbeing of his tenants, Price urged the government to impose a more comprehensive set of controls over building and planning to safeguard the health and the future growth of Victoria. To this end, Price issued further detailed instructions to Li and his architect on ways to improve the tenements and indicated that these recommendations should be adopted for all new buildings.

After seeing Price's recommended changes to the proposal, Li was alarmed. He immediately met with other Chinese landlords and together they sent a petition to the governor.[22] This petition subsequently found its way to the Colonial Office in London as the battle over the building plans continued, with Governor Hennessy lending his support to the Chinese landlords and Price and other officials pressing for stronger imposition of sanitary regulations. In the petition, the property owners argued that Price's proposed "improved tenements," which could accommodate far fewer inhabitants than the existing ones due to the inclusion of additional alleyways, backyards, and windows, were not suited for the Chinese at all. Chinese people, they claimed, were essentially different from Westerners in their living standards and health practices, and thus would not appreciate the new sanitary provisions that were designed for a "very superior class of residence." Furthermore, they claimed that

> Chinese habits were the outcome of a lengthened experience among the Chinese living in large and crowded cities, and are as deep rooted as most of their social customs, so that it is quite certain that the tenants for whom these houses are intended as they would not understand the reason, would in no way avail themselves of the facilities for the free access of light and air which the Surveyor General's proposed alterations would provide for them.
>
> The windows looking out into the proposed alleys would be kept closed and the alleys themselves not being intended for use as thoroughfares, would be made receptacles for the deposit of refuse and filth which would beyond question be suffered to accumulate to an extent in itself dangerous to health.[23]

The petitioners also claimed that back-to-back housing, which was from the point of view of Western sanitarians unhealthy due to the lack of light and ventilation, had been a legitimate form of housing throughout Chinese history. Citing as examples areas from mainland China that were free from epidemic diseases, they argued that "it has been the practice from time immemorial to build houses back-to-back." The petition then went on to state that the new proposal would lead to a waste of land resources, and that since land had become extremely valuable in Hong Kong, it was necessary to make the best use of space in order to make their investment profitable. Meanwhile, since Chinese tenants were "as a rule unwilling to pay high rents, it was only by dividing the houses into cubicles that many families and individuals could find suitable shelters."[24]

Although the petition was obviously aimed at preserving the interests of property owners, its main argument was structured around a generalized claim about racial difference. Building on the existing discourse of the cultural divide between Chinese and Europeans, it sought to discredit the sanitary regulations—now cast as a quintessential product of 'Western science'—by affirming that it was wrong to apply these standards to the Chinese race, which possessed a different, but no less sophisticated system for managing health and environment. The assertion that the Chinese were fully capable of taking care of themselves also had the effect of arousing a sense of collective pride and nationalistic sentiment, even though the ultimate goal was, ironically, to reinforce the status quo of colonial laissez-faire practices. By framing the sanitary debate around notions of race and culture, the petition also sought to evade the simmering discontent about speculation and the housing problem, as well as the inequality between the propertied class and the property-less, in a fast-expanding colonial capitalist city.

Towards Universalism? The Controversy over Water Supplies

In addition to the provision of light and ventilation, another issue that occupied the sanitary debate was the supply and distribution of water. Although the introduction of running water and an underground drainage system was hailed as representing a new phase of modernization in the nineteenth century, the actual functioning of these services was for many years fraught with problems due to inadequate supply and difficulty in maintenance. Instead of fulfilling their promise to make cities more healthy, these infrastructures were soon criticized for doing exactly the opposite: the prevalence of leaky pipes, choked drains, and dysfunctional water closets was blamed for breeding diseases and endangering public health.[25] These conditions also became the perfect excuse for those who opposed large-scale sanitary reforms, as it had been argued that the more elaborate these systems became, the more vulnerable they were to collapse and disaster.

The situation in Hong Kong was an extreme example of this paradox. Because of the constraints of its island geography, water shortage had been a constant threat as the colony depended entirely on rainfall for its water supply. This was partially mitigated by the construction of hillside reservoirs and gathering grounds for holding water reserves. However, the supply was never able to meet the demand of a rapidly expanding population.[26] Compounding the problem was Hong Kong's hilly topography, which made it difficult and expensive to channel water to different parts of the city.[27] Although hydraulic technology at the time was able to make the distribution system more efficient, the government was unwilling to invest money in the required infrastructure. So while engineers had repeatedly drawn up detailed proposals for improving the water supply, many components in their plans remained unrealized.

To economize on the use of water, the Water Authority (a branch of the Public Works Department) operated an intermittent system that restricted supply to certain hours of the day during the dry season. But this operation had been criticized by the sanitary engineers, who pointed out that, once emptied, the water pipes were prone to the entry of foul air and disease-causing germs.[28] From this perspective, informed by the miasmatic theory of disease, the intermittent system appeared to be injurious to health and had to be replaced by a constant system. However, the latter could only be made possible by increasing funding to expand the distribution of water.

Besides arguing from the standpoint of sanitary science, the engineers also provided an economic justification for the provision of a constant supply of water. Contrary to the prevalent logic of conserving water by limiting supply, they argued that a constant system could prevent waste if each house was installed with a meter that monitored water consumption. Once the usage exceeded a certain volume, charges would be applied to households on a progressive scale, thus encouraging people not to use more than they needed. But this initiative, which followed the operation in place in England at the time (and which eventually became the model for the present-day system), was not well received when first introduced. Not unlike the controversy over the improvement of the tenement houses, competing justifications for the demand for water were put forward by various stakeholders. And not surprisingly, race and culture came to the fore once again.

Before discussing the debate over the proposal for a universal water supply, it would be useful to provide an overview of the water consumption pattern in Hong Kong. By 1882, close to 2,000 European houses were provided with running water services connected to the public mains.[29] Many of these houses also had water closets installed (even though most were not fully functional). In contrast, very few Chinese houses were connected to services, and water closets were typically non-existent. Despite this vast discrepancy, water was charged at a uniform rate to all of the buildings.[30] Those living up in the hills often had trouble getting a stable supply due to imperfect channeling. But many

Europeans believed that this was due to water being used up by the Chinese living in the lower part of the city, and they therefore opposed the latter applying for new services.

Those without services (including most people living in the tenements) had to fetch water from the public standpipes that operated only in the early morning. This inconvenient arrangement created job opportunities for several hundred 'water coolies,' who made money by collecting water from the public standpipes and delivering it to individual households. Many people also obtained water from shallow wells and even rainwater drains. Although the water from these sources was unsuitable for drinking and cooking purposes, it was regularly sold, disguised as fresh water, to households. As the newspapers from this period indicate, scams involving the sale of contaminated water were common, and quarrels over such matters were a daily occurrence on the streets. These scenarios were regularly condemned in the local English press as a nuisance. But owing to the inadequacy of water supply, the government nevertheless continued to tolerate these practices.

To justify the unequal distribution of water between the European and Chinese districts, the government maintained that it was inappropriate to provide services to the tenements due to the lack of control over usage by multiple households. But a more significant reason was an underlying prejudice that held that the Chinese, especially the many 'lower-class coolies,' tended to waste more water than average Europeans. This ascription of 'native ignorance' about modern technologies was frequently invoked in legislative council meetings. As one government official once caricatured them, "Chinese coolies were always ready to turn on a tap but had a horrible horror of turning it off."[31] For this reason, it was argued that the best way to prevent waste was to make the Chinese get their water from the public standpipes, because they could not carry away more than they needed.

The idea of using meters to monitor water consumption and reduce waste can be seen as a major attempt by public health advocates to transform regulatory practice. Following the operation in Britain, it is believed that by assigning a value to water and turning it into a payable commodity, individuals—both Europeans and Chinese—would be willingly inclined to use less of it. Another major advantage of a universal supply was that it would eliminate the use of contaminated wells and the illegal sale of water. In this way, bringing the 'free' circulation of fresh water to every house would not only help prevent diseases and improve the health of the population, but would also foster a new set of social and economic relationships that would in turn redefine the boundaries between the private and public spheres. Like the regulation of the tenements, the initiative was grounded in an emerging liberal universalism that suggested lives could be bettered by the provision of the right material conditions. In this view, the expansion of urban services could mediate individual conduct and transform social norms. However, the creation of such "liberal infrastructures"[32] in a colonial society was stymied by the government's long-standing reluctance to spend money on public goods, on the one hand, and Europeans' demands that their privilege be protected, on the other.

The debate over Hong Kong's water supply intensified in the early 1880s amid growing concerns over epidemic outbreaks. Internal tensions within the colonial administration reached their peak in 1881, when a dispute between the 'pro-Chinese' Governor Hennessy and the colonial surgeon over the improvement of drainage turned into an impasse, eventually prompting the secretary of state to send Osbert Chadwick, a consultant engineer of the Colonial Office, to Hong Kong to investigate the situation. Chadwick's visit resulted in the production of a landmark report that mapped out a series of drastic measures to improve the colony's sanitary conditions.[33] Among the major recommendations was the provision of a universal water supply that included all the tenements. To ensure equity of water distribution, the city would be divided into districts based upon altitude to allow the water supply to be turned on in succession. Meters would be provided by the government and rented to property owners. To prevent waste, Chadwick urged that stricter regulations be set up to ensure the proper use of pipes and fittings. The "evil" intermittent system would be replaced by a constant system after the completion of a new reservoir that was expected to vastly increase the water supply.[34]

Under pressure from the Colonial Office, the Hong Kong government proceeded to carry out Chadwick's plans. In the 1880s and 1890s, hundreds of tenement houses were connected to the water supply. But the installation of meters lagged behind due to the heavy expense involved. The problem of water shortages came to a head again in the late 1890s when the colony experienced a prolonged drought. A report released in 1902 showed that the waste of water had not been reduced.[35] The capacity of the new reservoir at Tai Tam proved insufficient to alleviate the water shortage and, despite the potential danger it posed of contaminating the public mains, the intermittent system continued to be in use by the Water Authority. Meanwhile, European residents protested fiercely against providing water to the tenements, as the number of applications for the service continued to soar.

In the face of these problems, the government drafted a new Water Consolidation Bill in 1902, aiming to disconnect all services to the tenements.[36] In his letter to the secretary of state, Acting Governor Gascoigne reiterated the claim that it was inappropriate to provide running water to the "lower-class" Chinese, who were inclined to abuse such services for their own gains. In addition, he further alleged that, once provided with the service, the Chinese landlords would raise the rent to cover the water charges, thus further increasing the hardship of poorer tenants. Speaking in a familiarly paternalistic and self-righteous tone, Gascoigne argued that, because the priority of the government was to ensure the smooth functioning of Hong Kong's entrepôt economy, it had a duty to "protect" its "lower-class" laborers from being exploited by their landlords, whose only concern was to secure their rental profits.

After the bill was publicized, the Chinese property owners sent a lengthy petition to the secretary of state, Joseph Chamberlain.[37] Referring to Chadwick on the imperative of health, they warned that the new bill would defeat the government's ultimate goal of improving sanitation, because the cutting of supplies to the tenements would "induce the Chinese not to cleanse their dwellings." The property owners further underscored the necessity of water supply by citing clauses from the English Public Health Act, asking,

> If an adequate supply of water is considered a vital necessity for sanitation in a temperate climate like England, how much more should not a constant supply of water be considered an absolute necessity to every tenement house in a tropical climate like Hong Kong?[38]

To solve the problem of water shortage, the petitioners suggested the government provide a subsidiary "rider main" system to be connected to the tenements. This operation was originally conceived by Chadwick as a temporary measure to allow the Water Authority to provide an intermittent service without the risk of contaminating the public main. If the government could agree with this initiative and suspend the new water bill, the petitioners promised that they would share the expenses incurred in the construction.[39]

In his response, Chamberlain expressed his support for the Chinese property owners, contending that he was inclined to reject the new water bill because "when the great majority of the resident taxpayers of a colony protest in this manner against a measure, normally considered of a very reactionary nature, and given willingness to bear the expense necessary to meet their views, they should if possible be met halfway and must certainly be treated with great consideration."[40]

Unlike the earlier petition in which 'cultural difference' between the Chinese and Europeans was emphasized, this time the Chinese property owners were fighting for their right to water access by appealing to the "universal need" for sanitation and public health. Conversely, the colonial administration, in struggling to deal with the multiple challenges involved in supplying water to the population, resorted to a racial argument that blamed the "lower-class" natives for misusing urban services. But despite the contrasting perspectives in these narratives, all were nevertheless claiming that their initiatives would preserve the best interests of Hong Kong. The oscillating positions of the property owners and the colonial government in these cases also illustrate the ambiguous relationship between health, culture, and the built environment, and the fact that economic considerations always played a central role in reshaping these discourses. These contestations were played out in an even bigger controversy over sanitary reform: the resumption of a large number of tenements after the bubonic plague outbreak.[41]

The Taipingshan Resumption and the Discourse of Property Rights

The bubonic plague outbreak in Hong Kong, referred to elsewhere in this volume by Peckham, Pomfret, Richard Harris, and Robert Lewis, was a disastrous episode that killed over 2,500 people in the summer of 1894. As in other cities that experienced epidemics in the nineteenth century, the event led to wild speculation over the causes of disease and much finger-pointing at those held responsible for the catastrophe.[42] The fact that a majority of the victims were Chinese sparked intense fear among Europeans of contracting diseases from the "dirty natives." Meanwhile, the militant measures imposed by the Sanitary Board to combat the plague, including forced removal of patients from their homes, compulsory closure of many "unsanitary houses" for disinfection, and the eviction of thousands of tenants, led to widespread anger among the Chinese community. The resulting mass exodus of laborers to China and the drastic decline of trade brought the colonial economy to a standstill. As Governor William Robinson contended, "as far as trade and commerce was concerned, the plague had assumed the importance of an unexampled calamity."[43]

As the plague began to subside, the government appointed a Housing Committee to investigate ways to prevent any future recurrence of the catastrophe. From the outset, the focus of the committee was Taipingshan—the Chinese district where most of the plague cases were located. By this time, medical experts had already identified the plague bacillus. But despite the general acceptance of germ theory, colonial doctors and engineers continued to explain disease transmission by referring to the principles of miasma, asserting that the plague was spread through air emanating from the ground where the bacillus flourished.[44] This belief fit well with the observation that the soil of Taipingshan was typically soaked with sewage discharged from dysfunctional drains and through the broken floors of the buildings above. After examining the situation, the committee concluded that the best solution was to demolish all the buildings by fire, cast away the contaminated topsoil, and redevelop the area with better built houses, ample open space, and a more efficient drainage system.[45] To this end, the committee recommended that the government enact a new ordinance to resume 10 acres of land for redevelopment. Compensation would be paid to the property owners via a government-appointed Arbitration Board.

This, then, was the background for the first major land resumption in Hong Kong—an episode hailed in colonial records as an historic turning point, as the government took a decisive step towards long-term planning to protect the wellbeing of the population. But this was far from being a straightforward, triumphal story of benevolence. The legitimacy of the resumption was challenged on every front throughout the process. When the proposal was announced, it immediately caused a stir in the press, fueling debates over the infringement of property rights and the spending of large sums of taxpayers' money on the destruction of private properties. While some praised the government for finally waking up to the call for sanitary reform, others argued that the initiative would be futile, because it was, after all, the "dirty habits" of the Chinese, not the buildings, that were responsible for spreading diseases.[46]

A prominent opponent of resumption was one Granville Sharp—a British builder and well-known philanthropist who owned a large number of rental properties in Hong Kong. In a series of articles titled "Plague and Prevention," published in the *Hongkong Daily Press*,[47] Sharp wrote that, although the conditions of some tenements in Taipingshan were so bad that they had to be rebuilt, many others could be made "sanitary" by disinfection and minor alterations, such as adding windows to bring in light and ventilation. He also challenged the committee's suggestion that the houses be burnt and the polluted soil removed, warning that such actions could reactivate the plague bacillus and thus invite unimaginable disasters. But above all else, Sharp argued that the wholesale demolition of Taipingshan should be avoided because of its negative impact on housing and public health. The tearing down of so many tenements, he asserted, would further limit accommodation for the poor and exacerbate the overcrowding that was the ultimate enemy of sanitation. Speaking in the voice of a philanthropist, Sharp urged that more attention be paid to the needs of the native laborers:

> Our dependence upon Chinese cheap labor is becoming everyday more manifest. The interests of the poorer classes of Chinese are now assuming an importance unknown before, and their necessities must be most carefully considered . . .
>
> Instead of [demolishing those houses], every square yard of existing roof in the Island needs to be preserved, for the protection of the people who resort here, who are essential to us, and who advance our welfare. We want much more accommodation instead of less. This is the only way to combat overcrowding. The destruction of Taipingshan will throw great difficulties in the way of carrying out the beneficent intentions of the Government and the real wishes of the Sanitary Board.[48]

Finally, Sharp pointed out that plague prevention could not be achieved by fixing one area alone. Instead of using considerable public funds to destroy all the properties, he suggested that the government provide incentives such as rent relief for property owners and tenants to carry out sanitary improvements themselves, because the best result could only be accomplished by "mutual help between landlords, tenants and the authorities."[49]

In hindsight, one could argue that these statements were somewhat self-serving, as it was clear that Sharp was trying to prevent the demolition of his own properties. But these comments also illustrate the uncertainties encountered in the struggle to combat a deadly disease whose cause and means of prevention remained unknown. Despite the racist overtones of some of his writings, Sharp's warnings against the destructive consequences of the resumption resonated with many Chinese landlords, merchants and shopkeepers, who became increasingly concerned not only with their properties' loss of value, but also with the negative impact that the exodus of Chinese laborers from the colony would have on economic conditions. This anxiety was also shared by some administrative officials, who were wary of public discontent over the government's handling of the crisis.

It is not clear to what extent Sharp was able to influence public opinion, but growing resistance against the resumption was apparent in the months following the publication of his articles—a time when the plague had already subsided. Editorials in major newspapers such as the *Hongkong Daily Press* and *Hongkong Telegraph* began to renege on their earlier support for the demolition and turned their attention to issues of property rights protection and compensation for the owners. Although the Chinese laborers were continually caricatured as villains for spreading diseases, Chinese and European landlords were united in their fight against the resumption and for compensation for the rental income lost during the plague (when their houses were shut down by the Sanitary Board for disinfection). Their view was shared by a majority of the unofficial legislative council members, who had attempted to organize a committee to inquire about alternative ways to improve Taipingshan.[50] Although their initiative ultimately failed and the resumption ordinance was pushed through by the official majority (who outnumbered the unofficial members by proportion), the government was subjected to heavy criticism by the press and was eventually forced to reconstitute the legislative council by increasing the number of its unofficial members.

The opposition to the resumption by the unofficial legislators was not surprising; after all, most of them were directly connected to the largest property firms in Hong Kong.[51] The highly mixed pattern of property ownership in Taipingshan arguably defied the long-standing stereotype of the area as a purely 'Chinese district' disconnected from the 'European town.'[52] Somewhat ironically, the only unofficial legislator who supported the ordinance was the Chinese barrister and physician, Kai Ho Kai (knighted in 1912), who was also a longtime member of the Sanitary Board. Trained in England as a physician and later as a lawyer, Ho had long sought to educate the native Chinese about Western knowledge of medicine and public health.[53] Although he had previously opposed some of the building regulations on the tenements, on the basis that these would exacerbate the housing crisis, he was adamant about the complete reconstruction of Taipingshan for plague prevention.[54] To this end, unlike his European counterparts in the legislative council, Ho stood firmly with the colonial doctors and engineers who believed that nothing less than razing all the houses would allow the government to carry out a proper planning agenda, which was essential for remaking Taipingshan into a healthy district along modern sanitary principles.

After months of negotiation, the property owners of Taipingshan finally accepted the compensation offered by the Arbitration Board. All of the 384 houses in the plague-ridden district were razed the following year.[55] However, the contestation over property rights was far from over. In January 1895, a petition jointly signed by a large number of European and Chinese landlords who owned tenement houses outside the Taipingshan district was sent to Secretary of State Chamberlain.[56] The petitioners demanded compensation for rental income lost during the plague on the grounds that this amount was included in the payment to the Taipingshan landlords. They also petitioned to suspend a regulation that required them to maintain their buildings in accordance with several new standards introduced by the Sanitary Board, which would take possession of their properties if these rules were not observed.[57] The petitioners protested that such a regulation constituted a fundamental violation of their property rights, and that it was not the landlords' duty to supervise the conditions of the tenements:

> A landlord having once let his house has no right to be visiting and inspecting it at all hours of the day and night, and the only possible way of preventing the erection and maintenance of illegal floors and partitions is by appointing proper sanitary inspectors with statutory power to visit and inspect the various buildings from time to time, and the same remarks apply to the number of persons inhabiting a building.[58]

The petition ended with a somewhat threatening statement, that if the new regulation was put in practice it would devastate the colonial economy:

> [I]t will necessarily deter capitalists from investing either as owners or mortgagees of leaseholds in Hongkong, and will cause those who have already invested to withdraw their money at the earliest possible moment. The shock to confidence and good faith which the confiscation clause of this ordinance must cause will inevitably tend to drive the investing public away and thus cause most serious detriment to the Colony.[59]

The war of words between the administration and the property owners over the sanitary regulations was to continue for many more years (a new Public Health Ordinance was not enacted until 1903), all along fueling more questions not only about the protection of property rights, but also the legitimacy of a non-representative government that had long been accustomed to pushing through its policies without regard for public opinion. Meanwhile, the razing of Taipingshan had not prevented the return of the plague (which became an annual affair well into the early 1920s), and the problems of high rent, housing shortage, and the lack of urban services would continue to haunt Hong Kong for another three-quarters of a century.

Conclusion

The three controversies examined in this chapter have shown how discourses of health and sanitation, which had provoked intense public debate amidst the growing fear of epidemic outbreaks in Hong Kong in the late nineteenth century, had been re-appropriated and constructed anew by different social actors for specific purposes. By tracing the debates over public health, property rights, and the obligations of colonial authorities in the preceding cases, I have illustrated some of the underlying tensions in colonial capitalist development, in which the entanglement of public and private interests in property repeatedly thwarted attempts to implement building regulations and sanitary reform. These conflicts point to the unstable frameworks of colonial segregation and the multiple forces that shaped colonial space, which, as identified by Peckham and Pomfret, was inherently "fraught with tensions and contradictions between ideology and practical exigencies, between local and central government, indigenous resistance and colonial indigenization."

Notwithstanding prevalent European prejudice against the Chinese for their incivility and "dirty habits," the highly mixed ownership of the tenements had helped unite Chinese and European property owners in their resistance to policies that affected their interests as rentiers. As their economic power grew, Chinese landlords became increasingly assertive in exercising their rights under the colonial rule of law. Although their actions can be seen as evidence of 'native agency,' so to speak, they also indicate a process through which the Chinese propertied class was being incorporated more tightly into the colonial governing regime. Meanwhile, the advent of the public health movement, predicated on the provision of universal urban services and betterment of the lives of laborers, exerted further pressure on the colonial authority, which had been struggling with its simultaneous obligations to ensure the smooth functioning of a laissez-faire economy and to protect European privilege in an exclusionary colonial society.

The examination of the convergence of interests between the Chinese and European property owners and their shifting allegiance to the colonial state also reveals the complex power relations between these agencies, thereby unsettling the long-assumed divide between 'colonizers' and the 'colonized.'

The comparison of the different ways in which 'race' and 'culture' were invoked in the sanitary debate further illustrates the malleability of these categories, which were continuously re-articulated to support very different agendas. At the same time, the constant appeal to preserve the 'collective interests' of Hong Kong—most notably property rights, the rule of law, and the laissez-faire economy—suggests that, behind all the contestation and conflict, there was nevertheless a growing consensus in support of a particular rationality of development that was believed to have enabled Hong Kong's economic success under colonial rule.

Although questions about vested interests in property were not lost in public debates during the period investigated in this chapter, these issues have been largely absent from the mainstream historiographies of Hong Kong. Narratives of urban development have often focused on the antagonism between the Chinese and Europeans, whereas accounts of the history of public health and urban services have tended to highlight technological advances by medical experts and engineers. By looking closely at the competing claims over health and sanitation, this chapter has opened a window onto some of the contradictions inherent in the colony's sanitary and housing reforms. It has sought to explore the cracks and fissures within colonial discourses of planning—"frictions" that have been, for the most part, overlooked, despite their critical role in Hong Kong's development.

2

'Tropicalizing' Planning: Sanitation, Housing, and Technologies of Improvement in Colonial Singapore, 1907–42

Jiat-Hwee Chang

Introduction: Sanitizing Fervor

> . . . the plain unvarnished truth is that Singapore is a disgrace to British administration. There is no fouler, less-cared for place in the Empire. If it were not for the constant heavy rains which automatically wash out the side channels, there is not a street in the more closely populated portion of the city where life would be supportable. Even with all the natural advantages we have a death-rate that is positively scandalous.[1]

The passage above, extracted from a 1910 newspaper report on "Insanitary Singapore," reflects a prevalent sentiment towards the British colony in the early twentieth century. It was a view that persisted, prompting major housing and sanitary reform in the post-World War II period. Indeed, perceptions of Singapore as a singularly "insanitary" city and a "disgrace" to the colonial administration underlay what might aptly be called a 'sanitizing fervor', the subject of the present chapter.

The aim in what follows is to explore the extent to which preoccupations with sanitation and fears of contamination shaped colonial housing and town planning improvements in pre-World War II Singapore, particularly the housing of the 'native' population.[2] More specifically, the chapter focuses on issues at stake in the circulation and translation of sanitary knowledge and practices within the context of British colonial networks. The purpose is to develop a theoretical framework for rethinking colonial circulations, engaging with three interlinking concepts—'traveling theory,' 'governmentality,' and 'tropicalization'—in order to demonstrate the congruencies and incongruencies between, on the one hand, ideals of social order and, on the other, the implementation of policy 'on the ground.' As the reporter concluded with evident frustration in the report quoted above from *The Straits Times*, "there has been too much talk already, and it is time to begin work."[3]

Traveling Theory, Governmentality, and Tropicalization

A sanitary movement emerged in England in the mid-nineteenth century, motivated in part by outbreaks of cholera from the 1830s.[4] During the course of the century, public health initiatives in Europe led to improved standards of urban housing for the poor. However, these metropolitan sanitary and public health reforms had little impact upon and made minimal headway in the colonies during the same period, at least in relation to the housing of the 'native' population. Most sanitary improvements initiated in the British colonies were confined to the European population and their socio-spatial enclaves.[5] This inaction began to change at the turn of the twentieth century, particularly with outbreaks of bubonic plague and malaria in various parts of the British Empire. Another impetus for the shift in policy was the series of colonial development initiatives associated with the colonial secretary Joseph Chamberlain. Under his "constructive imperialism," the Colonial Office funded research in tropical medicine and sanitation as a means of eradicating some of the problems that were deemed to be inhibiting the socio-economic development of Britain's tropical colonies.[6] Experts in tropical medicine and sanitation, for example, were dispatched from the metropole to various colonies to investigate the causes of disease and to recommend remedies and preventive policies.[7] These measures contributed to the aforementioned sanitizing fervor in the early twentieth century and gave rise to a veritable proliferation of discourses on urban sanitation in the tropics.[8]

It was against this background that William Simpson, an imperial sanitary expert, was appointed by the government of the Straits Settlements in 1906 to investigate the sanitary conditions in Singapore. Prior to Simpson's appointment, the high mortality and morbidity rates of the native population in Singapore, especially the increasing number of deaths from tuberculosis, had been brought to the attention of the Straits government. Following reports from his medical officers and after his own inspection, Straits Governor John Anderson ascribed overcrowded and insanitary housing as the principal cause of the high mortality and morbidity rates. He appointed a committee consisting of the principal civil medical officer, the health officer and the municipal engineer, to look into the problem and to advise him on the appropriate course of action. In its report, the committee recommended that the sanitary conditions of these areas be rectified by rebuilding the houses according to a new town and housing plan. As the power conferred by the municipal ordinance was insufficient to execute the clearance and improvement of these insanitary houses, a new bill for dealing with the insanitary areas was considered by the legislative council. The council decided that an independent expert from the metropole should be appointed to investigate the sanitary problem in further detail and to furnish the Straits government with supporting evidence and recommendations for introducing the new bill.[9] On the advice of the Colonial Office, Simpson was therefore appointed and he issued a report that was to shape housing and town planning in pre-World War II Singapore in significant ways. Among other things, the report established the technical framework for sanitary improvement and led to the formation of the Singapore Improvement Trust (SIT) in 1927.

Given that Singapore was a port city and a nodal point in the British Empire, the broader colonial connections and the attendant movement of people, ideas, and practices—a major theme in *Imperial Contagions*—were especially significant to the colony's history of housing and sanitary improvements. Indeed, sanitary and town planning experts, administrators, engineers, and architects involved in the planning of other British colonial cities came to Singapore in the early twentieth century and influenced subsequent housing and town planning practices there. As other contributors have demonstrated elsewhere in this volume, when populations migrated transnationally and within empire, they introduced ideas and practices into new settings. These could be translated into institutional forms such as the SIT. The Trust, with its improvement legislation and practices, had precedents in other parts of the empire, such as Glasgow, Calcutta, Bombay, and Rangoon.[10] This mobility extended to the circulation of building types. Under the SIT, for example, building types common in the metropole and other parts of the empire, such as cottage houses, artisan quarters, and flats, were built in Singapore in the 1930s.

Bearing in mind the significance of transnational and transcolonial circulations in the development of Singapore, what kind of conceptual framework might best be deployed to elucidate these processes? Certainly, the Eurocentric diffusionist narrative of traditional architectural historiography, in which architecture and planning theories and practices supposedly disseminated from the center to the periphery, has been convincingly discredited by those working in postcolonial studies. Assumptions that architecture and urbanism in non-Western settings were "almost the same, but not quite"[11]—in other words, that they were based on Western models but were inferior copies trapped in perpetual backwardness—have been conclusively challenged.[12] In place of the Eurocentric diffusionist narrative, scholars of the architecture and planning histories of non-Western cities have used conceptual frameworks such as 'hybridization' and 'transculturation' to understand the circulation and translation of ideas and practices between the metropole and the colonies, and between colonies.[13]

Drawing upon these theoretical contexts, in this chapter I bring together three interrelated concepts. The first is Duanfang Lu's notion of 'traveling urban form,' which develops Edward Said's concept of 'traveling theory,' usefully extending its scope to illuminate the complex processes through which urban ideas and practices are appropriated, translated, adapted, and re-invented when they are circulated from one sociocultural context to another.[14] Lu's focus is predominantly on the Chinese domestication of the neighborhood unit scheme as a model layout for an integrated residential district, a model first formulated in the United States in the 1920s. However, techno-scientific knowledge and practices of sanitation and housing approximate to what Stephen Collier and Aihwa Ong have termed in another context "global forms" that are "limited or delimited by specific technical infrastructure, administrative apparatuses . . . *not by vagaries of a social or cultural field*" (my emphasis).[15] Collier and Ong suggest that, in order to understand such global forms, "a careful technical analysis—a technical criticism" is required, rather than sociological reduction or cultural relativization.[16] To be sure, the aim is not to posit a false dichotomy between the sociocultural and the techno-scientific, nor to posit a form of techno-scientific exceptionalism. Rather, my point is that in studying the circulation and translation of medical and sanitary knowledge and practices, which were central to the architecture and urban history of Singapore in the early twentieth century, one has to modify useful cultural concepts such as 'traveling theory.'

Second, this chapter draws on Michel Foucault's concept of 'governmentality,' which denotes a new rationality of government concerned with "the welfare of the population, the improvement of its condition, the increase of its wealth, longevity, health, etc."[17] In contrast to old sovereign power, which was about the right "to take life or let live," governmentality saw the introduction of new biopower to "'make' life and 'let' die,"[18] in the sense of administering, multiplying, and optimizing the biological life of the population. According to Foucault, governmentality entails the use of a *dispositif* or an apparatus that groups multiple authorities and agencies, and employs a variety of techniques and forms of knowledge to first define and specify targets of government, and then regulate and control them.[19] Foucauldian scholars also describe the *dispositif* or apparatus as a "strategic bricolage." It is a 'bricolage' in the sense that the elements deployed are multiple and heterogeneous, and 'strategic' in that the focus is on the 'logic' and 'tactical economy' of domination through which this bricolage is assembled and dissembled.[20] In other words, the emphasis is on the 'how' of government, particularly how specific technologies of government render problems of government visible, facilitate political calculations, and constitute 'rational' government.[21] As Richard Harris and Robert Lewis argue in this volume, the 1901 census in Bombay and Calcutta functioned precisely in this way as a means of visualizing the subject Indian population and, at the same time, rationalizing colonial authority. In this case, architecture and the built environment might be understood alongside statistics, censuses, maps, photographs, biomedical knowledge, and sanitary practices as part of the larger strategic bricolage of governmentality. This bricolage allows the combination of the social with the technical and the cultural with the scientific in the understanding of how knowledge and practices circulated and were translated.

Finally, the notion of 'tropicalization' encapsulates some of the tensions I have sought to delineate above in my discussion of governmentality. In his study of techno-science in colonial India, Gyan Prakash notes that colonial governmentality "could not be a tropicalization of its Western form, but rather was its fundamental dislocation."[22] Here, 'tropicalization' implies the superficial modification of governmentality's Western form to suit tropical conditions, rather than a substantive transformation. However, in his medical and environmental histories of the colonial tropics, David Arnold argues that the tropics were not merely a natural variation of the temperate zone. Rather, the tropics need to be understood along the line of Said's Orientalism as 'tropicality'; that is, as an environmental 'Other' deeply entwined with various forms of sociocultural alterity that contrast in fundamental ways with the normality of the temperate zone.[23] My use of 'tropicalization' in this chapter consciously draws on these tensions and contradictions in order to show how sanitary and housing improvements in colonial Singapore were understood, on the one hand, as extensions of metropolitan techno-science and technologies of government and, on the other, how they were construed as mutations of metropolitan forms that had been fundamentally modified by their emplacement in tropical Singapore.

Seeing like a Sanitary Expert: Rendering Technical, Making Visible

The Sanitary Conditions of Singapore was a landmark report in Singapore's housing and planning history.[24] Its author, William John Ritchie Simpson (1855–1931), Professor and Chair of Hygiene at King's College, London, and one of the co-founders of the London School of Tropical Medicine and the Ross Institute, was regarded as one of the foremost sanitarians in the British Empire at that time.[25] Simpson's report was the first comprehensive study of the housing and town planning problems of Singapore's native population— in other words, primarily the immigrant Chinese laborers. It made visible the seriousness of the problem and recommended a set of improvements that shaped subsequent colonial housing policies in important ways. Simpson did so by deploying what scholars of governmentality have called technologies of identifying and 'knowing the governed' and the built environment they reside in, so as to facilitate state interventions.[26]

These technologies involved techniques of quantifying, surveying, mapping, photographing, and drawing. Simpson examined the statistical information on the population, especially that pertaining to mortality rates, and concluded that the mortality rates of Singapore's native population were excessive and extraordinary, particularly since the immigrant population of Singapore was "essentially a population at the most vigorous period of life, viz. between fifteen and fifty-five years of age."[27] He attributed the high mortality rates to over-crowded and insanitary housing. One of the main causes of death was tuberculosis; Simpson mapped the number of deaths from tuberculosis recorded over a period of five years at two blocks of shophouses in Upper Nankin Street and Upper Chin Chew Street. The map Simpson produced shows the spatial distribution of death and disease, and illustrates his argument that the insanitary housing conditions, particularly the deficiencies in light and air, of some of the houses led to the greater recurrence of tuberculosis. Simpson also inspected and described in detail the dark, gloomy, and squalid conditions of the interiors of the shophouses. His descriptions were augmented with photographs of the interiors (Figure 2.1) and measured drawings of the plans and sections of the shophouses.

It has been argued that numbers have the power of "turning a qualitative world into information and rendering it amenable to control."[28] Numbers do not merely describe a pre-existing reality; arguably, they constitute the very

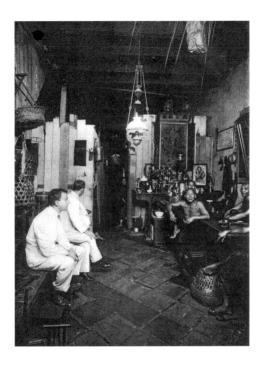

Figure 2.1

Photograph of the interior of the insanitary shophouse in Simpson's report.

'objective' reality they purport to describe. Likewise, the photographs have been described as operating in the manner of the Foucauldian gaze that "penetrated the hidden recesses"[29] of the insanitary housing, exposing the visual disorder of the overcrowded and insanitary interiors. In a similar manner, the drawings and maps rendered the disorder legible through selectively identifying and representing certain aspects while suppressing others. The interiors were simplified and represented in scaled drawings as geometrical spaces. Thus, the photographs, drawings, and maps were visual tools that operated in a similar manner to statistical enumeration—they represented reality in ways that facilitated the disciplining of that reality.[30]

The recurring themes in Simpson's enumeration, visual representation, and description of the insanitary shophouses were overcrowding and the deprivation of sunlight and fresh air. For example, Simpson noted that the shophouse interiors were subdivided into cubicles that had no windows to admit sunlight and fresh air; additions were made that further cramped the small courtyards and obstructed the entry of light and air; and the shophouses were so tightly packed that there was insufficient open space within and between them. As a consequence, Simpson put forth a list of recommendations that aimed at "opening up the dark and airless portions of the houses."[31] These included building back lanes of between 15 to 20 feet wide to separate the existing back-to-back shophouses and to open up the center of the shophouse block. Simpson also proposed that new bylaws be drawn up to limit the depth of buildings to not more than 45 feet, and he stipulated that at least one-third of the building plot should remain as open space. In addition, Simpson recommended that the proportions of open spaces and courtyards in relation to buildings be regulated by the new bylaws; he noted that the height of a building next to an open space or courtyard should not be more than one and a half times the width of that open space or courtyard, and that the minimum width of the courtyard should be kept at 10 feet.

This preoccupation with light and air was a feature not just of early twentieth-century sanitary discourse as practiced by Simpson but of architecture and town planning discourses of that time in general. The concern with air and ventilation could be traced to the miasmatic theories of disease transmission of the nineteenth century, in which diseases were thought to be transmitted through poisonous miasma. Miasma was associated with both the natural and built environment, such as marshlands, insanitary houses, and any place where decomposing waste matters could be found. Miasma was also believed to be generated by people through breathing and sweating and was understood to accumulate in overcrowded interiors, especially when the air was stagnant.[32] Thus, ventilation, which was thought to dilute the concentration of miasma in the air, and the prevention of overcrowding through the allocation of sufficient 'air space' per person were the typical remedies prescribed to deal with miasma. In the tropics, these measures were especially evident in the design of bungalows, military barracks, and hospitals in the nineteenth century, where minimum space standards and design strategies to facilitate ventilation were stipulated.[33]

Although miasmatic theories of disease transmission were supplanted by germ theories in the later part of the nineteenth century, the concerns with air and ventilation continued. Spacious and well-ventilated bungalows and quarters continued to be built as they were endorsed by British imperial scientists and medical experts, such as Ronald Ross and Patrick Manson.[34] In fact, these concerns were extended from the design of buildings to the planning of towns.

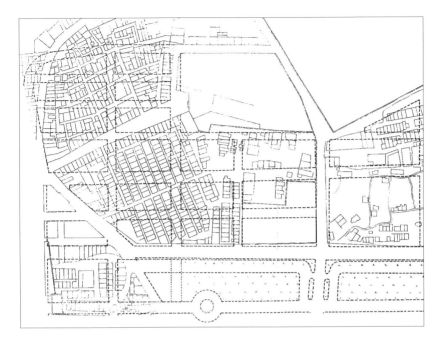

Figure 2.2

Wide, straight streets intersecting at right angles as "ventilating conduits" in dotted lines on top of what appears to be an insanitary city with narrow, irregular streets.

In his manual on tropical sanitation, Simpson noted that streets should be wide, straight, and intersecting at right angles, with the main avenues oriented in the direction of the most prevalent and healthy winds so that they would "act as ventilating conduits to town or village"[35] (Figure 2.2). Besides streets, the open spaces between and within buildings were articulated in the sanitary discourse as 'lungs' that should also be regulated according to ventilation needs.

One oft-repeated quote in early twentieth-century sanitary writings captures the significance of light and sunshine for sanitarians: "Second only to air, is light and sunshine essential for growth and health."[36] Although the rationale for the medical benefits of light in miasmatic theories was unclear, light was nonetheless valued by Victorian sanitary reformers for aesthetic and moral reasons.[37] With the advent of germ theories, light—specifically direct sunlight—was discovered to have antiseptic properties and to be particularly useful for treating diseases such as tuberculosis.[38] Thus, the presence of direct sunlight in both interior and exterior spaces became desirable for health reasons. This perceived desirability of direct sunlight in the built environment from the late nineteenth and early twentieth centuries onwards led to studies on how buildings could be designed and towns planned to benefit from solar radiation (Figure 2.3). Such studies also explored how these benefits could be systematically codified into a set of abstract design guidelines or bylaws. For example, Boston architect William Atkinson produced a series of visual studies of the distribution of sunlight on both the exterior and interior of buildings at different times of the year to obtain, among other things, the ideal orientation and proportion of building to street.[39] The renowned British town planner Raymond Unwin used sun path diagrams to study the relative advantages and disadvantages of different building orientations in order to rationalize the housing layout in his town planning projects.[40]

By using the 'natural' variables of light and air as the common denominators for evaluating sanitary conditions, buildings from different parts of the world could be compared. Their specific sociopolitical differences could be suppressed and their sanitary conditions evaluated on the purportedly objective

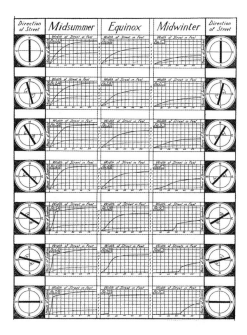

Figure 2.3

Chart showing hours of sunlight in streets of different widths and orientations.

variables of light and air. This was especially valuable for an imperial sanitary
expert like Simpson, as he moved between different parts of the British Empire,
advising the various colonial governments on how to improve the sanitation
of their towns and villages. In one of his manuals on tropical sanitation, drawings of both the Chinese shophouse from Singapore—culled from his sanitary
report on Singapore but unidentified in his manual—and another unidentified house, were presented as instances of the typical insanitary dwelling in
the tropics: both failed to provide sufficient open space between buildings that
could fit the 45-degree imaginary line known as the light plane (Figure 2.4).
Besides the use of light planes, Simpson also recommended other solutions, as
discussed earlier, based on the codification of light and air requirements into
simple numerical rules. These rules could be used as technical design guides or
legislated as building bylaws to regulate built form for securing the health of
the inhabitants. These codified rules could be said to behave in a manner akin
to Bruno Latour's "immutable mobiles," allowing planning theories to travel
without distortion.[41]

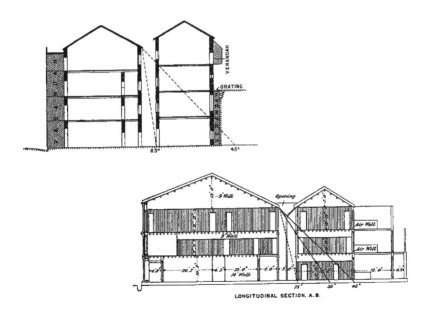

Figure 2.4
Sections of two houses that have open spaces that could not fit the 45-degree light plane.

Acting like a Colonial State: Belatedness and Inadequacies

The recommendations in Simpson's report were enthusiastically embraced by Singapore's legislative council. The municipal ordinance was amended and a special financial arrangement made to facilitate the recommended improvement works. However, no improvement work was undertaken for more than 10 years and, in 1917, Straits Governor Arthur Young had to appoint a new housing commission to re-examine the acute housing problem. The new housing commission, which published its report in 1918, relied on methods of investigation similar to the ones employed by Simpson, to the extent of reproducing photographs from Simpson's report. Unsurprisingly, the commission reached similar conclusions.[42] Like Simpson, they found that there was severe overcrowding and inadequate housing; indeed, that the conditions had been further exacerbated because of the population increase since 1907. Their recommendations were largely similar to Simpson's except that they reiterated the importance of having an improvement ordinance and the need to form an Improvement Trust along the lines of those in other British colonial cities such as Bombay and Calcutta.

The 1918 Housing Commission's recommendations were accepted by the colonial government, which, the following year, decided to appoint a technical expert to be the deputy chairman of the future Trust (DCIT); this person would "investigate the city problems and get to work prior to the creation of the Trust, and passing of new legislation to endow the Trust with efficient powers to carry out improvement, housing, town-planning and development."[43] This led to the appointment of Captain Edwin Percy Richards, a founding member of the Town Planning Institute and chief engineer of the Calcutta Improvement Trust between 1912 and 1913.[44] Richards was best known for the voluminous 400-page report *On the Condition, Improvement and Town Planning of the City of Calcutta and Contagious Areas*, published in 1914. This influential report was summarized and commented upon by Henry Vaughan Lanchester in *Town Planning Review*;[45] renowned town planner Patrick Abercombie hailed the report as "a fine achievement" that demonstrated "a good grasp of a problem of amazing intricacy."[46]

Not unlike the appointment of the previous technical expert, William Simpson, Richards' arrival in Singapore did not lead to any immediate and significant changes to the status quo. His attempts to draft "equitable, up-to-date legislation" to empower the SIT with "the *sine qua non* for reformation of present evils and for the future healthy, orderly, prosperous growth of Singapore"[47] were repeatedly thwarted; he resigned in 1924, three years before the Singapore Improvement Ordinance was eventually passed and SIT was formally established.[48] Likewise, Richards faced many challenges when he attempted to plan for town and housing improvements. As other science and technology scholars have noted, the implementation of any technical practice requires a specific socio-technical network of people, 'things,' knowledge, and practices to be in place, just as governmentality scholars have noted that intervening in the governed necessitates 'knowing the governed.'[49]

One of the key challenges Richards discovered was the lack of an up-to-date contoured survey map of Singapore, as the survey department had been understaffed for many years and lacked the resources to carry out a new survey. Without contoured surveys, Richards was unable to plan accurately, as Singapore was "four-fifths hilly."[50] He had to establish his own team to carry out the surveys.[51] Although his team managed to complete a four-chain contoured topographical survey of the city in 1924, after four years of work and much financial outlay, it was still insufficiently accurate for preparing a detailed layout of roads.[52] Moreover, the problems faced by Richards were compounded by the lack of accurate census information, which had been highlighted in both Simpson's Report and the 1918 Housing Commission's Report.[53] Like the lack of reliable statistical information on the governed in the case of the census, the absence of accurate spatial information on the environment in the case of the map could be attributed to the want of an operational socio-technical network, or what Collier and Ong have described as the "technical infrastructure" and "administrative apparatuses."

In the absence of new legislation and the necessary survey map for comprehensive town planning and housing improvement, W. H. Collyer, who replaced Richards as the DCIT, could only propose "a very modest programme of works" in the mid-1920s on an experimental basis and as a stopgap measure to address the worsening overcrowding and insanitary conditions in the colony. Back lane schemes were introduced in 1924. Open space schemes (Figure 2.5) for creating "lungs to let a little fresh air into the city" were also proposed for houses in the Chulia Street–Church Street block and Beach Road, where houses were described as "a rabbit warren of dangerously insanitary structures."[54] These schemes were proposed for areas deemed improvable by health officers, where partial demolitions to create back lanes or open spaces were considered sufficient. For areas where the insanitary conditions were deemed beyond redemption, more drastic measures of total demolition and rebuilding were necessary. These more drastic schemes, which also entailed clearing the slums and re-housing the affected population, were called "improvement schemes," as differentiated from the back lanes and open spaces schemes.[55] Although they adhered to the improvement schemata in Simpson's report, they were not part of any comprehensive plan of wholesale change as originally envisioned by Richards, because of the uncertainty surrounding the proposed improvement bill at that time. This piecemeal approach to housing and sanitary improvement was primarily undertaken to gauge the funds required for more comprehensive improvement works.

After much delay, the SIT was finally founded in 1927 with the passing of the Singapore Improvement Ordinance. The ordinance provided the Trust with some of the executive power it needed to carry out improvement schemes and to prepare the general town plan.[56] However, glaringly missing in the ordinance

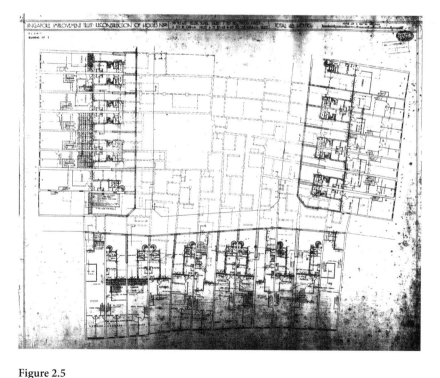

Figure 2.5

Plan showing an open space scheme at a block of shophouses bounded by Telok Ayer Street, Pekin Street, China Street, and Church Street.

was anything on the provision of housing for the general population besides those displaced by the improvement schemes. Furthermore, there was also a lack of clarity in terms of funding. Although in 1926 the colonial government committed a sum of 10 million Straits dollars for the purpose of dealing with Singapore's slum problem, a commentator noted that "the fund was never clearly defined in nature and purpose, and has not been operated as a 'trustee fund.'"[57] Up until the mid-1930s, SIT only built to accommodate those displaced by its improvement schemes. According to one estimate, housing erected by the mid-1930s housed only about 4,500 people.[58] As such, these housing measures did little to alleviate the problems of housing shortage and overcrowding. The original plan of addressing the housing shortage through private enterprise with the assistance of the Trust—by having the Trust improve lands outside the town and then selling them to private enterprises—did not come to fruition. By the mid-1930s, the housing problem was further aggravated by the rapid increase in population.

In the early years of the Trust's existence, it faced many challenges. What came to be known as the "Bugis Street case"[59] was a defining challenge. One of the powers conferred upon the Trust by the 1927 ordinance was the right to declare a building "unfit for human habitation," which would require the building to be demolished by either the owner or the Trust. In such a case, the Trust would need only to compensate the owner for the price of the site but not for the building itself. The evaluation of the fitness of a building for human habitation was to be based on the sanitary assessment by the municipal health officer using the technical—and thus purportedly objective—criteria of determining whether the light and air (or ventilation) in the interior was adequate, and if the water supply, sewage, drainage, and refuse and nightsoil disposal arrangements were satisfactory.[60] However, even such technical and supposedly objective evaluations did not go unchallenged. In 1933, when the Trust declared a few buildings in the Bugis area unfit for habitation, its decision was contested by the owners of the buildings. This challenge subsequently developed into a prolonged saga known as the "Bugis Street case,"[61] which was resolved only in 1937. The owners' appeal against the Trust's decision went all the way to the Privy Council in London, which ruled against the Trust. As there was no 'insanitary calculus' in the 1927 improvement ordinance, the health officer's assessment of unfitness for human habitation was based on the standard established by the Ministry of Health in England. The Privy Council ruled that

England's standard was not applicable to Singapore, and thus the Trust had no legal right to declare the buildings insanitary.[62]

The Bugis Street case brought into focus various issues surrounding slum clearance and helped to transform the Trust from an improvement agency into a proper housing agency. These issues were debated heatedly in the legislative council. Instead of demolishing insanitary housing, the building of more housing as a way to alleviate the overcrowded and insanitary conditions was deemed a better option. Langdon Williams, the SIT manager, submitted a key report that addressed these issues after he attended the International Town Planning Congress in London in 1935. From his survey of the housing policy in Britain, he argued that affordable housing for the working class could be built only by the authorities with state subsidies, not by private enterprises.[63] Public opinion expressed in the local newspaper also advocated the use of public funds to subsidize housing for the poorer classes of the native population.[64] All these led the Straits Governor Shenton Thomas to declare in 1936 that SIT should put up a 10-year housing program that would take "concrete shape in much larger schemes than have been attempted hitherto."[65] The use of public funds to subsidize housing was endorsed by the Weisberg Committee's Report and became the official policy in 1938. The Weisberg Committee argued that slum eradication was not just about "destroying bad houses," but about building housing that the poorer classes could afford.[66] Since private enterprises expected a return on their financial outlay that the working-class housing could not possibly yield, the Weisberg Committee saw "no alternative to the provision by Government of subsidized accommodation for the poorer working class."[67] With the recommendations of the Weisberg Committee, SIT became the official housing agency of the colonial state, empowered to build subsidized housing.

Following these changes, SIT started to be more involved in housing construction. It "experiment[ed] with various types of houses to suit different classes"[68] of the native population. One of main sites that the Trust built housing on from the late 1930s onwards was the Tiong Bahru estate, located at the edge of the congested Chinatown. Between 1937 and 1941, when building activity stopped due to the imminent Japanese occupation of Singapore, the Trust built 784 flats, 54 tenements, and 33 shops on the estate.[69] As the main building type in Tiong Bahru, the flats were regarded as some of the most modern buildings of their time (Figures 2.6 and 2.7). Not only were they built using modern materials such as hollow concrete blocks and steel windows,[70] they were also designed in a simple and abstract architectural language that accentuated clean lines and streamlined curvilinear forms. They were planned in such a way as to let the residents enjoy plenty of light and air, featuring individual flats with balconies for "sitting out," light wells in the middle of the blocks, and a "children's grassed playground" for the children to enjoy fresh air. Williams, who was also the architect of the flats, proudly claimed that they provided "modern comfort" and were comparable to similar schemes in Britain. These flats were, however, not intended for the poorest classes. They were meant for the "clerical class" that could afford a monthly rental of $25.[71] Despite their modern appearance, the Tiong Bahru flats were obviously influenced by the shophouse, especially in terms of the types of improvement that Simpson had proposed. Individual units were narrow and deep and the layout of the units made use of light wells, around which rooms were grouped.[72] Furthermore, the rear of the units lined black lanes in almost the same manner as the reconstructed rear of the shophouses after back lane improvements.

Besides the flats, another type of housing that catered to the 'clerical class' was 'cottage housing.' The first cottage housing scheme was a 'model village' with 65 double tendency houses erected in 1925 on 10 acres of land owned

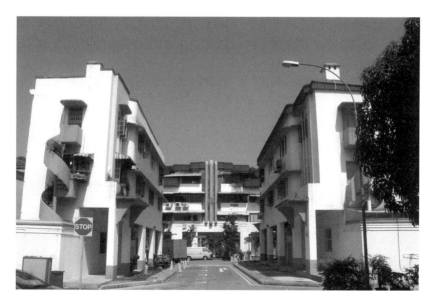

Figure 2.6
Clean lines and streamlined curvilinear forms of the SIT flats at Tiong Bahru.

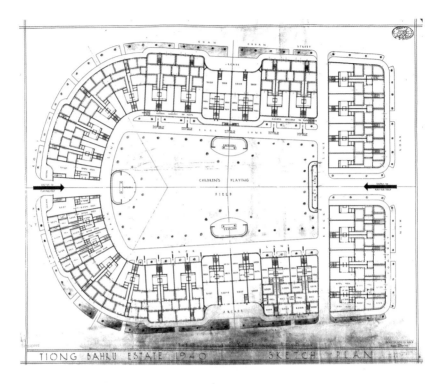

Figure 2.7

The horseshoe shape might be unique—light wells and back lanes—enclosing a 'Children's Playing Field' in the middle.

by the municipality at the junction of Alexandra Road and Henderson Road for people displaced by the Trust's improvement schemes.[73] The second was the Lavender Road Housing Scheme of 1928, in which 118 units of cottage housing were built for the clerical class and people displaced by the Lorong Krian Improvement Scheme.[74] According to Robert Home, the cottage housing type in the British colonies was probably derived from the British garden sub-urban single-family dwelling, which was popular in the early twentieth century because it helped to secure more 'light and air' for the inhabitants. Home also noted that town planners such as Richards considered the built environment of cottage housing to be more conducive to the production of "good citizens" than the "block dwellings" of the tenements.[75] Likewise, Williams contrasted the "cottage type of house, one room deep with ample kitchen, living room accommodation and all rooms well lighted and ventilated" that he designed for the Lavender Road scheme with the 'long narrow barrack' built form of the shophouse.[76] Besides these two schemes, the other SIT 'cottage' housing scheme was a very small scheme in the Old Race Course area, where 17 two-story houses were completed in 1941 (Figures 2.8 and 2.9).[77]

A third type of housing, known as 'artisan quarters,' was erected at Balestier, a suburban area a few miles away from the city center, in different phases during the 1930s (Figure 2.10).[78] They were one-or two-bedroom terrace houses, each with its own kitchen, toilet, and backyard. The units were arranged in blocks of six and eight, clustered around open spaces that doubled up as children's playgrounds.[79] The Balestier artisan quarters were first built as part of an improvement scheme for the Balestier insanitary area, 75 acres of swampy agricultural land "covered with filthy wood and attap houses and densely overcrowded."[80] They were designed to replace the attap huts, against the "squalor" of which their modernity, particularly their "atmosphere of brightness and spotless cleanliness," was contrasted.[81]

Although the artisan quarters were regarded as the "cheapest form of permanent housing," there was another category of housing built by SIT that was even cheaper.[82] This was the 'tenement housing,' first built as part of the 1920s improvement schemes discussed earlier, such as at Dickinson Hill, Albert Street, and Lorong Krian. As the tenement housing was rented out at low rates to the poorest classes, they were designed according to bare minimum

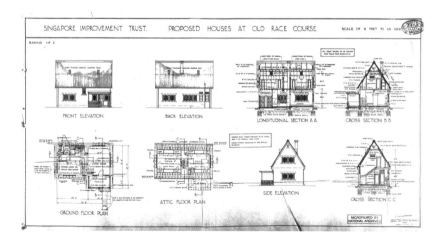

Figure 2.8

Sections and elevations of the SIT cottage housing at Race Course Road.

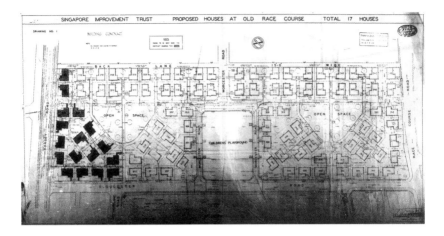

Figure 2.9

Overall site plan of the SIT cottage housing at Race Course Road. Only those colored in black were built.

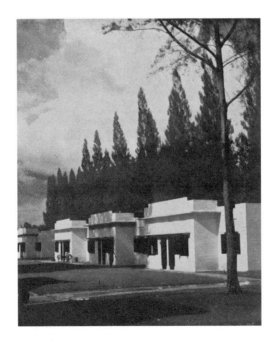

Figure 2.10

SIT artisan quarters at Balestier.

standards. In fact, one could even argue that they were substandard, as each family was typically allocated only a single room, with the kitchens and toilets as common facilities to be shared among the various families. Putting a whole family into a single room or cubicle was one of the main criticisms directed at the cubicles in the shophouses as they purportedly did not allow privacy for the adults in the family.[83] The compromising of this standard in the tenement housing was perhaps an indication that the other types of SIT housing discussed above were not sufficiently affordable for the poorer classes of natives. This was a point repeatedly raised in many reviews of pre-war SIT housing; it was not adequately addressed until the post-war housing reform.[84]

'Tropicalizing' Planning: Differentiation and Fragmentation

How can the various delays and partialities in the implementation of sanitary and housing improvements in colonial Singapore be explained? The colonial state's inaction between 1907, when Simpson's report was first issued, and the 1920s, when SIT was formed and the first steps towards housing and sanitary improvements were taken, could be attributed to the colonial state's concern about the financial commitment required. Despite the colonial development initiatives, British colonies received minimal financial support and were expected to be fiscally self-sufficient. As scholars studying the history of sanitary improvements and housing provisions in other British colonial cities have noted (including Cecilia Chu, who examines housing reform in Hong Kong in Chapter 1 of this volume), housing and sanitary improvements for the native population were typically underfunded.[85] The lack of funding and the chronic insanitary conditions of native housing were justified through colonial discourses of racial and cultural difference. It was frequently reasoned that, due to their fundamental 'Otherness,' the "ignorant and habitually uncleanly natives,"[86] who were "filthy in their habits beyond all European conception of filthiness,"[87] were incapable of observing hygienic practices and maintaining the environment in a sanitary condition. Thus, the limited resources of the colonial state were typically disproportionately invested in the improvement of sanitary and housing conditions in the districts where Europeans resided, such as their 'park-like' suburbs and cantonments.[88]

Although scholars of colonial cities have recently argued that spatial boundaries between the European and native towns were not clear and distinct but blurred,[89] the enclave nature of colonial cities—the clear separation of the cantonment and civil lines from the populous native town—that Anthony King first theorized in the 1970s is further reinforced if one considers the discrepant sanitary provisions and housing conditions.[90] In the context of British India, Sumit Guha describes these enclaves as "little islands of purity in the miasmatic landscape."[91] Instead of improving the sanitary and housing conditions of the native town, it has been argued that the colonial state implemented the more economical practice of leaving the native towns in many colonial cities alone and segregating the European enclaves from their contaminating influences instead.[92] This fragmented and splintered urbanism was especially apparent in colonial Singapore, even though it was one of the wealthiest colonies in the early twentieth-century British Empire, with sizable surplus revenue from the rubber and tin industries and opium taxation. In the planning and construction of the various military cantonments in Singapore from the 1890s to the 1930s, substantial resources were invested by the colonial government to ensure the provision of spacious barrack buildings with ample light and air, proper sanitary infrastructure, and large open spaces.[93] These were built with hefty military contributions drawn from the Straits Settlements' annual revenue.[94] Not only was the colonial state unwilling to invest in improving natives' insanitary housing while investing heavily in improving the European soldiers' lives, it also refused to abolish the use of opium, a major "tainted source" of the colony's revenue that was widely criticized, as it brought about much suffering among the native population.[95]

Scholars have argued that when governmentality, a concept developed to understand the "liberal modes of government"[96]—in other words, governing by working through the freedom of the governed—was transplanted to the frequently coercive and illiberal settings of colonial rule in the tropics, it took on coercive, racialized forms.[97] Ann Laura Stoler has argued that, though largely silent in Foucault's writings, racism was central to the metropolitan conception of biopower.[98] In the recently published transcripts of his lectures at Collège de France, Foucault noted that the intervention of racism introduced "a break into the domain of life that is under [biopolitical] power's control: the break between what must live and what must die."[99] In other words, racism introduced exceptions to the governmental rationality of optimizing lives. Racism, in fact, justified the exercising of the (sovereign) power to "take life" under modern governmental rationality. In Foucault's lectures, he looked at modern wars and massacres waged in the name of securing the biological existence of one population, most notoriously those waged by Nazi Germany.

However, to 'take life' did not necessarily mean intentional killing or the suspension of rights; it could refer to any governing activity that wittingly or unwittingly exposed a segment of the colonized population to considerable risk of ill health and death.

It is perhaps not unreasonable to argue that the use of opium revenue to pay for the improvement of European soldiers' lives, as described above, fits this model of colonial governmental rationality. Such an interpretation would also construe the tropicalization of sanitary and housing improvements as its 'Othering'—in other words, its racialization—in the way Arnold discusses tropicality. However, the 'Other' in the case of colonial Singapore was not a monolithic entity. While certain colonial discourses constructed the natives as habitually filthy and incapable of sanitary improvement, there were others who refuted these stereotypes and argued that "there are very few inveterate, incurable [native] slum-dwellers."[100] Those who advocated sanitary and housing improvements for the natives argued that "people will observe clean habits if only they are properly housed."[101] Moreover, the different types of housing built for various classes of native population, such as the clerical class and artisans, suggest that the colonial state's perception of the natives was not only shaped by race: the natives were invariably divided into different classes with varying capacities for improvement.[102]

3
Colonial Anxiety Counted: Plague and Census in Bombay and Calcutta, 1901

Richard Harris and Robert Lewis

Introduction: Data-gathering and Empire

Decades before equivalent data were published for New York, London, or Toronto, the 1901 censuses of Calcutta and Bombay produced a wealth of information relating to specific localities within two major colonial cities.[1] In this chapter we address a number of interrelated questions. First, why was this information gathered and published? Second, how was it interpreted or mis-interpreted, acted upon or ignored by colonial authorities? And third, what do the 1901 censuses of Bombay and Calcutta reveal about colonial govern-mentality, the social geography of these two cities in particular, and of colonial cities in general? In engaging with these critical issues, our aim is to contribute to wider debates articulated in *Imperial Contagions* about the interconnections between local situations and national, transnational, and imperial contexts, as well as contributing to ongoing discussion about colonial governmentality, modernity, and empire.

One compelling explanation for the publication of the 1901 censuses is that British administrators feared the plague. Its identification in October 1896, and the ensuing deaths in the following years, prompted widespread concerns on the part of colonial officials about their safety and authority.[2] As Cecilia Chu demonstrates elsewhere in this volume, in a chapter on housing reform in colo-nial Hong Kong, the plague brought to the fore industrial unrest, social discon-tent, and political conflict, while it served as a major impetus for the British to enumerate and plan on an unprecedented scale. As several writers have also suggested, the colonial state used the censuses to regulate and improve recalci-trant populations. To be sure, the British had long sought to secure information about their Indian subjects through intelligence-gathering activities.[3] However, the nineteenth century saw an intensification and centralization of such activities, and a growing interest in social statistics and census-taking, together with the development of new technologies, including the telegraph, that enabled faster and more efficient diffusion of information.[4] Indeed, some writers have suggested that data-gathering was pioneered, and carried furthest, in colonial settings, where state control was uncertain and where the cultural and geopolitical stakes were high. If this was indeed the case, it would make sense that India, the 'imperial jewel,' was at the forefront of a new informational drive. Certainly, 1901 was a moment when British efforts to 'know' the Indian population reached a new height. The panic induced by the plague triggered a frenzy of counting that resulted in a monumental census undertaking, unprecedented in its scope, thereby confirming Arjun Appadurai's suggestion, that data-gathering tells us much about the underlying anxieties of colonial rule.[5]

An Extraordinary Census

By 1901, the idea of a decennial survey of population was well established in India. The first national census was undertaken in 1872, and many basic procedures were soon worked out.[6] Its administration became more professional, while the scale of operation grew. More importantly, its purpose shifted away from making a simple assessment of resources and population to a view of the census as a means to better understand the character and dynamics of Indian society. This paralleled a broader shift in thinking. In the United States, for example, a simple count was replaced by "a full-fledged instrument to monitor the overall state of American society."[7] In Egypt after 1882, the British used the census to acquaint themselves with the country's agricultural resources, to promote good government, and guide policy.[8] In India, the invention of the census as a tool of social engineering required a more extensive administrative system, a large labor force, and the use of small-scale statistics. The enumerations and tabulations of 1881 and 1891, for example, required half a million people each, and elaborate communications between the Home Office in London, the various presidencies, and the numerous local municipalities.

The results seemed impressive. In 1881, the published report for Bombay included information on caste, education, language, birthplace, religion, occupation, and buildings, in 32 "sections" (subdivisions of the seven wards). The report also produced a listing for each city street, showing sex and religion.[9] Ten years later, the report for Calcutta contained statistics for 25 city wards.

These showed population, religion, sex ratio, house construction (masonry, other), occupancy status (vacant, occupied), age distribution, marital status (tabulated by religion), together with horses and cattle.[10] In addition, information on sex was reported at the finer, block scale. By the turn of the century, then, there was a tradition of generating statistics for small areas.

The 1901 census, however, took this practice to a new level. A wider range of information was gathered, including religion, caste/occupation, employment sector, sex, civil condition (marital status), dwelling condition, crowding, literacy, and country of origin. The 1891 census had contained inaccuracies, and great efforts were made to eliminate these. Building on the British preoccupation with classifying ethnic and racial groups, as well as social hierarchies, attention was given to identifying castes and subcastes. Intriguing to anthropologist and administrator alike, these were re-conceptualized and made the subject of a separate ethnographic survey.

Perhaps the most striking feature of the 1901 census was the extent to which information was tabulated, in some cases for small areas, in the two leading cities. In Calcutta in 1881, the tabulation of results had accounted for 34 percent of the total cost of the census. This proportion had risen to 41 percent in 1891, but then jumped to 52 percent in 1901.[11] Cross-tabulations were produced at what may be referred to as the district scale for both Calcutta and Bombay. In Calcutta, this consisted of 18 wards in the Old Town, 11 wards in the recently 'Added Area,' Fort William and Maidan, the 'Water Area,' and three distinct 'suburbs,' for a total of 36 areas. In Bombay, the district remained the 32 'sections.' The persistent decentralization of census operations ensured that there was little comparability between the two cities.[12] Many tables were unique, and only basic data were published at the district scale for both cities: area, population, number of houses, population trends since 1872 by sex (Tables I and II), and Christians, tabulated by race and age (Table XVIII).

Beyond the basics, each city featured unique—and extraordinary—information.[13] Forty years before the United States and 55 years before the United Kingdom published data for tracts with an average population of about 5,000, the British in India produced detailed information at a finer scale.[14] Bombay's tables were the most exhaustive. They showed, for example, civil condition by age, sex, *and* religion (Table VII); language and literacy by age, sex, and religion (Table VIII); and caste, tribe, race, and nationality by sex (Table XIII). Such information was not published for Calcutta. Nor were Bombay's eight 'special tables' on housing conditions produced for the Bombay Improvement

Trust. These reported information for 'circles,' of which there were about 200, averaging a population of 4,000. These tables showed dwelling conditions and occupancy. Special Table 6, for example, reported the number of persons by number of persons per room, while Number 8 showed population, by religion, showing tenement size (number of rooms), and number of occupants. Nothing comparable was published for Calcutta, where the lobby for the production of housing data was weaker: an improvement trust was not established there until 1912.

But Calcutta was not to be outdone. Although the range of district-scale tabulations for Calcutta was limited, it did include several unique items, including the number of Christians by race and age. At the circle scale, of which there were about 500, each with a population of about 2,000, information on overcrowding was tabulated against number of rooms, number of stories, and quality of construction (*pucka, kutcha*).[15] More remarkably, in a separate 'register,' religion was tabulated against sex at the scale of the block, of which there were about 5,000, each with a population of only 200. Most striking of all, however, was Table 15, surely the most remarkable published table of any city census for any place and time. Extending over 406 pages, it reported occupation by employment sector by sex *and* by religion, using no fewer than 516 occupational categories. Its production would be remarkable today, but was a stupendous achievement, given that cell counts had to be generated by volunteers who literally had to pigeonhole millions of 'slips,' one for each person. It took 13.9 person-years to produce—unusually, many of the clerks who helped produce it were women—and it accounted for over a fifth of the total costs of all tabulations in Calcutta.[16] Nonetheless, for all its data, detail, and innovative organization, one question about the 1901 censuses remains conspicuously unanswered: Why did the census-takers go to so much trouble?

Why States Enumerate Populations

In the nineteenth century, Europeans learned that populations could exhibit regularities, while individuals remained subject to chance. To 'tame chance,' many states began the systematic collection of social information in ways that changed how people thought about society and the individual.[17] Data-gathering reflected, and contributed to, the rise of the nation-state as a particular type of 'imagined community.'[18] Nations were communities with sharp geographical limits and sovereign powers, whose members mostly remained strangers. New technologies of communication, vernacular print literature, censuses, maps, and museums showed individuals the nature and shape of their host societies. By the late nineteenth century, censuses that were "profoundly novel," because systematic, became vital to the national project. According to Dipesh Chakrabarty, India's was simply "the most dramatic" example of a colonial government's concern with measurement.[19] It had become one of the indispensable "cultural technologies of rule" that a nation-state could deploy.[20]

From the early nineteenth century, states had used censuses to control and improve their populations.[21] In this sense, whether colonial or metropolitan, censuses should, perhaps, be viewed as a representative state-sponsored strategy of modernity. As Nicholas Thomas suggests: "Modernity itself can be understood as a colonialist project in the special sense that both the societies internal to Western nations and those they possessed, administered and reformed elsewhere, were understood as objects to be surveyed, regulated and sanitized."[22] As Bruce Curtis shows for Canada, governments assumed the right to imagine, represent, and in effect to 'make' their own populations.[23] At the simplest, there were two audiences. For those outside the nation, a census counted adults, especially males, a labor force and potential army, and perhaps factories and commerce too. For those inside, it served a normalizing function, showing (the range of) what was typical in terms of ethnicity and family size, for example, or of housing conditions.

In colonial settings, the audiences were complicated and multiple. Colonial powers were mindful of three, while they themselves constituted a fourth. The first audience consisted of other colonial powers, to be impressed by the size and riches of the colony, and by the capacity of the colonizer to enumerate and perhaps mobilize those resources. The second was the local population, in relation to which the colonial state could use the soft power of the census to maintain their subordination.[24] This colonizers did by presenting themselves as the source of 'authoritative knowledge': they showed the people—in their economic and cultural diversity—back to themselves.[25] As Stephen Legg has argued for India, the census was in part a "tool of domination."[26] Several writers have suggested that the census influenced the way Indians thought about themselves, not least because it engaged hundreds of thousands of enumerators, drawn from literate and influential elements of the population.[27] The third audience was composed of the citizens of the colonial power itself, who might need to be persuaded that their taxes (not to mention sons and husbands who served in the armed forces) should support colonial ventures. Indirectly, but perceptibly, the census of India informed the politics of the imperial as well as the colonial capital.

The fourth audience was the colonial administration itself. In any country, governments make surveys to reveal new facts about, or to construct specific understandings of, those they govern. But this is doubly true in a colonial setting. Few administrators were locally born, and many were resident for only a few months or years. Almost all were sheltered, attending school back home, living in European enclaves. At best, they learned fragments of the colonial culture. This was especially true in a place as large and diverse as India. Some went out of their way to learn the local culture, but most were largely ignorant. And so, as Gyan Prakash has argued, the British "hungered for more accurate data to enhance the 'taming of chance' in the alien and hostile environment of India."[28] In that context, as the commissioner of the 1891 Indian census noted, censuses were doubly important in the colonies, since other types of data, including registers of births and deaths, were deficient. More than back home, census data were seen as vital for government.[29]

Directly and indirectly, in developing their ideas about statistics and social surveillance, many writers have drawn on arguments sketched by Michel Foucault. For Foucault, the extreme model of surveillance was Bentham's panopticon, from which prisoners might continuously, but unobtrusively, be observed. Later writers have invoked this symbol, but Foucault's discussion of "the plague town" is relevant to a much wider range of situations.[30] Foucault takes as exemplary the military orders for Vincennes during a plague outbreak at the end of the seventeenth century. These called for minute scrutiny and regulation of social behavior. In the end, supposedly, the "plague-stricken town [was] traversed throughout with hierarchy, surveillance, observation, writing," making it a "utopia of the perfectly governed city." But such utopias could not exist: the state lacked the necessary resources.[31] Municipalities and nation states struggle to inform themselves about, and to regulate, their citizens, but evasion and resistance are the norm. The relevance to colonial India, and above all to Bombay and Calcutta when the plague recurred, is obvious.

As Foucault's treatment of the plague town also indicates, however, he inferred too much from the rhetoric of historical agents.[32] The corollary is that he paid too little attention to what those agents actually did, and to the reactions of those who did not wish to cooperate. The census, as an instance of Western science and rationality, is a case in point. Ambitious in conception, its implementation was a huge project, with all sorts of ramifications and consequences.

In colonial settings, statistical and scientific projects were double-edged swords.[33] They were designed as tools of rule, but they could be appropriated by those who sought to resist. In the census, the manner in which the British conceptualized several categories, including caste and house, was influenced by Indian understandings. In particular, the nascent Indian middle class influenced the manner in which they were positioned within the census and, by implication, Indian society.[34] Similarly, the native population changed, and was shaped by, the colonial conception of caste.[35] Then, too, unlike in the political arena, in the census everyone was counted in one sense as equal. Tabulations of people underlined the extent to which the British were outnumbered. This did not matter much as long as the British could take popular acquiescence for granted but, as riots showed in the 1890s, they could not.

In various ways, the British position in India was fragile, giving rise to a sense of cultural anxiety.[36] The colonial administration had to negotiate the chasm between their simplified understanding of Indian culture and the way this played out on the ground. The social realities of India did not fit administrative categories. Even under the easiest of situations, the discontinuities between what the British believed should be the case and what they actually found was problematic, and often incomprehensible. Under more trying conditions, such as during the plague outbreak, this rupture produced anxiety and fear. It was this "fear and panic generated by the plague" that was to lead the British to channel their anxieties into the creation of an extraordinary project.[37]

Indian Censuses in the Late Nineteenth Century

As the British refined it, then, the Indian census was directed at the four audiences relevant to any colony: rival powers, the indigenous population, the home audience, and colonial administrators. The difference was that the stakes could not be higher. India was the world's greatest colony, and its effective government was vital. In London, it merited its own India Office, and a separate civil service. Documenting its size and resources mattered enormously, and the accomplishment was itself a source of pride for such a large and diverse territory. It is easy to understand why the British administration there made the effort. The stakes were raised by the Great Revolt of 1857–59. After this turning point, the responsibility for administration was transferred from the East India Company to the new India Office. The rebellion underlined the fragility of British rule, and showed its ignorance of popular sentiment. It underlined the need for better information that might then be used for military, as well as civilian, purposes.[38] The first general census of 1872 was the belated result.

But the challenges of census-taking in India were huge, as Reginald Hooker noted in a comparison he made of the British and Indian censuses in 1894. Speaking to the Royal Statistical Society in London in his role as assistant secretary, Hooker observed that "the population of India is, probably in every single respect, the most difficult in the whole world to enumerate."[39] The challenges, he suggested, were "the enormous number of people, the variety of races, [and] the comparative illiteracy of the masses."[40] It was reckoned that only two percent of Indians could both read and write, while the additional necessity of translating census materials into the 17 languages that were understood by enumerators itself posed a major task.

A further complication was that many social categories were alien. The mixture of Muslim, Hindu, Sikh, and Jain was strange to British minds, but at least the concept of religious difference made sense. The very idea of caste, however, was bewildering. The Indian census of the late nineteenth century gave more attention than its British equivalent to questions of ethnicity and caste. The latter became a symbol of the exotic and primitive character of Indian culture.[41] Census administrators repeatedly wrestled with the concept. In 1881 they linked it to the idea of *varna*, or hierarchy, abandoned this in 1891, but then revived it from a different angle in 1901. Generating useful information was not easy.

Fortunately, support for the Indian census came from British professionals, notably statisticians and anthropologists. The former were fascinated by the logistics of enumeration and tabulation, and attended talks such as that given by Hooker.[42] The latter were intrigued by the issues of race and caste. By the 1890s, in the name of science, they were urging census-takers to redouble their efforts.[43] In December 1899, speaking for the British Association, M. Forster told the secretary of state for India that the forthcoming Indian census was "a special opportunity . . . for collecting valuable ethnographic data concerning the races of the country." Slyly, he added that H.H. Risley, the new census commissioner, was himself "an accomplished ethnographist [*sic*], well known by his publication on the Tribes and Castes of Bengal."[44] By autumn 1900, representatives of the Indian Finance and Commerce department, which was footing the bill, agreed that a survey could have a general "scientific importance" for the understanding of race. "It has come to be recognized of late years," they observed, "that India is a vast storehouse of social and physical data which . . .

[might] contribute to the solution of problems which are being approached in Europe with . . . inferior materials."[45] For a combination of reasons, then, the Indian census became part of "a model of the Victorian encyclopedic quest for total knowledge."[46]

Risley deflected pressures to extend the census, instead promoting a separate, subsequent, and specialized ethnographic survey.[47] This began in the summer of 1901, after the spring census. These surveys were complementary. As the British secretary of state observed, "the census provides the necessary statistics; it remains to bring out and interpret the facts which lie behind the statistics."[48] For the latter tasks, anthropologists as well as economists were needed. In 1901, an article in *Man*, the journal of British anthropologists, argued that "an ethnographic survey of India and a record of the customs of its people is as necessary an incident of good administration as a cadastral survey of the land and a record of the rights of its tenants."[49] Both surveys were of interest to scientists and administrators alike.

The need for all types of information had grown with the expanding complexities of administration and as the local expertise of officials became attenuated. In the fall of 1900, Finance and Commerce informed the secretary of state that "of late years there have been complaints that the English officials . . . know less about the people than those of an earlier generation."[50] The reasons were complex. In the past, "leave and transfers were less frequent, and office work was lighter than it is now." The Rebellion of 1857–58 had created a social divide that administrators found difficult to cross. To avoid mistakes, they needed facts and interpretations on a growing scale. These considerations played an important background role, but explain only part of the extraordinary efforts taken for the census of 1901.

Special Efforts for 1901

The flurry of activity that produced an ethnographic survey was paralleled by efforts to upgrade the decennial census. The tone was set in the early planning. In summer 1900, as schedules and methods were being devised, J. P. Hewitt, secretary to the government of India, made his employer's views clear to the government of Bombay. This was the agency that would be responsible for supervising census operations throughout the presidency, as well as in the city itself. Hewitt urged that "the coming census should be conducted with special care," and that tables should be produced "in full detail for the purpose of comparison."[51] Because detailed city-level data had not been produced for 1891, he also required a written history of the city. This was later published along with reports that summarized the 1901 data, and that reported how the census was actually carried out.[52] A similar history and reports were published for Calcutta.[53] As with the ethnographic survey, then, British administrators saw the need for interpretation as well as facts. The municipal governments of Bombay and Calcutta readily agreed that new information was needed. Hewitt noted that "in Bombay, as in Calcutta, the Corporations themselves are desirous of collecting some information bearing upon structural and residential conditions within municipal limits."[54] In Bombay, this had been urged by S. Rebsch, chair of the Bombay Improvement Trust, a planning agency established in 1898.[55] The presidency agreed. In September, J. Atkins, secretary to the governor, told Hewitt that "the Governor in Council is strongly in favor of the incorporation of the special information in the Census Schedules."[56] All levels of government, then, spoke with one voice about the need for better data.

The inadequacy of the 1891 census was agreed. Writing to his staff on February 1, 1901, a month before the count, Risley urged that "it is [all] the more necessary" that the city's responsibility for census supervision be clearly realized, "as the statistics of the last Census for Calcutta are practically worthless."[57] This was easy for him to say, since he had not been responsible, but his opinion was widely shared. As a result, detailed guidelines regarding the conduct of the census had already been distributed. These covered definitions, the delineation of small-area boundaries, and proper numbering of houses; the assignment of responsibilities within the administrative hierarchy, including methods of staff recruitment and training; the conduct of the two-stage enumeration process, which involved enumerators making a preliminary inventory, which they checked and updated on census day evening "after the lamps were lit"; and laborious methods of tabulating results using a "slip" system, with cross-checks in local returning offices both before and after results were sent in to central offices.[58] Risley had discovered that everything had not been going exactly to plan, and so he explained in detail what needed to be fixed. Each ward must have its own superintendent; new blocks should be established, each with its own supervisor; the drawing of block boundaries "will require much attention and some judgement," and so should be supervised by the citywide census officer; supervisors, who should be government officials, must show "every enumerator . . . round his block." And, since only 675 of the 825 necessary supervisors had already been appointed, "there is no time to be lost."[59] The desire for accuracy, and the sense of urgency, is palpable.

Recognizing that illiteracy was common, census administrators in India had already fashioned a uniquely exhaustive method. Throughout the British Empire, as in Britain itself, the norm was for household schedules to be distributed ahead of time. These were completed by household members (or heads), and then picked up by enumerators after census day. In India from 1881, enumerators themselves filled in all census forms. Only residents of Bombay, Europeans, and others of high rank received a household schedule, which became a mark of status. Because there was insufficient time for enumerators to collect all information in one day, a system of double-enumeration was devised. A week or so prior to census day, enumerators compiled basic data which they merely updated on the day itself. For 1901, tightening up one loophole, Bombay adopted this door-to-door double enumeration, even though it involved more work.[60] This required the division of the city into circles and blocks, and a closer supervision of staff and so, with support from W. L. Harvey, the municipal commissioner (an unelected appointee), Enthoven, urged the presidency to appoint a census officer just for the city—a first.[61]

The point of these efforts was to gather new, accurate information, and also to tabulate it in detailed form. In the summer of 1900, directions to this effect came from London, where the secretary of state for India "expressed a wish that the statistics of the larger cities in India should be tabulated in full detail for the purposes of comparison." This entailed the production of two main sets of tables: "imperial," which were standardized for all of India (and indeed other colonies), and "provincial," being "what each province requires for administrative purposes in addition to the Imperial Statistics."[62] In addition, at local discretion, some cities could produce special tabulations to satisfy particular needs. And to improve accuracy, a German system was adopted, whereby information was painstakingly copied from enumerator schedules onto slips of paper that could be sorted and re-sorted. In sum, taking into account the extraordinary scale of the Indian census, and given tight financial constraints, administrators were aiming high. Why?

There is no great mystery as to why special efforts were made in 1901. In September 1900, Provincial Secretary J. Atkins wrote that "the occasion appears to Government to be peculiarly opportune for a Census of Bombay City." He continued, "the events of the past few years would seem to render it more than ordinarily important, in the interest of the city, that no effort should be spared to secure . . . reliable and accurate results."[63] Atkins probably meant to refer to a cluster of related events. Recently, both Calcutta and Bombay had seen substantial industrial development. This had attracted migrants, fueled urban growth, raised residential densities, and provoked industrial unrest.[64] The population of Bombay had risen by more than 10 percent a decade, growing from about 640,000 in 1872 to 820,000 in 1891; Calcutta's from 685,000 to 950,000.[65] The overcrowding was awful. Coolootola, the densest ward in Calcutta, contained 281 persons per acre, up from 226 in 1891, higher than the most congested of the working-class districts of London. And ward averages disguised smaller-scale variations. In 12 of Calcutta's census circles, densities exceeded 300 persons per acre, reaching 707 in Coolootola's Circle 3.[66] Conditions in Bombay were worse, as its Improvement Trust recognized. Even at the scale of sections, in 6 out of 32, densities exceeded 400 per acre, and reached 598 in Kumbharwada.[67]

But area-wide densities tell only part of the story. Their effects depended in part on the type of dwellings, and how much living space most people enjoyed. In Bombay and Calcutta, the level of domestic crowding was extraordinary. In Calcutta, there were 2.2 persons per room; that is, each person had less than half a room in which to eat, sleep, relax, and often work. One in eight had the use of less than a quarter of a room, and a disproportionate number of the most crowded households occupied inferior *kutcha* dwellings.[68] Again, Bombay was worse. There, four-fifths of the population lived four or five to a room in one-room tenements.[69] Although the figure is hard to credit, it has been estimated that in Bombay by the 1890s about 100,000 laborers—more than one resident in 10—routinely slept on the roads or sidewalks.[70] Streets are always a locus of social tension, and it is not surprising that Bombay saw major riots in 1893 and 1898, together with many minor outbreaks of mayhem. One way in which the municipality responded was to re-organize the police force. More generally, popular unrest underlined the need for better information about, and closer surveillance of, the population.[71] This in turn made the need for a more complete census even more pressing.

The Plague and the 1901 Census

If labor conflicts justified surveillance, so too did deteriorating health conditions. Of course, poor social and environmental conditions were part of everyday life in urban India. Cholera, malaria, and tuberculosis had long been scourges. For at least 40 years, the growth of industry, trade, and urban population had contributed to disease outbreaks that had made Bombay and Calcutta among the unhealthiest cities in the world. By the 1890s, half of all newborns in Bombay died before their first birthday, and in the next decade the ratio actually increased.[72] This was worse than Colombo or Singapore and far worse than Cairo, none of these being salubrious cities. General death rates per thousand rose from just over 23 in the period 1886–90 to more than 65 between 1886 and 1905.[73] Cholera was a major killer, devastating some neighborhoods, while malaria and tuberculosis killed large numbers of people.[74] The situation in Calcutta was little better. High death rates, then, were part of the fabric of urban life in colonial India.

The plague, however, was new, deadly, and frightening. Its appearance in Bombay, in October 1896, engendered a panic that forced colonial authorities to rethink its administration and to re-organize its enumeration of the urban population. The disease took hold on the European imagination, partly because it spread more rapidly in India than anywhere else. Worldwide, between 1894 and 1938, about 13 million people died of this disease, to which mortality India contributed 12.5 million, or 95 percent of the total.[75] To be sure, it affected Indians more than it did Europeans. In 1897, as an epidemic gained momentum, plague mortality ranged from a high of about 24 per thousand among lower-caste Hindus, through 10–16 per thousand for other Hindus and (mixed race) Eurasians, 6–8 per thousand for Jews and Parsis, down to 2 among Europeans.[76] A similar pattern persisted for several years, as plague deaths slowly declined, with rates for the different ethnic groups ranging from 22 down to 1 per thousand in 1900.

Although Europeans were not greatly affected, and although the plague killed fewer people than malaria or tuberculosis, it provoked great anxiety among colonial administrators.[77] It was the rupture between what the colonial authorities believed was typical and what was actually occurring that prompted panic. The causes of the plague were widely debated but undetermined, undermining the authorities' sense of control over urban space. The plague called into question their strategies for separating themselves from the native population and from disease, both contagious and otherwise.

The main British strategy for controlling risk was segregation. Notably in Africa, but also elsewhere, they insulated themselves by setting themselves apart. In India in the late nineteenth century, social unrest, poor housing, and epidemic diseases encouraged them to redouble such efforts.[78] One problem, however, was that they relied on servants for many domestic tasks, including cleaning, cooking, and childcare. In India, the challenges were greatest in

Calcutta and Bombay, where rapid urban growth, and the very size of the cities, made it difficult to enforce consistent land use planning. In 1914, E. P. Richards, an English planner with Indian experience, prepared a report on Calcutta in which he claimed that in most Indian cities "we find fairly well demarcated separate Hindu, Brahmin, Mohammedan, Eurasian and European quarters."[79] He contrasted this with the situation in Calcutta (and Bombay). "The first unpleasant thing that usually strikes an Indian newly-arrived in Calcutta," he suggested, "is the enforced mixture of castes, creeds, and races found in every street, and in nearly every dwelling-house or place."[80]

Richards was right about the intermixing. To be sure, contemporaries and later writers pointed out that Calcutta, like Bombay, had a European quarter. This fact is noted by A. J. Christopher, the only scholar to use small-area data from the Indian census for this period. But Christopher points out that, in both the city and the suburban districts that were thought of as European, "other communities [ethnic groups] dominated both as resident servants and householders."[81] Overall, he suggests, "Calcutta . . . presents a remarkably complex pattern within which the European population occupied a position of political dominance, but did not convert this into legally based structural segregation."[82] If, as Richards claims, Indians were distressed by this, the British were doubly so. It may be that British administrators and businessmen were better prepared to put up with this situation because many could return to family property in London or pursue a career elsewhere.[83] It may also be that living conditions in Calcutta, "an incredible cesspool" at this time, encouraged them to view the city as only a temporary home.[84] But the plague must have made them feel vulnerable.

Apart from public safety, there were economic considerations. There was a real concern that the British imperial trading and manufacturing system would be disrupted. Calcutta and Bombay were centers of industry, especially in jute and cotton, and also major ports, shipping manufactured and agricultural goods around the world. As both cities became plague hot spots, the danger arose that their trade might be shut down.[85] Indeed, for a time, goods shipped from Bombay were quarantined. The plague, then, soon proved itself to be "disastrous to trade."[86]

A second and even more immediate concern was that, as plague cases rose in 1897–98, Indians exited the cities. At the height of the Bombay plague, it was estimated that between a quarter and a third of the city's population left town. That is why, contradicting other evidence, the census registered a decline in

Bombay's population during the 1890s. This mass exodus was possible because many residents had only limited local ties. During the late nineteenth century, high death rates would have reduced the populations of Calcutta and Bombay except that both received huge numbers of rural migrants. The 1901 census was to find that a majority of residents in each city had been born elsewhere— fully 77 percent in Bombay.[87] Most migrants were men, who returned seasonally to home villages and who could leave town at short notice. An astonishing number did so, more even than the number of plague deaths could have justified.[88] This exodus undermined the production of cotton, drove up labor costs, threatened profits, and left the elite without servants. Anxious about business conditions, the Chamber of Commerce and Industry urged drastic action.

Popular fear was driven by several factors. Experts were only beginning to figure out the etiology of the plague bacillus, connecting its life cycle with that of the rat. The inadequate state of knowledge was especially felt in Calcutta (as opposed to Hong Kong and perhaps Bombay), where the local health officer, William Simpson, was criticized for incompetence.[89] The mood was one of uncertainty about causes and solutions.[90] As Gyan Prakash has argued, it was this uncertainty that made the British hunger for more accurate data with which to tame chance.[91] Something had to be done.

Administrators acted in ways that approximated Foucault's description of the plague town.[92] In Poona, the chair of the local Plague Commission declared that measures taken there "were perhaps the most draconian that had ever been taken to stamp out an epidemic." In Bombay, they initiated what Rajnarayan Chandavarkar terms "a vigorous, indeed draconian programme."[93] Inevitably, inspectors concentrated on the areas where plague cases were most common. They searched, disinfected, and sometimes burned houses, quarantining people in isolation hospitals where castes were mixed, willy-nilly. Their approach was systematic and ruthless, and disruptions to domestic life were dramatic. The response was immediate and forceful. Indians resented the intrusions, and resisted the removals.[94] They hid infected and dead bodies; more than one British plague official was assassinated. Rumors abounded. And, in 1898, a major riot was triggered by a party searching for concealed plague victims. David Arnold has pointed out that the result of strict regulation was "the greatest upsurge of public resistance to Western medicine and sanitation that nineteenth-century India had witnessed."[95] They could also be read as an expression of dissatisfaction with British rule as a whole.

These plague events framed the census of 1901. The riots of 1898 were put down, but administrators could not persist with drastic measures. In his history of Bombay, written for the city census that he directed, S. M. Edwardes suggested that one side effect of the plague was to encourage Indians to accept more official intervention.[96] If so, his comment was valid only for mild intervention, exemplified by the census. After 1898, health regulations and inspections were relaxed, as administrators reverted to cheaper and less intrusive measures.[97] In their place, and because of the plague outbreak, the idea for a new planning agency in Bombay was developed and pushed through.[98] A similar agency was proposed for Calcutta, but this project was not realized until 1911. In 1898, the Bombay Improvement Trust received wide powers to develop new sites and redevelop old ones. Its mandate was to demolish overcrowded and plague-infested tenements, and also to facilitate the segregation of Europeans. In the end, the Trust only ever undertook projects to house Indians, and so Europeans had to find their own way into the suburbs.[99]

But the Bombay Improvement Trust did become active, and added its voice to those who sought acceptable ways of shaping the health of city residents. Its concern about what was taking place in the city's neighborhoods, and how plague spread from street to street, encouraged an interest in data-gathering. Anxious that disease and deteriorating houses were a lethal brew, the Trust identified new, and better, social surveys as its second-highest priority. In August 1900, its chairman wrote to the provincial superintendent of the Census, pleading for the compilation of "very detailed statistics" for small areas, which would provide "a very valuable guide for our operations."[100] This request received support from the highest quarters. In July 1900, when J. P. Hewitt wrote to the government of Bombay, urging that "special care" be taken about the census, he gave three reasons.[101] First, that government needed to know "the real effect of the plague upon the various classes of the population and the several quarters of the city." Second, that better data would "throw light upon the prospects of the schemes now being undertaken by the Improvement and Port Trusts." Only the third reason—the possibility that better data might also "furnish the Corporation with a precise statistical basis for any financial or administrative measures that might be contemplated"—spoke to more general matters. Timing was everything. If turn-of-the-century Bombay was "rendered into an object of knowledge in the form of maps, surveys and censuses," it was because of the personal anxieties, economic disruptions, and social tensions that recent epidemics had precipitated.[102] To a lesser degree, the same was true in Calcutta. Above all, we owe the extraordinary city censuses of 1901 to the British anxiety about the plague.

Conclusion: A Hostage to Fortune

In July 1900, a prescient warning was sounded by the department that funded census operations. While census administrators were thinking up new projects, the Home Department sought to apply the brakes. "Without wishing to interfere unduly with the discretion of Local Governments," it commented, "the Government of India are [sic] constrained to point out that there is a tendency to multiply statistics out of all proportion to the use that will ever be made of them."[103] It urged that, especially "for smaller [geographical] units . . . definite proposals for their completion should first be submitted to the Government of India."[104] Their concerns were with the timely publication of results and, even more obviously, the cost.

In one respect, the concerns of the Home Department were misplaced. Population counts were published in newspapers within a week of the census night, March 1, 1901. All statistical tables, even Number XV for Calcutta, were published within about a year, which puts many modern censuses to shame. But the Department had good reason to doubt that the data would actually be used. By the turn of the century, even Britain had made little use of census data for the development of national policy, and this appears to have been equally true of India.[105] This certainly seems to have been the case for the 1901 data, despite the thought and effort that had gone into its tabulation.

Indeed, very few of the small-area data for 1901 for Calcutta or Bombay were ever used. In the short run, local administrators did consult some of the numbers. In 1902, the administrative report for Calcutta suggests that tabulated data had already been used by "Plague, Engineering and Health Officers," though it is not clear how, or how much. More than a decade later, the head of the city's newly established Improvement Trust made some use of section-scale data on density to trace trends from 1891, while planning reports on Calcutta and Madras drew statistics from the 1911 census. But these ignored the analytical possibilities that enumerators had created in 1901, and there are notable silences. In Calcutta, where a plague outbreak in 1901 presaged several years of elevated mortality, a 1905 report included ward-scale statistics on plague cases and "rat returns" (by then the connection with rats was coming to be accepted). But the author did not connect this evidence with the small-area evidence on occupation, religion, or crowding in the published census. Similarly, annual reports of the Bombay Improvement Trust do not indicate that the agency used the tables that it had specifically requested. And in 1909, when he assembled a three-volume gazetteer for Bombay, S. M. Edwardes cited only aggregate census material for the whole city.[106] He had lived and breathed the census for a year, but could find no use for most of the information that his staff had collected and tabulated. And, perhaps most revealingly, later censuses did not attempt to reproduce the sorts of tabulations made in 1901. Here, indeed, is a conundrum.

In short, one perplexing feature of the 1901 census is not that so much information was gathered but that so little was done with it. Why was this? One reason is that, in fact, some of the data were unhelpful. The detail in Calcutta's Table XV, for example, was quite unmanageable. It was more reckless than admirable, indicative of a state of mind rather than of calculation. But useful data *were* gathered, on crowding, housing conditions, and social patterns, that could have guided municipal officials, planners, and newly established planning agencies. Some information may have been employed in ways that escaped the written record. If so, such usage must have been piecemeal and incidental. It seems that it was the gesture of the 1901 census, not its results, that counted. Massively precipitate, it revealed the colonial government's immediate fear of the plague, and the larger anxieties of colonial rule.

II

Hygienic Enclaves

4
"Beyond Risk of Contagion": Childhood, Hill Stations, and the Planning of British and French Colonial Cities

David M. Pomfret

Introduction

This chapter highlights the significance of European children and ideals of childhood to colonial authorities' efforts to rethink and refashion spaces of sanitized and hygienic 'nature' in the urban contexts of 'tropical' colonies. Though the actual number of European children remained small, and their presence has often been overlooked by historians of empire, they were deeply implicated in the managed expansion of segregated spaces and neighborhoods. These 'enclaves' were in turn integral to the re-ordering of imperial authority in empires' hegemonic phase.

Moving with their families within and across empires, European children formed an unstable presence, connecting and rupturing, buttressing and breaching the boundaries between the intimacy of the private, domestic environment, and the burgeoning colonial 'public sphere.' Many recent studies have demonstrated the significance of the domestic environment to the fashioning of colonial subjectivities, and have emphasized the roles played by women, and the 'intimate' realm of the family, in defining the racial membership of colonial communities.[1] As the presence of women in colonial space grew from the turn of the century, so too did that of children. Meanwhile, foreign communities' assertions of their own cultural superiority vis-à-vis colonial subjects came to rest firmly upon domestic norms. Children's gendered identities were similar to those of women in that they also occupied a liminal position in empire, and were often defined in terms of vulnerability. Yet, as they came to embody an especially powerful set of anxieties about racial and cultural reproduction in the tropics, children and childhood emerged at the forefront of discussions over health, disease and (dis)order and informed a series of colonial urban planning interventions.

Ideas about how to manage childhood in the so-called *zones torrides* had long been influenced by ideas about disease causation and transmission; as laboratory research afforded new insights into the microscopic world of contagion, childhood—a life stage coming to be connected with ideas of human "interiority"—was to provide a language through which fears of contagion and arguments for enhanced prophylactic barriers between colonial elites and subject peoples could be expressed.[2] In the early twentieth century, as the rising status, wealth, and political engagement of local elites challenged European colonial rule in Asia, childhood emerged as a key theme—and children became a critical consideration—within colonial urban planning.

This chapter examines the links between contagion, colonial childhoods, and urban planning by focusing on the case of the hill station. It builds upon an argument set out in the introduction to *Imperial Contagions*, namely that the new era of colonial public health did not produce the demise of enclavism but its re-conceptualization and 'embedding' in new forms in the strategies through which sanitized spaces of 'nature' were extended into the pathologized places of the colony. 'Hill' or 'altitude' stations in Asia provide a useful focus for this study, as their histories have been used to illustrate claims for a more general shift from enclavism to public health in European empires. Hill stations had emerged from the 1830s as part of a response by the British (in India) and French (in the Caribbean) to the high mortality rates suffered by colonial troops, informed by climatological interpretations of disease transmission. However, as declining mortality rates and the challenge posed by germ theory saw environmentalist paradigms become increasingly unfashionable in the early twentieth century, hill stations have also been seen to have fallen into a "swift decline as centres of colonial influence," serving as little more than "nurseries of the ruling race."[3]

This interpretation fits within an important argument in the history of medicine, which posits biomedicine as an integral element within the European colonizing process during the late imperial era, or as a 'tool' of empire applied by authorities to the tasks of safeguarding commercial traffic, managing indigenous populations, and maintaining social order.[4] During the early twentieth century, in particular, historians have argued that new laboratory-based knowledge of infection and its associated practices played an important role in colonial states' advancement of programs intended to improve the health of colonial subjects.[5] With the onset of this new era of public health, earlier 'enclavist' approaches to health, institutionalized in barracks, sanatoria, and hill stations with the principal intent of maintaining colonial armies, were largely superseded.

This perspective has not gone unchallenged, and recent studies have begun to examine how older models persisted alongside, and were combined, in new forms with understandings of microscopic pathogens as primary agents of disease.[6] By examining the case of children in colonial hill stations, this chapter aims to build on recent scholarship showing that the shift from older enclavist models of colonial medicine to a newer emphasis on the prevention and treatment of disease was by no means straightforward. It does so by looking across empires to focus upon two such enclaves: the Victoria Peak Hill Reservation, an equivalent of the hill station in the British crown colony of Hong Kong, and the hill station of Dalat, on the Lang Bian plateau in the French 'protectorate' of Annam. By examining the ways in which British and French fears of contagion, mapped onto the bodies of European children, played a fundamental role in shaping the built environment of colonial cities, it seeks to demonstrate that colonial medicine was not homogeneous 'on the ground' but was riven with tensions, contradictions, and cross-cutting impulses.

The Laboratory, the City, and the "Hill District Reservation" in Hong Kong

In January 1912, Dr John Mitford Atkinson hosted medical experts from the Straits Settlements, the Philippines, French Indochina, India, the Netherlands-Indies, Japan, and Johore at the second congress of the Far Eastern Association of Tropical Medicine held in Victoria, Hong Kong. As president of the association, Atkinson proudly led delegates on a tour of the key sites of the colony's anti-contagionist infrastructure, the development of which he, in his time as chief medical officer, had overseen. The group inspected a series of hospitals, the colony's bacteriological institute, and its disinfecting stations. These were important sites in the ongoing struggle against contagion and the advancement of public health. Built upon a series of breakthroughs in the laboratory, emblematic of the newfound influence of bacteriologists within the colonial state, they were closely connected with the process of managing and making legible colonial subjects.[7]

Atkinson himself had drawn his authority from a position created in response to the bubonic plague epidemic that ravaged Hong Kong in 1894. Following the diagnosis of the first case of the plague on May 8, 1894, this highly virulent outbreak had paralyzed the port city of Victoria. The intensity of the epidemic and the highly visible, public nature of the debate over the rival claims by Shibasaburo Kitasato (Robert Koch's former student) and the Swiss-French bacteriologist Alexandre Yersin (a student of Emile Roux) to have identified the plague bacillus raised awareness of bacteriological interpretations of contagion within the colonial state.[8] From here it informed a remarkable range of coercive interventions, discussed by Cecilia Chu in Chapter 1.

Those with a stake in the managed exploitation of colonial possessions were attracted to the idea that bacteriologists, in their mobile laboratories, might alleviate the economically damaging obstacles to trade produced by contagion in the short term and make empire more cost-effective in the long run.[9] As Robert Peckham explains in Chapter 6, the laboratory was an ambivalent space, defined by the very 'nature' it purported to exclude, but also deeply politicized. It was a space yielding knowledge that contained a potential challenge to carefully defended hierarchies of race. For, as much as 'race' was present in the laboratory, under the bacteriologist's lens the microbe could potentially become a race-blind agent and invader of bodies. This perspective jarred with a British vision of imperial authority grounded in older environmental interpretations of racial vulnerability. Hence, while the work of Ronald Ross, who in 1897 identified the mosquito as the vector for malaria, and its potential to reduce the cost of colonial administration, fascinated the colonial secretary Joseph Chamberlain, the new paradigm never entirely overcame resistance and indifference within the Colonial Office. Bacteriology, connoting as it did planning at one remove, sat uneasily alongside the "quintessentially British" approach to empire, supposedly based on pragmatism and 'experience' acquired in the field.[10] Ross's research (notably in Sierra Leone) inspired not the application of urban planning tools to the elimination of disease from indigenous populations under British rule, but rather the imposition of greater social and physical distance between colonizer and colonized.[11]

As bacteriologists began to identify microscopic pathogens as the primary agents of disease the new paradigm influenced planners' efforts elsewhere to reorder neighbourhoods within colonial cities along more socially segregationist lines. While laboratories produced knowledge of specific microbes, parasites, and vectors, this in turn underlined the need for enhanced prophylaxis.

'Tropical' endangerment was coming to be seen as residing not only in the climate and environment but also in native bodies and populations that, as an extension of the environment, were recast as reservoirs of disease.[12] While the institutional structures of the new anti-contagionist orthodoxy, proudly displayed in Hong Kong in 1912, evidenced an official commitment to the notion of expanding 'colonial public health,' this did not supersede, but rather stimulated new engagements with, the older technology of the hill station enclave. At the very moment when the older medical rationale for hill stations was being challenged, these spaces began to look more valuable than ever in the eyes of British colonial elites.

This was especially true of those in Hong Kong, where, as Cecilia Chu shows elsewhere in this volume, from the 1870s attempts by the rising Chinese elite to acquire residences in 'European' areas of 'Victoria' triggered anxious protests over 'encroachment' and the impending 'subsumption' of white communities. Demands for a formal re-ordering of space along racial lines stimulated a series of official engagements. Under the governorship of Sir George William Des Voeux, the European Hill District Reservation Ordinances (1888) declared illegal the construction of "Chinese-style" tenement buildings within a demarcated "European district." These failed to allay anxieties over so-called encroachment. In May of the same year, a funicular tram line connected Victoria with the Peak. At an altitude of around 1,800 feet (550 meters) the land on Victoria Peak had begun to be developed decades earlier under the governorship of Sir Richard MacDonnell, who built a summer house there, and had also been the focus of a sanatorium project. Anxieties over the declining residential homogeneity of elite European neighbourhoods saw the Peak emerge as the focus of a campaign for the formal exclusion of Chinese through the creation of a "reservation" in law. Owners of property on the Peak petitioned Governor Francis Henry May for the closure of the "Hill District" to Chinese. May (who also resided on the Peak) supported this request on the grounds that (as he advised C. P. Lucas at the Colonial Office) "if [the Peak] is not reserved it will be overrun by Chinese in the course of years."[13]

The use of planning tools to effect racial segregation in Hong Kong formed part of a more widely observed trend in turn-of-the-century colonial urban planning informed by decisions made both in colonial contexts and in the Colonial Office. Joseph Chamberlain, influenced by the Rossian shift, had made racial segregation official policy in the planning of sub-Saharan African colonies.[14] Yet the planning of neighborhoods in accordance with the 'cantonment' policy used in British India, while considered appropriate in Africa, did not translate as easily to Hong Kong, where the exclusion or relocation of wealthy Chinese from existing, high-prestige neighborhoods, as May's proposal entailed, was to prove deeply contentious. The potential for such a move to risk offending increasingly powerful local elites made Chamberlain reluctant to accede to the demands of Hong Kong's foreign community and within the colonial government for segregation on a racial basis.

Chamberlain had objected to the efforts of Governor Sir Henry Blake to introduce European-only schools in 1902, and also opposed Blake's efforts, the same year, to use the contagionist orthodoxy (and specifically the pretext of controlling malaria) to prevent Chinese from residing within a reservation designated for European use in Kowloon.[15] Indeed, the home government only sanctioned the Kowloon Reservation in February 1903, after the Hong Kong government agreed to add a clause permitting persons "of good standing" to reside there too.[16] The first effort to restrict residence on Victoria Peak in law had been made in 1902 and described intended residents in similar terms, and made approval conditional upon the governor.

When Governor May broached the idea of an ordinance explicitly excluding Chinese from the Peak Hill District with Chamberlain's successor, Alfred Lyttelton, in 1904, he did so at an inopportune moment. Lyttelton was mired in a controversy over the use of indentured Chinese laborers in South Africa, which had inflamed liberal sensitivities over questions of race in empire. In April, as the Colonial Government prepared a bill excluding Chinese from the Peak for its first reading, Sir Henry Blake wrote to the Colonial Office to advise that such a move would be politically dangerous.[17] The need to tread delicately was more than evident to May. So, too, was the fact that arguments about inferior hygiene among the "Chinese" provided scant leverage when it came to excluding wealthy Chinese from the Peak.

Germ theory had gained currency in Hong Kong after 1894, partly because the plague epidemic seemed to corroborate beliefs about the connection between disease, space, and class.[18] On these grounds, some sections of the Chinese elite had even supported the Taipingshan resumption scheme discussed by Cecilia Chu in Chapter 1. However, as May frankly admitted, "one cannot plead Sanitary necessity for the [Hill District] Ordinance for there is no danger of coolie houses being built."[19] Seeking a language of authority with which to convince the Colonial Office of the need for immediate action, May also struggled to mobilize climatological tropes of white vulnerability.[20]

Appeals to white racial vulnerability as somehow fixed in the environment ran up against a long-observed statistical decline in European mortality rates and administrators' frequent claims for Hong Kong's much improved sanitary condition. Notwithstanding these constraints, the second reading of the bill on April 19 was followed by the passing, on April 26, 1904, of the Hill District Reservation Ordinance, which included a clause allowing the governor to exempt "any Chinese" from it.[21]

May's ability to push through the legal enforcement of racial segregation turned to a significant extent upon his ability to connect the older orthodoxy of the threat posed by tropcial living to European health with specific fears for the physical endangerment and cultural contamination of European children. In dispatches to the Colonial Office, his emphasis on the need to protect the "rising generation" played to a new congruence of interests between the colonial administration and a home government reeling from the disastrous performance of the British Army in the Boer War, a series of gloomy reports upon physical 'deterioration,' and eugenicist condemnations of the failure of the state to act to enhance or protect racial efficiency. The fate of the imperial nation was coming to be linked to the health of British children as never before.

Colonial officials sought to wield the same argument in negotiations with Chinese elites over racial segregation on the Peak. For example, during the second reading of the bill on April 19, 1904, the governor repeated the familiar argument for segregation in the interest of the health of European "families."[22] While it seems unlikely that the "leading Chinese" were convinced by this line, at a time when the ability of foreign communities to protect their most vulnerable members had emerged as a crucial index of authority the defense of childhood nevertheless carried considerable weight. Significantly, the Western-trained physician, Dr Kai Ho Kai, one of the two Chinese representatives on Hong Kong's Legislative Council and liaison with "leading Chinese," interpreted his willingness to endorse the bill in precisely these terms. Though detecting "a decided savour of the nature of class legislation" in the ordinance, Kai Ho Kai endorsed it on the grounds that such precautions were "necessary for the health of Europeans," and "especially the children."[23]

By summoning the sentimentally charged issue of children's health to support the racial segregation of space, the colonial government used assumptions about childhood to connect medical science with the cultural domain of racialized identity.[24] Though there were only a few dozen children living on the Peak in Hong Kong in 1904, children's bodies served as sites of a racial vulnerability no longer so easily attributed to white bodies in general. As an admissible point of vulnerability, the colonial 'child,' constructed as perennially between bouts of sickness, embodied an abject rupture, a 'natural' enclave within the white colonial community (and within the individual, according to the new science of psychology). The construction of the reservation as a 'space of childhood' within the colony in some sense mirrored the internal breach within the rational, governing, adult, colonial body.

However, the enclave could never be completely 'sealed' against contagion. When in 1917 members of the colony's culturally 'Chinese' Eurasian elite sought to exploit a legal loophole in the 1904 ordinance to purchase properties on the Peak, May, once again serving as acting governor, repealed the ordinance, removing overt reference to 'Chinese' but renewing his emphasis upon the language of contagion when making *all* applications to reside conditional upon the governor's personal approval. The need to legislate was again explicated with reference to the health of children, who constituted a contagious constituency requiring protection behind a reinforced *cordon sanitaire*.[25] In this way, Chinese continued to be barred from residing on the Peak in Hong Kong (with the notable exception of Robert Ho Tung), while the Peak came to symbolize British power in the region (in contrast to India, for example, where as Dane Kennedy has shown indigenous elites' relocation to hill stations during the interwar years led to their identification as a symbol of the decline of the Raj).[26]

As the laboratory, near invisible in the field, yielded a striking new perspective—through the lens of the microscope—of the microbe within the enclave, the menacing danger posed by the microbe, and the 'teeming' masses of the Chinese city below could now be imagined as more remote. Magnified many times, the objectified invader and pestilential host loomed large in the language of colonial governance. However, for the ruling elites, the view from the Peak had the effect of inverting the microscope, and diminishing the microbial threat below. In Hong Kong, with the dilemma of elite residence resolved, the early momentum built in the field of public health was lost. Government sponsored public health initiatives between the wars were limited, piecemeal, and poorly funded. A Town Planning Committee, for example, was created only in 1939. By the end of the period, reformers criticized the colonial government's record in this area for its tentativeness, even in comparison with other British-administered commercial centers such as Singapore, Bombay, and Calcutta.

Yet, this was no straightforward 'retreat' to luxurious indifference in the heights. The sentimental defense of alien childhood was enlisted in a series of coercive interventions re-ordering colonial space along segregationist lines. Indeed, focusing on the family allowed the enclave to be extended coercively into the 'Chinese city' below. On October 23, 1918, the secretary of state for the colonies, Walter Long, agreed to the establishment of another reservation, this time for the benefit of British and American missionary families on Cheung Chau Island.[27] Modeled on the Peak District Reservation Ordinance, the bill proposed that no person should reside within the southern portion of this island without the consent of the governor-in-council. This time, Chinese representatives on Legislative Council, Lau Chu-pak and his brother Ho Fook, expressed their opposition in the strongest possible terms. Ho dispensed with the references to "class" preferred by Ho Kai and denounced the Bill as "nothing more or less than racial legislation."[28] Lau pointed out that, since Cheung Chau was far from commercial or residential quarters and was hardly overcrowded, its reservation through law was unjustified. Both proposed that the bill be held in abeyance.

The lawyer, Mr C. Grenville Alabaster, a member of the Legislative Council, commenting on the amendment, countered with the following:

> Cheung Chau is an island which has been developed solely by residents who belong to a race which finds it necessary to take their children to the sea-side as much as possible in the summer and who are separate themselves from their children by sending them home for education . . . They desire that their children should play on these beaches.[29]

Alabaster's line of argument was heavily informed by the defense of a racial-cultural vision of childhood. In his view, the bill was a matter of some urgency, since, while it remained under consideration, "all sales of land in Cheung Chau were held up for one year, and other missionaries who desire to build like their friends have been held up for that period—one year nearer the time for sending their children Home."[30]

The defense of vulnerable childhoods within the enclave proceeded alongside efforts to push hygienic nature beyond the temperate heights into the pathologized plains, in the form of the racially exclusionary enclave. Neither environmentalism nor the elision of Chinese with the marauding microbe were sufficient to secure segregation at sea level in Cheung Chau. But through appeals to childhood, an intrinsically mobile 'natural' condition, the enclave was itself made mobile and expanded into the plains. There it mediated between the inconveniences of (outdated) climatology and (politically inexpedient) bacteriology and allowed new interpretations of the etiology of disease to be transposed onto a discourse of cultural contagion. Childhood as a cultural category was, of course, far from being fixed and monolithic, but shared assumptions about this mutable life stage could nevertheless, far from the Peak, productively cloud debates over access to space in the colonial city, naturalizing British officials' inclinations to push the enclave out into the colony at large. In response to Chinese representatives' bitter complaints about the Cheung Chau ordinance, Acting Governor Claud Severn could brazenly declare, "I cannot observe anything in the Bill of a racial kind at all."[31]

Colonial Childhoods, Pastorianism, and Planning in French Indochina

When the eminent bacteriologist Alexandre Yersin traveled to Hong Kong in 1912 to attend the second congress of the Far Eastern Association of Tropical Medicine hosted by J. Mitford Atkinson, he did so not only as the organization's vice-president but also, in spite of recent squabbles with the Government General, as a high-profile associate of the French colonial state in Indochina. Though the major urban centers of 'French Indochina' (which comprised the formal colony of Cochinchina, the protectorates Tonkin, Annam, Laos, Cambodia, and the leased territory of Guangzhouwan) had not suffered an epidemic incident of equivalent magnitude to the Hong Kong plague of 1894, the Government General of the Indochinese 'Union' pursued the development of a far more ambitious system of public healthcare than that which emerged in Hong Kong.

This system was built up at a time when colonial theorists were re-interpreting French overlordship in terms of the exploitation of underutilized resources for the benefit of colonizer and colonized alike. As *indigènes* were also referred to in terms of their productive potential, their protection against disease was considered critical. Officials envisaged a colonial politics of medicine radiating from modernizing urban centers, winning the hearts and minds of subject peoples and permitting the more effective exploitation of colonial labor markets. To this end, Paul Doumer (governor from 1897 to 1902) appointed local directors of health, a Conseil supérieur de santé des colonies, and added a *directeur de la santé* to the *corps de santé colonial* created in 1890. Disease prevention was defined as a responsibility of the colonial government in the law of February 15, 1902, and a national health code was established. In 1905, Doumer's successor, Paul Beau, set up the Assistance Médicale Indigène, which focused upon the further expansion of preventive public health in Indochina.[32]

In developing this state-led drive to safeguard public health, the colonial administration drew upon Pastorian bacteriology, and upon the expertise of Yersin in particular.[33] Following his return in 1894 from Hong Kong, where he had discovered the plague bacillus, Yersin had established a laboratory in Nha Trang with the help of the colonial government, and in 1902 he accepted Governor Doumer's request to create a medical school in Hanoi.[34] Though Governor Beau's tendency to meddle led to the transfer of direct authority for Indochina's two Pasteur Institutes back to Paris in 1905 (with Yersin assuming directorial control over both), Pastorian laboratories continued to proliferate; in his book of 1922, the Institutes' biographer, Noël Bernard, could openly celebrate their "role in the extension of French influence."[35] So significant was the work of these productive enclaves that at times the distinction between the institutes and the colony collapsed, and metonymical references were made to the latter as a 'laboratory' of French colonialism.

Before the 1920s, major urban areas were the main focus of efforts to expand the reformist colonial politics of medicine and its supporting bacteriological infrastructure.[36] Notwithstanding the lip-service paid by administrators to universalist ideals, the uneven application of healthy planning defined and delimited neighborhoods in which segregation was a striking feature. In Hanoi, as Michael Vann has shown, the expansion of the French quarter left the 'native quarter,' an unhygienic residuum within the borders of a city, built on soil declared 'French.'[37] Nevertheless, the internal borders of the *quartiers blanches* remained porous, and were continually breached by migrant workers. In consequence, the disease threat, and the debate surrounding it, remained deeply racialized. A powerful set of anxieties cohered around locals' penetration of 'hygienic' French neighborhoods. These anxieties intensified further during and after the Great War, when Chinese and Vietnamese elites used newly accumulated wealth to purchase residences in such areas. As in Hong Kong, the growing racial heterogeneity of elite neighborhoods was to coincide with the launching of efforts from within the colonial state to re-invigorate the hill station through appeals to the needs of a specific colonial constituency— the vulnerable white 'child'—in a period marked by the further expansion of state-led public health campaigns.

Childhood, Hygiene, and the Planning of Dalat

In the interwar years, Dalat, located at an altitude of 5,000 feet (1,500 meters) on the Lang Bian plateau in the southern highlands, emerged as the focus of plans to re-inscribe French authority far from the febrile atmosphere of the major urban centers. Yersin, widely credited with having "discovered" Dalat during a mission undertaken in 1893 to survey and map the Lang Bian plateau, had been impressed by the temperate climate that he encountered there. He recommended the site to Governor Paul Doumer, who was keen to establish a British-style hill station sanatorium. Doumer sent 'missions' to survey the area and to set down general principles for the site's future development as a seasonal administrative center. Though these initiatives lost their impetus after Doumer's departure from office in 1902, in the following years the military continued to take an interest in the site as a potential sanatorium for the armed forces.[38] In 1906, Paul Champoudry, who had been named 'administrator' of Dalat, devised an urban plan that foregrounded the needs of the military. However, a lack of funding ensured that these plans remained unrealized, and the hill station project languished. A decade later, Dalat still possessed a mere handful of chalets, and one building which served as a hotel with just six rooms.

It was only in wartime, with leave to the metropole canceled or curtailed, that surging demand for these accommodations stirred a revival of interest in the hill station project.[39] Dalat's supporters now reprised earlier arguments by Doumer and Beau and identified not only the military but also civil authorities as its chief beneficiaries. The inspector-general of public works in Saigon advised the governor in Hanoi of the need to "endow the colony with a sanatorium where administrators and *colons* may spend a month or two with their family for the benefit of their health."[40] He advised that a new hotel would also be essential to accommodate "families travelling with their retinue of servants."[41] By 1919, the need for a new development plan was already evident, and in 1921 Governor Maurice Long commissioned the chief architect and city designer in Indochina's Department of Urbanism, Ernest Hébrard, to draw up plans for a seasonal administrative center capable of accommodating higher-ranking administrators and their families and children in Dalat.[42]

When Hébrard, well-known for his work on Thessaloniki, eventually produced his master plan of 1923, it revealed a striking segregationist intent.[43] The plan used strict zoning requirements to divide the town into an administrative quarter, a European residential quarter (where villa-type accommodation surrounded by gardens was planned), and a more compact *village annamite*, which would be located some distance from the French quarter in order to guarantee "harmony."[44] Contemporaries identified the lake and the new hotel (the "Lang Bian Palace," which opened in 1922) as key 'poles' in the plan, but were also struck by the care taken to designate space for the exclusive use of French children whose families it was hoped Dalat would accommodate. The Lang Bian Palace Hotel was, for example, to include gardens and spaces designed specifically for children's games while, around the lake, a *collège de garçons* and *collège des filles* were intended to become the most important "public institutions."[45]

As construction costs increased, Hébrard's plan for a large administrative quarter (like much else in his scheme) was left unrealized, but Long's successor as governor, Martial Henri Merlin, doggedly pursued the provision of space for the exclusive accommodation and schooling of European children. During his time in office, Paul Doumer had initiated a vast increase in Indochina's administrative cadres. As the new generation of administrators rose in seniority, and were promoted, they married and brought their families to live with them. With children accompanying their parents in larger numbers, protests over the quality of education services in Indochina intensified. These were skillfully orchestrated by pressure groups such as the *Ligue Populaire des pères et mères de familles nombreuses de France*, which had established offices in Indochina during the war and boasted a burgeoning membership within the colony's administrative cadres.[46]

It was in this context that Merlin reminded the *résident supérieur* of Annam, Pierre Pasquier, of the "urgent" need to identify buildings in Dalat suitable for "a French elementary school, with boarding [facilities], for the exclusive use of children of European origin."[47] The intention was to supplement the small mixed primary school that already existed in Dalat with one capable of accommodating the growing number of French children living in Cochinchina, Cambodia and further afield. Merlin set the project on a more formal footing through an *arrêté* of July 30, 1924, and allocated funds to cover the costs of construction.[48] But, in spite of the governor's exhortations, progress was slow.[49] In September 1924, Garnier, the deputy commissioner of Dalat, informed the high resident of Annam that the construction of school dormitories was behind schedule, and in 1925 the new governor-general, Maurice Montguillot, pushed once more for the realization of the boarding school project (described as "very urgent").[50] In January 1926, amid growing exasperation at these delays the *service de l'arrondissement* was swept away and replaced by a new municipal commission, whose inaugural members were charged with ensuring that the boarding school opened within 12 months.[51] The school, which offered elementary and secondary level classes for boys and girls, was formally created as the *Petit Lycée* by *arrêté* on July 16, 1927, and finally commenced its functions on September 16, 1927, and on January 7, 1928, its boarding section finally opened.

The significance of the school extended well beyond the few dozen students it initially admitted. Dalat had emerged at the heart of a drive to re-establish French health and authority in the heights. As debates continued to rage over the possibility of white settlement, an administration facing an increasingly confident indigenous elite and vociferous anti-colonial movement made the presence and acculturation of European children critical to substantiating a re-ordering of empire encapsulated in visions of a 'French' Dalat. However, desires for stability and permanence ran up against fears of contagion informed by the new orthodoxy of the Pastorian laboratory. Children's bodies emerged as key sites upon which the older claims of medical geography could be tested and, it was hoped, the ongoing dispute over Dalat's claims to sanitary status could be resolved.

Decades earlier, Yersin and others had identified the cooler temperatures of the hills as ideal for the restoration of energies dissipated by colonial living. Dalat's viability as a center for European residence had been linked to its potential to allow children and European youth, who would otherwise be "enfeebled" by the tropical climate, to thrive.[52] However, from the turn of the century, after Ronald Ross's findings cast doubt upon assumptions of the prophylactic benefits of the heights, the colonial press debated whether children in Dalat might really be able to live beyond risk of contagion.[53] In 1905, the governor of Cochinchina, François Rodier, sent the Pastorian bacteriologist Joseph J. Vassal, of the Nha Trang Pasteur Institute, to study the 'malarial index' on the Lang Bian plateau. Vassal conducted blood tests on Vietnamese children resident in Dalat. Those tested displayed signs of malarial infection, prompting Vassal to warn that highland regions were "not always protected by altitude" and that the plateau was in fact infested with Anopheles mosquitoes.[54]

Plans for the hill station were informed by the desire to accommodate children and to cater for their specific needs but amid ongoing concerns about salubrity the actual presence of French children threatened to compromise the entire project. As visions of Dalat as a sanatorium were superseded by grand ambitions for an administrative quarter, planners struggled to reconcile desires to relocate children to the heights (potentially the key to race survival in the tropics), with fears that the same group would constitute a sickly, dis-orderly presence and a potent internal threat to the realization of Dalat as a hygienic enclave. In 1923, a barrage of complaints identifying the infectious agency of sick children as a hazard for healthy adults in Dalat reached the letters page of the newspaper, *L'Impartial*, and attracted the attention of administrators.[55] The commission set up to oversee the development of the Lang Bian Palace Hotel lambasted the management's failure to implement plans to segregate children from adults in interior and exterior space. As the hotel renovations dragged on, it had emerged that the space designated to serve as an indoor play area for children was still being used as a makeshift workers' quarters, and in consequence the children in residence were playing on the ground floor of the building and disturbing the repose of guests.[56] This seemed to be symptomatic of a more general dis-orderliness. The children's gardens planned around the hotel had still not been laid, prompting demands from the commission that these be provided "as rapidly as possible."[57]

In the mid-1920s, as successive governors drove forward the French school project in the face of misgivings over contagious intruders, the entomologist Dr Joseph-Emile Borel was invited to conduct new studies of malaria infestation in the Lang Bian plateau. The stakes were high. The studies of malaria that Borel had undertaken in Indochina more generally had illustrated recently, as Laurence Monnais shows in Chapter 10, the extent of the failure of the State Quinine Service to stem the circulation of the disease through prophylactic quinine treatment. Mindful of the Government General's interest in the hill station project and guided by the prerogatives of the Government General (as Pastorians' work tended to be), Borel undertook a series of studies, in June 1925, March 1926, and December 1926. These produced, again from the blood of Vietnamese children, "proof" that no endemic malarial threat existed.[58] Borel read Dalat's salubrity off the bodies of children whom, he claimed, "enjoy a generally remarkable state of health, the like of which we have never seen anywhere else, South Annam and Cochinchina included."[59]

While Borel's vision of the healthy *Vietnamese* child usefully affirmed the school project, it was less useful to colonial planners committed to realizing an exclusively 'French' enclave. So it was through appeals to an older racial climatology that the colonial state gave official sanction to claims for Dalat's prophylactic benefits. A promotional brochure published by the Direction General de l'instruction Publique of Indochina in 1930 and distributed at the Exposition Coloniale International (held in Paris in 1931) explained that Vietnamese children had "no special reason to come to Dalat," because they could study in "their own climate" in Saigon or Hanoi and, moreover:

> Statistics collected by the residence-mairie show that the climate at altitude is, on the contrary, harmful to them. They show . . . among the native populations of the plains who move to Dalat, above all among the children, a very high increase in mortality, especially due to pulmonary infections which remain latent in the hothouse temperatures of Cochinchina, but which develop very rapidly among the natives in the cold climate of Langbian.[60]

In fact, the physicians who scrutinized the health of Vietnamese children attending school in Dalat noted little more than a slight predisposition to trachoma.

Having removed the Vietnamese child from this picture, education authorities enticed French parents to consider the *lycée* through a description of it as:

> The initiative of justly concerned authorities, well aware of the need to allow young Europeans, whom the climate debilitates and reduces to a state of inferiority in the plains, to undertake a full secondary education in comfort, and in climatic conditions favouring their physical and intellectual development and good progress in their studies.[61]

Within the carefully delimited space of the school, the climate acted upon children, the embodiment of a distinctly 'French' nature, in concert with modern hygiene. The laboratory overlapped with, and protected, vulnerable nature, but remained invisible. Readers of the brochure learned that certified European nurses assisted the chief doctor on his twice-weekly visits to pupils subjected to a regime of careful weighing, measuring, and general surveillance in order to ensure that they "take the medicine they have been prescribed."[62] As authorities explained with a Rousseauian flourish: "Our boarder is at home everywhere and, although there are monitors in each sector, the child is too immersed in his games to know that he is under surveillance."[63]

The desire to realize a 'French' Dalat, embodied in the segregated school project, proceeded upon a combination of climatology and germ theory, and hinged upon the key constituency of children. While climatology was used to validate the shift to the heights, and to stand in defense of segregation, experts who endorsed claims for Dalat as 'pristine' also appealed to the enduring danger of the malarial threat, its vector, the mosquito, and its 'reservoir'—the Vietnamese child—as they pursued the realization of this segregationist ideal.[64]

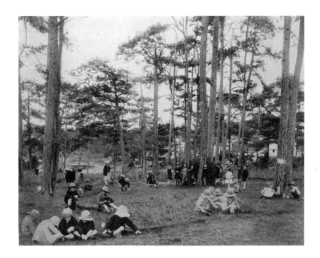

Figure 4.1

"Under the Pine Trees," Direction General de l'Instruction Publique, *Le Petit Lycée de Dalat.*

Appeals to the danger of infection grew more strident as the ideals set down in Hébrard's plan were challenged by the growing, and increasingly assertive, Vietnamese presence. Dalat's chief doctor, Marcel Terrisse, was determined that Dalat would function as "first and foremost, a sanitary city."[65] To realize this, Terrisse, as a member of the Hygiene Commission named by *arrêté* on July 24, 1924, and charged with monitoring the sanitary condition of Dalat, pursued a program of vector control, extending from drainage to the relocation of the "Annamite quarter" to the north of Dalat: "in such a way as to allow for its complete isolation in the case of an outbreak."[66] But in contrast to Borel, Terrisse contributed a deeply alarmist interpretation of recent studies of malaria and the disease threat posed by the Vietnamese child. He advised the deputy commissioner:

> It is now known that malaria is in Dalat among the native population. The clinical examination of 106 children (taken at random) from 0–12, children born in Dalat and who have never left—has revealed that 30% of the children have light malarial symptoms, 10% serious [symptoms]. Mosquitoes are numerous in Dalat in the annamite village . . . In certain quarters of the European city, in particular, at the Langbian Palace [Hotel] and in the vicinity of the new Public Works quarters, the inhabitants are very much troubled by the presence of mosquitoes.

Terrisse concluded that "malaria is a very serious threat to the hill station and we must engage in a very active struggle against it and against mosquitoes in particular."[67]

The close association of Vietnamese children with the disease threat, informed practical interventions in colonial urban space. The commission took steps to condemn the existing school for local children on hygienic grounds, rebuilding it further away from the European district.[68] In 1926, when Noël Bernard, director of the Pasteur Institute in Saigon, drew up a report defining the role of the municipal hygiene bureau, he identified the supervision of "childhood hygiene" and "school hygiene" as two of its principal duties.[69]

Dalat's development into a segregated enclave played out through and within debates over children and spaces of their acculturation. As stakeholders marshaled old-fashioned topographical determinism and bacteriology behind the multiply contested drive for segregation, evidence that white children thrived in the heights was used to buttress old-fashioned climatology. As in Hong Kong, when theories of disease transmission proved to have insufficient traction, colonial planners resorted to claims for expert knowledge of the management of children's health.

Nowhere was this clearer than in authorities' attempts to secure the coercive expansion of public health measures in the face of challenges from those representing indigenous people's interests. When Vietnamese members of the municipal commission protested vociferously in September 1928 at the comparative lack of investment in education for *their* children, and demanded the right for local students to enrol in French schools, the resident mayor, Chassaing, was well aware that appeals to medical geography or a racialized bacteriology would not mollify the disputants. He was willing to admit that "the beneficial influence of the climate of Dalat is felt as much by the native children as by the European children." However, while playing down racialized climatology, he went on to defend segregation by appealing to culturally essentialist interpretations of French childhood. For Chassaing, the admission of locals to the *lycée* was "impossible," owing to the fact that Vietnamese children would discourage the enrolment of "foreign children who do not possess the same sympathy for the *indigènes* as the French [children]." The solution of a separate, Vietnamese *lycée* was proposed, agreed to, and postponed indefinitely owing to a "lack of funds."[70]

While scholars have portrayed the period of the late 1920s as one in which Dalat failed to make the transition to either sanatorium, health retreat, or tourist resort, such an argument misses the important point that other projects, and in particular the military sanatorium, languished precisely *because* the presence of children burgeoned within the town's expanding school infrastructure.[71] The commission granted land to the Sisters of Saint Paul de Chartres at a vastly reduced price, conceded land to the Société Saint Augustin for the construction of a secondary school for girls, and commenced work on a *Grand Lycée* intended to permit the students in the *Petit Lycée* to complete their studies.[72] In August 1935, the resident mayor proudly reported on the commission's contribution to the 'baptism' of the *Grand Lycée*. An *arrêté* of May 10, 1935, had endowed the new Grand Lycée with the name 'Yersin.' At the same time, all work on barrack buildings was halted. Governor-General Pasquier informed Commander-in-Chief General Gaston-Henri Billotte that the introduction of a barracks was likely to present "the greatest of inconveniences in a hill station reserved primarily for women and children."[73] By the late 1930s, this left the military restricted to a presence of 100 men, and vastly outnumbered by children.[74] In December 1936, the resident mayor proudly reported: "there are in Dalat close to 450 European children, at the Lycée 'Yersin' the Couvent des 'Oiseaux' or at the Soeurs de l'Institution Nazareth."[75] The census of January 28, 1937, revealed that of the 697 Europeans in Dalat, 300 were children.[76]

The construction of the school infrastructure and the related debate about the nature and needs of children proved crucial to efforts to develop Dalat more generally into a segregated, hygienic city. Contemporaries explicitly connected the dream that Dalat might become a center of government with the existence of the schools and their pupils.[77] The realization of space for the accommodation and education of children prompted officials to contemplate the realization of a bigger project: the elevation of the segregated hill station enclave to a site of imperial governance. It was soon after the *Petit Lycée* began to admit students that Governor-General René Robin chose to declare that Dalat could now go on to become "Indochina's administrative capital."[78]

A Balm for the Plains: Childhood and Authority at High Altitude

In the early 1930s, frustration grew over the perceived gulf between segregationist ideals and the failure of planning to contain the Vietnamese within the areas designated for them. This tension found expression in the architect-planner Louis-George Pineau's new plan for Dalat of 1932.[79] Two years earlier, the Yen Bay uprising had sent shockwaves through the French community, evidencing the proximity of elite power centers to sources of anti-colonial 'contagion.' The desire for a more effective *cordon sanitaire* in Dalat, expressed in earlier proposals for a 'neutral zone' between the *village annamite* and the European center filled with a belt of gardens and public places, was formally enshrined in Pineau's plan.[80] Official desires to re-inscribe and defend the internal borders of this privileged community again found expression in the ordering of space for children.[81]

Yet, as the political landscape darkened, the Vietnamese elite proliferated in Dalat to the extent that doubts grew over whether an exclusionary approach was realistic, especially after 1936, by which time the Government General reported to the left-wing Popular Front government. The reforming governor, Jules Brévié, had been favorably impressed by Dalat during a visit, perceiving the value of the town's educational infrastructure in acculturating a 'French' elite that could of necessity no longer be restricted to those who possessed a 'pure European' or 'pure French' heritage. Around the same time, the admission policy of the *lycée* was revised, so that it was before a racially mixed gathering of students at the Lycée Yersin on July 12, 1938, that Jules Brévié declared:

> At points on the globe where there is contact between different races an incredible effervescence is developing. We must prevent this from degenerating into chronic disorder; we must re-establish the harmony essential for the wellbeing of men and the progress of societies in all aspects. This is the role vested in you, by the very fact of your presence in a place where these transformations are occurring.[82]

Precisely because race could not, in this vision, stand as the most significant referent of 'Frenchness,' a more intensive and carefully ordered cultural conditioning was required, and the *lycée* pupils' obeisance to cultural Frenchness required more stringent screening. Within the confines of the school, children from a variety of racial backgrounds could be placed at one remove and scrutinized. Like laboratories, they could thus serve as a cultural training ground and retooling site of key strategic significance in which 'harmonious development' could proceed. Officials drew upon the Pastorian infrastructure flourishing in contiguity with educational spaces to segregate and discipline children and to make them visible and legible.

The sorts of germs most closely associated with the Pastorian program were, of course, invaders transmitted to healthy individuals from the infected. Because children arrived in the "healthy" heights potentially infected by the cultural and political contagions of the plains, they were to be subject to special scrutiny. Paying tribute to Yersin at a ceremony held to inaugurate the *Lycée Yersin*, the school's science teacher, Rochet, described Dalat as a solution to "the unrest of the public squares" in the colonial cities below. Pupils who had been exposed to these *milieux* were potential carriers of *fleaux social*. They required immunization against not only the adverse effects of the climate but also political radicalization and a whole gamut of suspect "crazes" to which modern young people were judged susceptible.[83]

In Dalat, however, elite children were not to be merely passive objects, or recipients of Frenchness. Since childhood could when necessary flexibly accommodate race, they were ascribed the role of active agents of colonialism. By this time, vaccination had become the symbol *par exellence* of modern preventive medicine. In January 1936, in the same year that the *lycée* was named in his honor, Alexandre Yersin had opened a branch of the Pasteur Institute in Dalat. The Pastorian laboratory, of course, not only detected disease pathogens but also cultivated them, rendering them less virulent, and prepared them for re-injection as vaccines that would produce immunity. As the uncertain future of French colonialism forced elites to confront the need to redefine, preserve, and disseminate the *genie française*, a particular genre of childhood was rediscovered in the heights as a potential balm, a metaphorical vaccine, for the strife besetting the plains.[84]

The school-enclave recirculated a growing number of healthy, acculturated children into the plains. There, elite children were to perform, rather like laboratories, as small, active units, almost unseen yet capable of serving as metonymical representatives of the whole. Just as Kitasato and Yersin, by deploying the laboratory to investigate plague, had *made* the bacillus the essential thing about the plague by deploying the school as a space of observation and perfection the colonial government, drew children toward the epicenter of French colonialism.[85] And as the French colonial administration stepped up plans to transform Dalat into a federal capital of French Indochina, children, existing at the points of "contact between races," could easily be aligned with this key trope of colonial federalist thinking.[86]

And yet, this was a risky venture. Dalat was hardly immune to the political virulence of the plains. As protests focused around youth, the high concentration of children in the hill station stoked fears that the laboratory might inadvertently become a source of contagion. The need to signify Dalat's—and by extension Indochina's—'Frenchness' was heightened further by the fall of

France in May 1940. With the Vietnamese peninsula thereafter only nominally under French control, and colonials' mobility once again stymied by war, Dalat became an enclave from which the elite, however fancifully, dreamt of reclaiming the peninsula, and indeed the metropole. As mutable and mobile as the school/laboratory in which they were studied, children had emerged at the heart of elites' efforts to reassert their own durability and permanence. Now, just as work in bacteriology in the colonies had surpassed that of the metropole, so, went the forlorn hope, the graduates of Dalat's schools might outshine their defeated metropolitan counterparts in the nation's hour of need.

Facing this dire scenario, the pro-Vichyite governor-general, Admiral Jean Decoux, pushed forward the project of turning Dalat into an administrative capital. He tackled surging population levels in the town through plans for a *Cité Jardin* north of the center. Demand for residential space in Dalat again intensified, and 50 new French-style chalets were planned to house administrators in 1943. Priority was assigned to those "with a minimum of two children," and absolute priority was accorded to families with four children or more. In accordance with the pronatalist vision to which Vichy officials subscribed, the importance of children impelled the re-ordering of domestic space within the "garden city."[87] However, rather than amounting to a fundamental break with pre-war developments, this can be seen instead as the latest engagement in a long-running process whereby the re-ordering of colonial space to accommodate hygienic 'nature'—a concern integral to the transformation of Dalat from a handful of chalets into a center of imperial governance—was drawn upon the specific needs of children and childhood.

Conclusion

Children and childhood migrated to the epicenter of the cultural politics of colonial urbanism after the bacteriological turn. As elites re-ordered colonial cities, the older technology of the enclave was re-interpreted and integrated into 'public health' programs, as illustrated here in the case of the hill station. The re-ordering of space in colonial contexts proceeded through a series of situated encounters and struggles over the defense of childhood, or what adults defined as children's interests. As in the laboratory, a space characterized by porosity, where microscopic agents of contagion were identified and treated, so in the hill station children were removed from, but remained intimately connected with, developments 'in the field.' In the cultures of planning fashioned by colonial states, coercive public health infrastructures were intimately connected through the domain of childhood with the retreat to segregated hill stations. In this way, public health *and* the enclave were involved in the co-production of nature and society. Authorities grappling with the contradictions and controversies that the commitment to a 'public' health entailed worked childhood into a language of administrative command. The productively contagious body of 'the child,' abject and pathologized, embodied the enclave within the colonial community. It existed in a dialectical relationship with the tropical environment. As such, elites could invoke this constituency to undergird microbial theories of disease and older climatological discourses of peril—or, if necessary, to navigate beyond them.

Across empires, childhood was invoked in planning and urban policies launched at the highest level of the colonial state. In this way, during the early twentieth century, enclaves moved in from the periphery to become new centers from which elite authority could be relaunched. While these maneuvers in themselves were born of a sense that European imperial power was on the wane, hill stations in these colonial contexts did not simply slip into a 'swift decline.' Instead, as the cases studied here reveal, they were invested with new significance as colonial elites, across empires, re-negotiated access to space, defined the limits of hygienic modernity, and strove in the face of a growing anti-colonial fervor to perpetuate their rule.

5
Planning Social Hygiene: From Contamination to Contagion in Interwar India

Stephen Legg

Introduction

The interwar period (1918–39) was one of rapid sociopolitical change in colonial India. It saw the emergence of mass-movement anti-colonialism, communal nationalism, and a thoroughgoing women's movement, as well as the scalar reorganization of the state through the systems of dyarchy (partial provincial self-government) and fuller regional autonomy through the Government of India Acts (1919 and 1939). Inflected by all these changes, but possessing a logic that was both its own and linked to broader international shifts, were trends in medicine and public health. These trends can be framed in various narratives: the shift from curative to preventative medicine; the movement from a colonial enclavist concern for the elite to a more nationalist concern with the broader population; or the diffusion of scientific spatial organization from medical institutions to the broader public sphere. These are questions of racial sociology, geography, and anthropology, but running throughout them all is a shift in the scientific episteme from that of contamination to that of contagion. This shift had been ongoing since the late nineteenth century, but in the interwar period it was refracted through the logic, and 'art of government,' of hygiene. This emphasis had effects not just on parasitological understanding and pathogenic theories, but also on the planning of cities and the way in which international campaigners focused their social reform efforts in India. This chapter will open with some reflections on contagion theory and urban planning, and will then move on to consider the emergence of hygiene theory and its effects on colonial biopolitics. It will demonstrate this shift through, first, an analysis of changing public health policies in Delhi, including those regarding venereal diseases and prostitution, and second, a study of international campaigns against venereal diseases. These two examples will provide valuable case material, but will also shed light on broader processes due to their wider significance. Delhi became the capital of colonial India in 1911, and the transformations that took place there clearly show how urban planning was dependent upon the whims of colonial governors in this period. The regulation of prostitution, as Foucault famously argued, comes at the intersection of individual self-conduct and the regulation of the population.[1] Referencing concerns over 'racial' decline, birth rates, family life, fidelity, and imperial sexuality, the prostitute stands at the nexus of individual morality and demographic anxiety. In the interwar period, internationalist campaigning against sexual contagion, here studied via the British Social Hygiene Council's work, marked a transformatory shift in Indian public health policy. In surveying these developments, this chapter will hopefully encourage contemplation of the 'late colonial' period during which India continued to act as an epistemic, as well as military and economic, sub-imperial pole for the Indian Ocean arena.[2]

Contagion, Hygiene, and Colonial Biopolitics

In his classic work *Colonizing the Body*, David Arnold made it clear how intensely geographical Indian colonial medicine was.[3] One of these geographies was spatial and concrete: the institutions (the hospital, jail, and barracks) that allowed intense observation, and control, of disease. These spaces of colonial modernity allowed an aesthetic, a limited practice, and a boundless fantasy of control to spread through the imperial imagination (see, for instance, the images of King George's Hospital at Lucknow, opened in 1911, and the Mayo Hospital at Lahore, opened in 1871, included in the 1938 London publication *Social Service in India: An Introduction to some Social and Economic Problems of the Indian People*, Figure 5.1).[4] But a second, more exotic, geography was that of the tropical landscapes of India within which European health was presumed to be more at risk.[5] This environmentalist paradigm was, of course, an ancient one, but its emphasis on *contamination* endured in the fecund tropical environment of India.[6] Colonial medicine was, therefore, long obsessed with medical topography—the mapping of diseased environments. The transmission of disease could be through direct contact, through rotting or infected matter, or through aerial miasmas or 'mal-arias' (bad air), while the tropical climate was thought to weaken the body.[7]

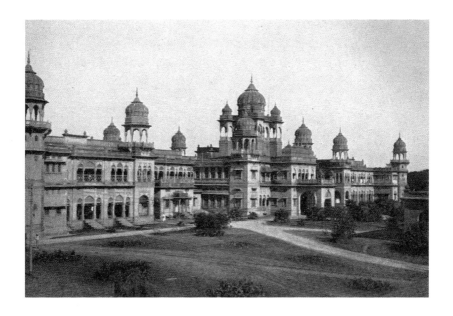

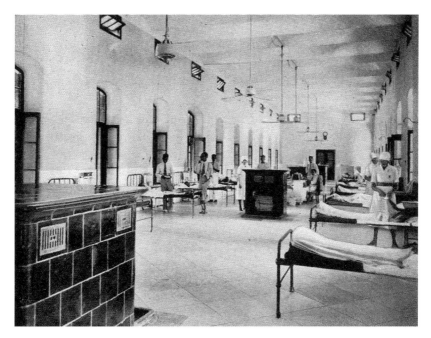

Figure 5.1
Spaces of medical modernity in colonial India.

The government of India proved resilient to *contagion* theory until the 1890s, even as international sanitary conferences and cholera outbreaks along pilgrim routes in India presented evidence to support Koch's bacillus theory.[8] Yet this eventual transition did not mean a significant and immediate shift in the types of interventionist spaces created through state medicine. Environmentalist understandings of pathogenic environments fueled demands for sanitary reform that were contrary to governmental financial preferences and the laissez-faire non-interventionism of the mid-to-late nineteenth century.[9] Outbreaks of disease in the imperial port of Bombay necessitated, however, major infrastructural sanitary improvements that had a major impact on its urban morphology, and on the approach to urban landscaping in India more broadly.[10] Such interventions targeted environmental conditions that made the spread of contagion more likely and, as such, carried forward the geographical imagination of the environmentalist paradigm, and also reinforced imperial claims to mastery over space (see Figure 5.2 for a typical contrast between disordered Indian towns and the glistening urbanism of colonial modernity).[11]

Prostitution policies provide a famous example of this approach to space and disease. While 'venereal diseases' had never been associated with miasmas, their genital origins being all too evident, they were closely associated with contagion. This was a metaphorical connection, drawing upon the Augustinian depiction of the prostitute as the sewer that cleansed humanity. But it was also a practical one; the Contagious Diseases Acts (1864–69 in Britain, 1868 in India) had allowed for the registration, inspection, and, if infected, compulsory incarceration of prostitutes.[12] The Indian act was repealed in 1888, which left colonial authorities scrambling for a way of safeguarding their military cantonments from venereal disease.[13] Only in the twentieth century would a broader concern with the Indian population lead to a more thoroughgoing policy regarding prostitution and urban health.[14]

The evolution of such geographical imaginations, and their inherent power relations, have been theorized by David Armstrong as "public health spaces."[15] The environmentalist, or miasmatic, model associated disease with particular places and led to quarantine and the eradication of the threatening elements of the environment. This medical measure can be associated with the 'sovereign power' to appropriate territory, and to use violence and force to re-order space.[16] The second model, of contagion, focused on flows between the body and the environment, and led to the establishment of *cordons sanitaire* between 'pure' and 'impure' people and places. This can be associated with a disciplinary

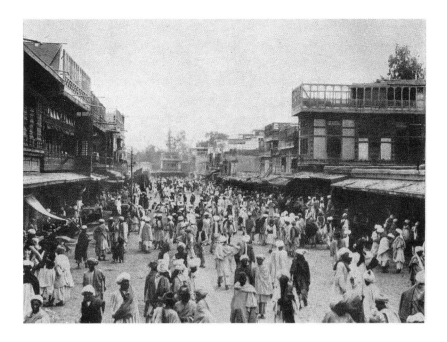

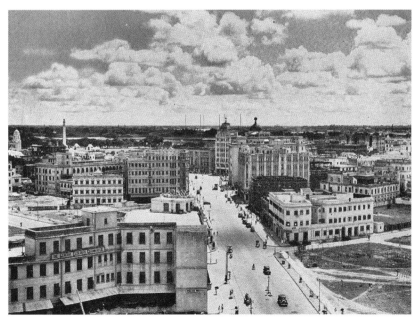

Figure 5.2
Contrasting urban forms in colonial India.

model of power that placed 'abnormal' (unhealthy, threatening) people or places under surveillance so as to monitor and reform infected people and places; a model of power based itself on the medieval European plague town.[17] In her work on colonial Singapore, Brenda Yeoh has shown that "[t]hrough the interplay of strategies and counter-strategies, negotiation over the control of sanitary aspects of the urban environment played a key role in describing the relationship of power between ruler and the ruled."[18] In attempting to lower the mortality rates of Chinese and Malay inhabitants of the island, disciplinary tactics of categorization, inspection, and surveillance were adopted, to limited effect. The impossibility of producing a self-disciplining "native subject," due to the limited funds of the municipal government and the radically different medical episteme of the local population, led to a shift in tactics:

> The municipal 'inspecting gaze' had shifted from overseeing the daily practices of the Asian population carried out in specific spaces (such as the house, street, market, or public place) to controlling the dimensions, arrangements, and legibility of particular spaces (such as the house, the building block, and ultimately, the city as a whole) in order to influence the practices of those who inhabited or used such spaces.[19]

This shift in emphasis to the practices, not just the movement or health, of individuals is the key change here, and marks the deeper influence of contagion theory on public health spaces. This final model was termed that of "hygiene" by Armstrong and marks a concern with the interlinkages between personal and public health, as mediated by personal conduct. The association of the health of the individual body and that of the body politic is a keystone of "biopolitics," and the concern with the "conduct of conduct" was central to Foucault's interest in liberal governmentalities.[20] This shift does not, however, make hygiene any less geographical. The emphasis on the personal brought the home into the purview of health officials, and led to a broader conceived "dream of hygienic containment" that came to dominate "the extensive culture of hygiene which we know as public health."[21] Contagion and hygiene are, therefore, not separate concepts or practices; instead, hygiene marked a distinct development in twentieth-century thinking regarding how to address the threat of contagion. But how would hygienist discourses play out in colonial arenas, which were marked by a neglect of individual care for colonial populations perceived as, at best, religious or ethnic communities or, at worst, an undifferentiated category of 'the native'?[22]

This question has been most directly addressed by Alison Bashford's ground-breaking *Imperial Hygiene: A Critical History of Colonialism, Nationalism and Public Health*.[23] Bashford showed that the boundaries, borders, enclosures, and interventions associated with hygiene and public health were also spatial tactics deployed by colonialism, nationalism, and racial administration: "All these spaces—these therapeutic, carceral, preventative, racial and eugenic geographies—produced identities of inclusion and exclusion, of belonging and citizenship, and of alienness."[24] Yet in the twentieth century, such policies had to apprehend an emerging emphasis, even in the colonies, on health and welfare and, later, citizenship, in which hygiene was not just a public health responsibility of the state, but also a duty of each individual. This marked, for Bashford, a clearly new stage of biopolitics, the administration of the life of a population through encouraging new conduct, but also through collecting new statistical information about a population. As Deana Heath has put it: "Hygiene connected the governance of the self to larger governmental projects and thus became a means of imagining and embodying the strength and purity of the individual, community, nation, and empire."[25] Yet she also acknowledges that imperial projects to manage the flow of polluting material (whether of the mind or body) around the empire often came into conflict with colonial models of hygiene that took on national, and unique, inflections. There were colonial logics at play that *depended* upon undermining the self-governing capacities of Indians so as to justify colonialism, to refute anti-colonial nationalist claims for *swaraj* (self-rule), and to further obfuscate the fact that so much Indian ill health was created by the conditions of colonial modernity (the overcrowded town fostering tuberculosis and venereal disease, or the newly cultivated paddy field conducive to malarial mosquitoes). David Arnold's recent work has demonstrated how beriberi (a condition caused by deficiency of vitamin B1 [thiamine] related to an over-dependency on polished rice) exposed the precarious vulnerability of laborers' bodies.[26] The cure, vitamin injections or tablets as well as changed diet, suggests a nutritional governmentality outside the scope of the growing body of work on colonial biopolitics.[27]

Warwick Anderson's work, for instance, on American colonialism in the Philippines, examined the abstract depiction of American laboratory and public health spaces and bodies in relation to Filipino embodiment and impure spaces.[28] As against programs of immunization, which made war on a diseased population, hygiene marked a biopolitical engagement with individual health, though modified to take into account presumed native capacities.[29] Similarly,

Laura Briggs has examined American policy in Puerto Rico, showing how the 'difference' of the latter was reproduced through women's bodies and sexuality.[30] Inspired by British anti-contagious diseases legislation, a series of moral panics were mobilized to stoke fears over syphilis and the threat it posed to the American navy, women and children, and to Puerto Rican claims to U.S. citizenship and status.

Sarah Hodges has most directly addressed late colonial biopolitics in India, through her work on birth control and the related debates linking health and governance.[31] Vitally, she stressed that such debates should go beyond the boundaries of the state, as governmentality studies have insisted, taking in social action and knowledge production regarding food or housing. Hodges also contrasts 'top-down' immunization with 'bottom-up' projects aimed at improving health in general through behavioral changes. Yet the latter were filtered through Indian 'difference' by the 'strange beast' of colonial welfare:

> Succinctly, in the colonial Indian context, there existed neither institutions nor the desire to gather the kind of totalizing knowledge about the Indian subject population, nor was there either the political will to engineer large-scale transformations in the overall health profiles of the population.[32]

Through such a lens, Hodges' interest in sex and sexuality is less concerned with the micromanaging studied by Ann Stoler and others.[33] Rather, "[i]n the 'welfarisation' of colonial sexuality, sex remains significant but less in terms of the precise acts and parties involved and more in terms of how sex was mobilized to connect individual practices to a broader social body."[34] This was exactly how prostitution came to be re-envisaged through the lens of hygiene, not as a perversion, or even as an urban nuisance, but as a risk to the population and, as explicitly rendered, the race. The demand that Indian women, both prostitutes and wives, be treated and cared for was part of a welfare push from Indian representatives that clashed with attempts to hem back the colonial state and reduce expenditure. This led to increasingly outward-looking Indian scientific elites, who looked to bodies like the League of Nations for inspiration in their project to "decolonize international health."[35] Understanding the development of contagion theory and its influence on planning and governmental policy, therefore, demands an appreciation of diachronic historical change and legacies in specific places, as well as a synchronic appreciation of imperial and internationalist networks. The rest of this chapter will attempt to convey some of this complexity through a summary of the evolution of public health in Delhi as explored through debates about urban living in general, and venereal disease in particular. Second, an examination of the work of the British Social Hygiene Council will give an insight into some of the internationalist influences on sexual regulation in interwar India.

Delhi: Municipality, Province, and Capital

After the uprising of 1857, Delhi was apportioned to the Punjab Province but was administered by its own chief and deputy commissioners. In 1863, a Municipal Committee was established, consisting of the deputy commissioner, three Europeans, and seven nominated Indians.[36] The municipality immediately set about a series of infrastructural improvements to create a healthier environment in the city. These included road repairs; drain and sewer clearance; the creation of public latrines; the removal of encroachments on public lands; the removal deposits of offal and filth at Ajmeri and Turkman gates; the opening of a dispensary in Sadar Bazar by a hakim for those classes who ". . . though poor, have no faith in English medicines;"[37] the removal of a cremation ground to a site "less objectionable" on sanitary grounds; and the closure of burial places near the (European) Civil Station, while all burials within 500 yards of the city walls were banned. An elaborate system was also put in place to track the population of the city, both for planning purposes and to better calculate rates of mortality. The registration of births was initiated through binding mullah sweepers to report within 24 hours all births and deaths, for which they were paid a fee, but would forfeit their job should they fail. For the first four months, all relatives were ordered also to register births, to check if the system was working. While it is highly unlikely, given the Municipal Committee's track record of urban governance, that this system worked, it gives a sense of the intent, at least, to understand Delhi as both a place of disease and of a variable population. Such efforts continued over the following decades: wells were cleaned and the city ditch cleared; the slaughterhouse was moved outside of the city walls, as were other "offensive trades"; the city and suburbs were divided into *ilaka* subdivisions and were regularly inspected for problems, mainly with conservancy. However, as with Singapore, it was found that about a quarter of the municipal budget was being spent on the police.

In 1878, a sanitation subcommittee was established in line with broader trends across larger municipalities throughout India. Many of the ideas informing the logic of the committee were crystallized in a publication by the vice-chairman of the Calcutta municipal board, Reginald Craufuird Sterndale's

1881 *Municipal Work in India; or, Hints on Sanitation, General Conservancy and Improvements in Municipalities, Towns and Villages.*[38] In fitting with contemporary Orientalist discourses, Sterndale praised India's ancient texts for embodying the principles of municipal rule, yet claimed these traditions had become extinct, until revived by the "liberal minded administrator, the late Sir Cecil Beadon, during his Lieutenant-Governorship of Bengal."[39] One of the key duties of a municipal committee was to apply sanitary science so as to remove the sanitary evils associated with departing from the rules of nature. While later hygiene science would emphasize the importance of domestic and personal health, the sanitary mindset condemned the Indian for prioritizing such concerns and failing in infrastructural science and public health: "Ancient, however, as sanitary laws may be, they do not seem to have been in vogue at any time among the Hindus; and this, although the Hindu shastras teem with laws for the purification of the body and household cleansing."[40] Such laws were said to be appropriate for scattered dwellings but not for cramped urban living. Liberal sanitary laws and regulations were said to be based on three simple principles:

1. That the protection of health and comfort was as much a right as that of security of life and property;
2. That property brings duties and responsibilities as well as rights and privileges; no one should cause offence to their neighbors;
3. That individual interest must be subordinate to the interests of the community at large.

   . . . in the present day it is necessary to base our sanitary regulations upon a [more] utilitarian foundation,–*viz.*, that the individual must be content to sacrifice a small part of the possible profit or pleasure he might derive from the unrestricted use of his own estate for the general benefit or enjoyment of the community.[41]

What this makes exceptionally clear is that sanitary science was not just part of, but at the vanguard of, liberal governmentalities that sought to craft out, in the name of contagion theory, possessive individualistic subjectivities through the manipulation of material space. This immediately, however, called forth the inherent tension in liberalism: give people individual rights and they can use them to block inconvenient projects for the common good. Liberal governmentalities relied upon these checks on state power, hemming back government to allow the free functioning of society and population. Sterndale also noted that certain writers on economics (J. S. Mill) oppose state interference on such matters. He could, however, fall back on the notion of *difference*; what he was detailing was not just *liberal* governance, but a particularly *colonial* governmentality:

> It must, however, be admitted that the State must protect those who are
> incapable of discriminating between what is and what is not necessarily
> for their own good; and this is undeniably the condition of the mass of our
> Indian town populations. In regard to questions of sanitation and hygiene,
> they are as ignorant and helpless as children or imbeciles, and it is, there-
> fore, the undoubted duty of the State, and under it the local authorities,
> to do for them what they cannot do for themselves, and what selfish and
> short-sighted landlords will not do for them . . .[42]

Despite the mention of hygiene, it was the environment of the poor land-labor-ing classes that was thought to represent the most urgent threat: quarters where soil and atmosphere reached the lowest depths of contamination; where subsoil and surface water went undrained; where houses were surrounded in filth and the air was burdened with "noisome emanations." This was the rallying call to municipalities across India and, while Delhi motioned towards suitable action, the money, motivation, or capacity was not supplied until a crisis and an opportunity presented themselves in the early twentieth century.

The crisis was that of the plague. Although anti-plague measures were most vigorous, and have been most commented upon, in Bombay, due to its status as an international port, the disease was actually more lethal in the Punjab area of north India from which Delhi had been carved.[43] In 1901–03, a few cases of the disease were reported each year but did not spread, while 1903–04 saw 11 cases, still way fewer than the 91 cases of cholera that year.[44] In 1904–05, however, the plague 'became indigenous,' with 637 deaths reported, although the actual number of dead would have been much higher. The worst suffering was in the poorer and cramped suburbs of Paharganj and Sabzi Mandi outside the city walls. Affected premises were disinfected free of cost and pamphlets on prevention were translated and distributed. There were over 300 deaths the following year and 35 in 1906–07, but the plague returned in 1910–11. Few agreed to be inoculated and the only measures available were to move people out of quarters where the disease was worst.

While these measures reflected the relatively modest health apparatus of the city at this time, a dramatic event in the winter of 1911 radically changed Delhi's prospects. At the imperial durbar in the city in December of that year, King George V announced that the capital of India would be moved from Calcutta to Delhi itself, and that a new capital would be constructed near the old city. Delhi would become a centrally administered province, and strenuous efforts were made by the municipality to match its new status as part of the capital region. A health officer was appointed in August 1912, charged with addressing the sanitary and general health of the city. As such, future epidemics were treated with much more intensity. In 1917–18, an outbreak of influenza was met with a rash of measures, including notices in English, Urdu, and Hindi throughout the city; lectures in houses and bastis; disinfection of affected houses; "Elphinstone Picture Palace" slides detailing preventative measures deployed; disinfection of trams and notices distributed against spitting; closure of schools and colleges; reductions in the gathering of people in cinemas and theaters; and the establishment of 18 street dispensaries and eight traveling dispensaries. The shift towards an emphasis on hygiene, conduct, and education is clear here, but these were largely curative measures. With regard to the plague, Delhi now worked towards a preventative science. In 1923, the central government of India's public health commissioner reported with satisfaction on Delhi's anti-plague measures. The city's geographical position and railway connections left it open to the plague, prevalent in neighboring provinces, from all sides. An outbreak in 1922–23 had killed 1,510 in the city and 1,185 in the district, but the significance of these statistics was made very clear:

> The proximity of the Imperial City with its 30000 inhabitants and of the winter headquarters of the Government of India made it imperative that the progress of the disease be watched closely; consequently the possibilities of a large 'carry over' of infection to the winter of 1923–24 had early engaged the attention of the Department of Education, Health and Lands and the local Public Health authorities.[45]

A similar emphasis on the capital can be detected in anti-malarial policy. In 1912 when the site for the new city was being determined, the "relative malariousness" of different sites was mapped. From this, recommendations emerged for combating malaria in the city: a canal to the north of the old city was to be cut off and filled up; the durbar area to the north of the city was to have flood protection measures installed; canals within the old city were to be treated; and, within New Delhi, proper storm channels were to be installed and open pits to be filled in. However, a report from 1927 showed that the only thorough action to have been taken was that in the new city. An examination showed that there were still seriously high levels of malaria in Delhi, so Rs50,000 were provided for action in 1930–31. A further report in 1936 acknowledged the lack of progress, but questioned whether efforts should focus on Delhi province, or just New Delhi. Were action to occur more broadly, it was, again, clear why:

> The following notes are based on the principle that anti-mosquito measures, if applied to New Delhi municipal area alone, will not in all probability suffice to control malaria in the New City, since the existence of an infected population in its immediate vicinity may from time to time induce outbreaks of malaria within the city itself and, moreover malaria carrying mosquitoes may under favourable meteorological conditions be brought into New Delhi from outside areas, however perfect the control of breeding may be within the New Delhi municipal area itself.[46]

Both of these reports represent the extent to which Old Delhi's administration was over-determined, and explicitly controlled, by the central government in New Delhi, and how the racial geographies of Delhi's health geographies were thereby implicitly fortified. The annual reports by Delhi's medical officer charted the growing frustration with this organization, as Delhi became more and more congested due to people flocking to the capital city.[47] One of the most passionate campaigners for health reform in Delhi was Dr K. S. Sethna, whose 1929 report charted and statistically tabulated the disease and congestion that wracked the old city. But the problem was as much one of medical approach as material conditions. He argued, "[a]lthough the Science of Hygiene has developed at a rapid rate, the public outlook on Health as opposed to Disease has not altogether changed."[48] Sethna wrote that the old idea of medicine was to cure. While still correct, hygiene also aimed to prevent illness, which was still under-appreciated in India. Health should accompany human progress and comfort:

> We have talked about a 'Sanitary Conscience' but we have not yet evolved what I should call a 'Health Atmosphere'. More and more responsibility is taken from the shoulders of the general public and placed on the Health Department, so much so that instead of acting and thinking for themselves many people require someone to act for them.

While there was ever-increasing demand for municipal sanitation, this need would lessen were people to act hygienically (to stop throwing refuse in the street, to use drains, to keep food clean, to notify rather than hide infectious diseases). In sum, the need was for popular *cooperation*.

Alas, nine years later, Sethna found that his calls had gone unheard. In the 1938 report, he argued that, while the cost of preserving public health was great, it was less than the cost of disease; reducing the cost of the latter depended on prevention. He chastized the public for not showing themselves worthy of such investment, for not knowing what they, as *citizens*, paid for: pre-natal clinics were not used; diseases not notified; women not given access to venereal disease clinics by their husbands. Sethna had gone so far as to hire health propaganda staff who went through the city singing "health songs" composed by his department. His object was that all members of public health departments be "disciples of hygiene" to guide the public. The benefits of this distanced yet intense conduct would be to remove the paralyzing fear of sickness. In his retiring address, after 24 years of public service in Delhi, Sethna pleaded:

> The evolution of public health work from the prevention of contagious diseases to the prevention of all diseases and further from the negative prevention of diseases to the positive appeal for health has resulted in a very complex health organisation . . . [but] Health, like Charity, begins at home.[49]

The home was thus returned to, but as the site for a revolution in health, not for Sterndale's sparing approval of Hindu domestic economy. Yet the domestic sphere, and individual conduct, was a realm that remained beyond the scope, or even desire, of the colonial government, whether the New Delhi authorities, the Delhi administration, or the Municipal Committee. While tuberculosis wracked the city, there were no effective measures to re-house slum dwellers, and the city extensions were taken up by the expanding middle classes.[50] Similarly, while rates of venereal diseases remained high in the city, thoroughgoing legislation was not passed until the 1940s.[51] This was, in part, the result of campaigning by Meliscent Shephard, the representative in India of the Association of Moral and Social Hygiene (AMSH).[52] But Shephard's objections to prostitution were dominated by the concerns of *moral* hygiene, namely, the unequal moral standard and the exploitation of women to satisfy the desires of men. *Social* hygiene focused more intently on science and medicine and proffered an alternative set of techniques for challenging the most infamous of the 'contagious diseases.'

The British Social Hygiene Council

> . . . contagion is always about contact. Thus through most of the nineteenth century 'contagious diseases' meant sexually transmitted diseases— transmission through the closest and most problematised contact of all.[53]

If hygiene marked a new peak in the intensity of biopolitics, it also marked a novel intervention in the governing of the sexual self.[54] Hygiene emerged as a key technology at several intersections of the domains of sexual conduct and population regulation.[55] These included the literature of sexology; Havelock Ellis, for instance, wrote both the six-volume *Studies in the Psychology of Sex* and *The Task of Social Hygiene*.[56] Another was that of public feminism, in which venereal diseases and the role of men and women were discussed, while a final intersection was that of eugenics and public health. Bashford has shown that segregation was *not* simply the spatial response of a contagionist mindset; "health detention," or the lock hospital model, continued into the twentieth century in Queensland, for example.[57] But she also shows how, in the pages of the British Social Hygiene Council's (BSHC) journal, *Health and Empire*, the "threat of compulsion" was highlighted and the need for voluntary healthcare for infected women prioritized, while also stressing the *imperial* threat that venereal disease posed.

As suggested above, while moral hygiene drew attention to the immorality of prostitution, social hygiene focused on the threat posed by prostitution to the health of the population. In the United States, it was closely associated with sexual regulation, prostitution, and the control of venereal diseases, while in the United Kingdom, at its broadest, social hygiene targeted birth control, family policy, nutrition, industrial efficiency, social policy, and 'mental hygiene,' especially of the poor.[58] The BSHC title was adopted in 1924 by the National Council for Combating Venereal Diseases (NCCVD), which had been formed to implement the recommendations of the 1916 report of the Royal Commission on Venereal Diseases.[59] It focused on extending free treatment for venereal diseases into the civilian population and was funded by the state. Yet its earliest reports show that it appreciated that venereal disease was as much an imperial and international concern. It contemplated not just the risk of venereal disease to the United Kingdom, but also of, for instance, diseased African soldiers returning home after the war. As such, a traveling commission of medical advisors was funded in 1920 to visit the East (Gibraltar, Ceylon, Colombo, Malta, Singapore, and Hong Kong) and the West (the Bahamas, St Vincent, Bermuda, Jamaica, Barbados, British Guiana, and Antigua). The BSHC had also established a branch and dispensary at Bombay in 1918, which registered 1,296 people in 1919–20, many of whom were prostitutes.[60] This branch was taken over by municipal authorities by 1923.[61]

Unlike the AMSH, which focused on working with and through local organizations, the BSHC wanted organizations throughout the empire affiliated to it and working upon the same general lines.[62] Perhaps with this in mind, the government of India declined the offer of a visit from the traveling commission, although a separate commission was accepted between November 1926 and March 1927.[63] The states of Bihar and Orissa pronounced themselves opposed to the commission and refused to cooperate, while the "political atmosphere" in Bengal made a visit impossible.[64] During the tour, Mrs Neville-Rolfe had an interview with the public health commissioner, who admitted that the large towns needed action, but that the government was wary of raising the question of prostitution. The resulting BSHC report on India highlighted what it viewed to be high levels of gonorrhea and syphilis, a low level of outpatient care, and a near total absence of full-course treatment for venereal diseases. This was attributed to a lack of medical staff, premises, and equipment. The BSHC made recommendations along three lines that bridged the medical concern with the "contagiousness" of venereal diseases with the hygiene concerns about their "socialness." Rejecting any notion of compulsory segregation or detention, the medical recommendations were all regarding in-or outpatient care and the establishment of teaching hospitals, child welfare centers, and drug distribution centers. In terms of social action, there was need for a campaign of "public enlightenment" that would explain the relationship between commercial prostitution, venereal disease, and the "racial effects" of syphilis and gonorrhea. The council also recommended cinema censorship, the penalization of commercial prostitution, and that hostels be provided for those undergoing treatment.

This bringing together of the social and the medical was in line with the BSHC's imperial vision. In 1924, the NCCVD published a report on its first Imperial Social Hygiene Congress, in which it declared its intention to tackle the social problems that lay behind sexually transmitted diseases.[65] The Congress was addressed by the Minister of Health, who stressed the need for collective action to challenge "Free Trade in disease," and by the president of the NCCVD, who outlined the "racial" threat posed by gonorrhea and syphilis. It was left to the late colonial secretary, L. S. Amery, to address the outside world, which he did through tackling "Imperial Questions," which were divided geographically. For dominions, the question was one of "securing the concentration of an intelligent and outspoken public interest on the great social and health problems connected with these diseases," preventing them, and curing them quickly.[66] For colonies and dependencies, however, the question was different, due to Britain's greater responsibility. This was no longer simply the responsibility for establishing law and order or eradicating those "grosser superstitions" through a form of negative trusteeship, as embodied in Sterndale's approach to Indians' (non-)capacities for self-governance. Rather, public opinion was acknowledging that Britain's trusteeship "has its very positive aspects and obligations, and that we are concerned not merely in keeping the peace but in endeavouring to make the very most out of the populations for whom we have assumed responsibility."[67] While Britain had come to terms with the need for political education in its colonies and dependencies, it had underemphasized training in "social life, health, and moral conduct." This struggle by the colonial state to acknowledge a form of governance that was positive, that went beyond the violent adjudication of peace to making the most out of populations through training in social life, health, and moral conduct, is by now a familiar one through the literature on late colonial biopolitics. It was a governmentality taken up by Dr Sethna in Delhi, it was acknowledged by the government of India as it extended its protective measures against venereal disease beyond the cantonment, and it was at the very heart of the AMSH's imperial campaign.

However, as the paper presented at the congress by Dame Rachel Crowdy on "international positions" regarding prostitution and trafficking suggested, the imperial perspective was already being augmented by alternative, yet also transnational, opinion.[68] This was acknowledged in 1934, when the British Social Hygiene Council published its first Empire Social Hygiene Year-Book. As with the Imperial Social Hygiene congresses, serving and retired members of the Indian Civil Service were well represented. The foreword was provided by Sir Basil Blackett, who had worked in India between 1922 and 1928 as a financial expert and served as the occasional president of the BSHC on his return.[69] He began by recalling the heady influence of imperialism in the "nineties," at both its best (Kipling) and worst (violent jingoism). However, in 1934, he admitted that catchwords such as "King and Country" or "white man's burden" were now deemed superior or insulting to fellow citizens in India or Africa. Echoing Amery's comments 10 years previously, he suggested the task of empire had changed from that of supplying law and order to demonstrating the best of Western civilization. In the post-war period of doubt, people were said to have turned to the "international" and not the "imperial." The League of Nations would come to have a significant impact upon prostitution policy in India, and it was thoroughly penetrated by hygienist literature. It was, however, swayed from its earlier social hygienist emphasis on science and the policing of prostitution to a moral hygienist interest in the traffic in women and children.[70] While the League contributed greatly to the global campaign against epidemics and for social medicine,[71] its effects in India were, as with nineteenth-century debates on municipal liberalism, mediated by racial difference and geographies of sovereignty and colonial governmentality.[72]

These internationalist conduits of hygiene thought were, therefore, as subject to colonial difference as former stages of contagionist thinking, and also had their effects on the planning of urban space. In terms of social hygiene, the major effect was to encourage the abolition of tolerated brothel zones and to outlaw soliciting in the street.[73] The laws that enforced these hygienist concerns displayed the historical and translocal influences that this chapter has tried to demonstrate; a contagionist but individualist concern with infection, as well as a newly internationalist concern both with imperial race and the potential of a postcolonial scientific modernity.

6
Matshed Laboratory: Colonies, Cultures, and Bacteriology

Robert Peckham

Introduction: Situating the Laboratory

The photograph of the bacteriologist Alexandre Yersin, discoverer of the plague bacterium in 1894, standing at the entrance of his makeshift laboratory in Hong Kong, has become iconic: emblematic of the ingenuity and stoicism of the late nineteenth-century 'microbe hunter,' even as it recalls the pre-eminence of the colonial laboratory as the site for defining infectious disease (Figure 6.1).[1] Yersin is both the adventurous explorer and the intrepid scientific traveler, while the provisional laboratory is a *scene*: of experience, action, and discovery.[2]

This chapter explores Yersin's temporary bamboo structure—hastily erected in the field by Chinese workmen for 75 piastres in June 1894—in relation, on the one hand, to an ideal of the Pastorian laboratory and, on the other, to a crisis of planning induced by an outbreak of bubonic plague in British Hong Kong. How might Yersin's 'matshed' relate to the Institut Pasteur (inaugurated in 1888), a Louis XIII-style brick and stone edifice built on some 11,000 square meters of land on Rue Dutot in Paris? In other words, to what extent did the metropolitan laboratory, conceived as a rationalized space for scientific research, coexist (or not) with the improvised colonial laboratory? What defined a colonial laboratory in the 1890s? Where were such laboratories situated? And, finally, as Peter Galison has formulated it: "How do the buildings of science literally and figuratively configure the identity of the scientist and scientific fields?"[3]

The negotiation and overt politicization of colonial space in 1890s Hong Kong, considered elsewhere in this volume by Cecilia Chu and David Pomfret, provide useful contexts for exploring the mobility of experimental research,

123

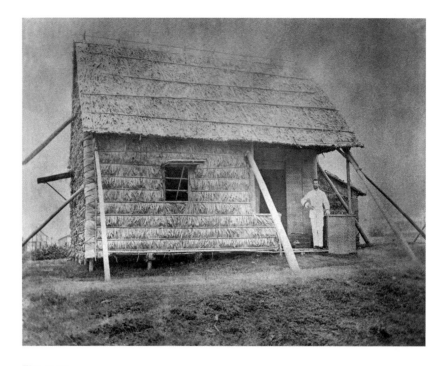

Figure 6.1

Alexandre Yersin in Hong Kong, 1894. Courtesy of the Institut Pasteur.

as well as the exportation and expansion of metropolitan "hygienic modernity."[4] The plague epidemic underlined the ways in which differences between
'national' sanitary and bacteriological approaches were reinforced and undermined in the field.[5] In the absence of a dedicated British bacteriologist, a
Pastorian (Yersin) and a Kochian (Shibasaburo Kitasato) worked to locate the
parasitical 'source,' collaborating to a greater or lesser degree with the British
colonial establishment.

Developing these themes, the chapter begins with a brief overview of the
circumstances surrounding the race to identify the microbe in Hong Kong, as
well as the reconfiguration of colonial medical spaces in the face of an epidemic
crisis. It then proceeds to investigate Yersin's 'matshed' in relation to British
and French colonial discourses on indigenous dwellings, exploring some of
the ideological contexts within which the mobile or makeshift laboratory was
produced. The aim is to offer a counterpoint to the growing body of literature that proclaims a laboratory 'revolution' in medicine and tends to overlook

the variety of laboratory spaces, focusing instead on a fundamental epistemic shift.[6] Finally, the chapter examines Yersin's 'discovery' of the plague bacillus in the light of his exploration and mapping of French Indochina, arguing that Yersin's dual role as scientist and explorer underscores the contested nature of 'exploration' as a field that is "riven with differences over the style, methods, and function of the explorer."[7]

While allusions to improvised laboratories pervade histories of colonial medicine in India—such as Mark Harrison's assertion that "until 1900 colonial laboratories were invariably makeshift, ephemeral affairs"[8]—scant attention has been paid to colonial laboratory practices, with a few notable exceptions.[9] To be sure, the notion of a singular colonial laboratory is itself problematic, suggesting an incontrovertible typology of experimental space, whereas laboratories—both metropolitan and colonial—were characterized by their diversity.[10] One further aim of this chapter is thus to stress the mobility of laboratory technologies and the specific ways in which laboratory practices were reconfigured as they migrated between sites.

In so doing, the chapter amplifies three major themes of *Imperial Contagions*. First, it considers the ways in which networks of exchange between metropole and colony determined the character of colonial and metropolitan science, architecture, and planning.[11] At issue, here, is the extent to which colonial science can be regarded as a form of "prefabricated" knowledge or as "the local enactment of fixed scientific procedures and vocabulary invented and ratified in a metropolitan centre."[12] Second, the chapter investigates the interrelations between different regimes of mobility, including the diffusion of disease, the circulation of air and sewage, the movement of 'native' labor, the dissemination of information, and the flow of commodities and capital in trade. And third, it examines the relationship between the 'field' and the 'laboratory' as a techno-scientific enclave for the production of new knowledge about disease. Although the emphasis is on colonial elites, rather than on laboring classes, the aim is nonetheless to re-situate the laboratory within a dynamic, transimperial, and transcolonial framework by drawing upon a growing body of scholarship concerned "with the spatiality of scientific knowledge" and "the migratory patterns of science on the move."[13]

Laboratory science is predicated on notions of controlled experimentation and replicability, as well as on the standardization of expertise, instruments, and procedures. However, as David Livingstone has argued, "spatial forces" are involved "at every scale of analysis—from the macropolitical geography of national regions to the microsocial geography of local cultures."[14] Furthermore, in her study of colonial botany and "bioprospecting" in the Caribbean, Londa Schiebinger has demonstrated the extent to which colonial science was produced in hybrid and contested "transcultural" or "biocontact zones."[15] In short, through an investigation of the provisional sites of scientific knowledge in Hong Kong in 1894—and, specifically, of Yersin's laboratory—this chapter aims to demonstrate the hybrid nature of colonial laboratory science as a particular form of 'exploration,' thereby illuminating the unstable borders demarcating field site and laboratory, "science in situ" and "science in motion."[16]

Makeshift Hong Kong and the Race for the Microbe

In the 1860s, plague epidemics broke out in southern China's Guangdong Province, reaching Hainan Island and southern Guangdong in the following decades and, by the 1890s, the port cities of the Pearl River Delta, marking the outbreak of the so-called Third Plague Pandemic.[17] On May 10, 1894, the government of Hong Kong, on the advice of the colony's Sanitary Board, issued a formal proclamation that the crown colony was an infected port, contemporaries ascribing the arrival of the disease to crowds of Chinese New Year revelers from Canton (Guangzhou) and attributing the speed of diffusion in Hong Kong to a number of factors, including drought and the unsanitary conditions of the Chinese districts.[18]

Given Hong Kong's nodal position as a British entrepôt and a commercial hub of empire, there was some urgency in containing the spread of infection. On June 12, 1894, the bacteriologist Dr Shibasaburo Kitasato, director of the Japanese Institute of Infectious Diseases (established in November 1892), arrived in Hong Kong as the representative of an imperial Japanese government commission to assist in the hunt for the plague microbe.[19] The Japanese team was promptly furnished with research facilities in the Kennedy Town Hospital. As Kitasato himself declared, Dr James A. Lowson, acting superintendent of the Government Civil Hospital, had "put everything needful at our disposal in the most friendly spirit. A room in the Kennedy Town Hospital (one of the plague establishments) was given to us and there we began our work on June 14th."[20] Specimens of bacilli were obtained from a corpse and the news appeared in the editorial pages of *The Lancet* on June 23.[21]

On June 15, the same day that the preliminary report of the Japanese breakthrough was wired to London, the Swiss-born, naturalized French physician and bacteriologist Yersin arrived in Hong Kong accompanied by two servants. He had been dispatched from Saigon by the French Colonial Service, which was fearful of the epidemic reaching French dominions in Indochina. Yersin brought with him basic laboratory equipment, including a microscope and autoclave for sterilizing instruments, although he was lent an immersion lens by Dr James Cantlie, dean of the College of Medicine for Chinese.[22] No formal space was made available to him by the authorities. Instead, after several days working in a gallery of the Kennedy Town Hospital, Yersin obtained permission to put up a makeshift laboratory in the grounds of the Alice Memorial Hospital, also known as the New Glass Works Hospital, a temporary matshed institution situated close to the infected Chinese areas. On June 20, a week after Kitasato, Yersin succeeded in isolating the plague bacillus.

The construction of provisional research spaces in Hong Kong in 1894 was part of a planning crisis produced by epidemic disease, which threw into relief the limits and extent of colonial authority and its ability to police and regulate space. Yersin's makeshift laboratory needs to be seen within the context of Hong Kong itself as a 'makeshift' free port since, as Cantlie noted in a lecture on the plague published in *The Lancet* in 1897: "The city was hastily built about fifty years ago, when all too hurriedly tens of thousands of Chinese sought occupation and habitation under the British rule."[23] Although, as the photographer John Thomson noted in the 1890s, the city presented an impressive view "with its solid granite buildings, its magnificent esplanade and palatial residences," this grandiosity was offset by the chaos of the island's "low-lying quarters," where "the poorest and most depraved class of Chinese" resided in areas that were conducive to "zymotic diseases," such as the plague.[24] Furthermore, as Osbert Chadwick had noted in his *Report on the Sanitary Condition of Hong Kong* in 1882, there was only "a small number of really permanent Chinese settlers," the rest being, like the Europeans, "only temporary residents" whose "first or principal wife remains at the home of their ancestors, in their native country."[25]

Legislation, in the form of the Squatters Ordinance of 1890, had sought to regulate the haphazard occupation of land and introduce a more rational system, since, as Cantlie asserted, "the city [had] never recovered" from the "feverish haste to build without proper control." Here, the association of the colony's makeshift and expendable character with the pathological ("feverish," "recovered") is made explicit: the colony is dangerously provisional and its lack of organized settlement renders it susceptible to infection.[26] By the same token,

in his study of leprosy in Hong Kong, Cantlie had warned of the threats posed
to the colony by the uncontrolled migration of "diseased" Chinese (1890):
Hong Kong's 'openness', upon which its mercantile success and wealth were
founded, exposed it to lethal pathogenic threats.[27]

The colony's improvised, laissez-faire character was further reflected in the
makeshift nature of its medical and research establishments. Thus, the smallpox hospital was variously described in the mid-1890s as the wooden 'smallpox hut' or the Temporary Smallpox Hospital. Similarly, the Government Civil
Hospital (1849) was established in a converted, private two-story bungalow.
On its destruction by a typhoon in 1874, it was then provisionally housed
in the Hotel d'Europe in Central, until finally moving into a new four-block,
purpose-built structure on Hospital Road (1879). This building had originally
been intended for the Lock Hospital, which was moved, temporarily, into a
former school and private houses.

According to the governor, Sir William Robinson, the bubonic plague in
1894 was an "unexampled calamity" that would likely result in the "destruction and re-building of one-tenth of Hongkong."[28] To control the infection
and to cope with the many Chinese dislodged from their quarters, "numerous
matsheds have been erected and Government has hired blocks of unoccupied
buildings and godowns [warehouses] for the segregation and isolation of those
whom it has been necessary to keep under observation."[29] Commercial and
institutional spaces were re-assigned as 'medical' locales: for example, a glass
factory under the supervision of the Tung Wah Chinese Hospital, the Kennedy
Town police station managed by doctors and nurses from the Government
Civil Hospital, and a slaughterhouse otherwise described as the new "pig and
sheep depôt" (Figure 6.2). At the same time, the extent of the crisis soon put
pressure on these provisional spaces, prompting the erection of additional
structures, such as the second New Glass Works Hospital, a matshed building also known as the New Alice Memorial Hospital or the Alice Memorial
Matshed, which was used for the spillover of plague victims between June 17
and July 21.[30]

Meanwhile, the existing Alice Memorial (1887) and Nethersole (1893)
hospitals (established by the London Missionary Society for Chinese patients
seeking Western treatment), which had closed due to their proximity to the
affected Taipingshan area, were converted into refuges for the Chinese who had
been forced to evacuate from their "unsanitary" housing.[31] Existing medical
spaces, such as the hospital hulk *Hygeia*, were designated for plague victims.

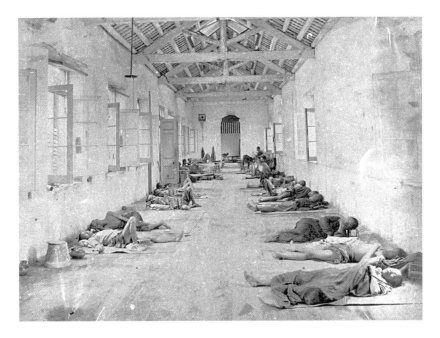

Figure 6.2

The Glass Works Hospital, Kennedy Town, 1894. Courtesy of the Public Records Office, Hong Kong.

Infection highlighted and amplified tensions between the colonial regime and the Chinese community over the definition and ownership of 'medical' spaces.[32] "No disease," the *British Medical Journal* announced somberly in 1897, by which time the disease had reached India, "necessitates more close and constant medical supervision than plague."[33] Indeed, this "supervision" required a new 'front-line' emphasis, wherein humanitarian and medical research institutions adopted the makeshift forms and operational modalities of the military encampment, with an emphasis on efficiency and mobility.[34]

Cabin Fever: The Politics of the Matshed

Yersin referred to his temporary laboratory as a *cabane à paillote*, a term which denotes an indigenous wood-framed hut of matting or bamboo: "I installed myself with my laboratory equipment in a small straw hut (*cabane à paillote*) which I had built."[35] In the narrative of the discovery of the plague bacillus in

June 1894, Yersin's ephemeral laboratory occupies a pivotal role and is variously described in English as a "matshed" or a "thatched hut."[36] The photograph of Yersin—reminiscent of the self-portraits of the white-suited poet and
'gun-runner' Arthur Rimbaud taken in Abyssinia in the 1880s[37]—has become
an indispensable part of the Yersin 'legend,' evoking simultaneously Yersin the
intrepid explorer, frontiersman, and physician-scientist, while intimating a
missionary dedication to French colonial *mise en valeur*. As Patrice Debré has
written of Yersin the 'explorer': "There were no medications in his bags; he took
with him only a gun, a microscope, a Chamberland filter, and some canned
food."[38] Furthermore, as Laurence Monnais-Rousselot has observed, in historical studies Yersin remains an emblem of "the new race of missionaries."[39]

In a letter to the *British Medical Journal* in 1897, in which he defended
Yersin's reputation from the aspersions of Lowson, who remained critical of
Yersin's claims about the efficacy of his plague serum, Cantlie praised Yersin
for the "care and indefatigable energy with which he dealt with all bacteriologi-
cal matters." For Cantlie, the supreme expression of such care and energy was
Yersin's construction of the makeshift laboratory:

> He built a laboratory for himself close to the Plague Hospital, and had
> a large assortment of animals and apparatus for experimental work. So
> earnest was he that alongside the laboratory he put up a mat-shed dwell-
> ing, so that he might not waste time going to and fro to his work.[40]

Crucial to the description of the matshed was the order of things and the
planning of space upon which this was predicated. The matshed was a locus
of scientific life as well as work, housing experimental equipment, including
Yersin's experimental animals: rats, mice, rabbits, and guinea pigs.[41] Household
and workplace conjoined, so that the makeshift laboratory suggested a radical
domestic economy: life that was work, work that was life.[42] As Yersin noted in
his journal for June 21:

> I quickly made a deal with a Chinese builder who, in return for 75 piastres,
> agreed to build me a bamboo house thatched with straw in two days (8
> meters by 3), comprising two rooms (one serving as a bedroom, the other
> as a laboratory), as well as a small cabinet for cultivating microbes.[43]

This conflation of work and life was not, of course, unique to the matshed:
it was the Pastorian *modus operandi*. Studying silkworms in the laboratory
at Pont-Gisquet in the late 1860s, there had been "practically no boundaries
between work and private life."[44] In Paris, Pasteur's living quarters had been

designed as an integral component of the Institut Pasteur, with easy access to the laboratories. Moreover, as Emile Roux's assistant, Yersin was the first to take up residence in the new institute on January 20, 1889, occupying a large room with two windows above the library on a floor specifically intended to accommodate the institute's assistants (*préparateurs*).[45]

As a temporary structure, situated in the field, the Hong Kong matshed laboratory was 'open' to the elements, causing Yersin considerable discomfort from mosquitoes, which kept him awake at night.[46] The hardiness, dedication, and resourcefulness which characterize this experimental life are also the qualities celebrated in accounts of Yersin the explorer, who camped in native *huttes* on his travels into the interior of Annam (see Figures 6.3 and 6.4). In 1895, the weekly *Journal des Voyages* featured an account of Yersin's travels to the hill-tribe country with a cover illustration of Yersin sitting down to a meal of rice with 'natives' outside a straw hut.[47] At the same time, Yersin's matshed suggests the Pastorian ascetic toiling in his laboratory-cell for the greater good of science. The laboratory constituted a homosocial and hermetic, bachelor environment. As one newspaper reporter expressed it, Yersin's "investigations had been conducted quietly and not *coram populo*."[48] In the 'legend' of Yersin, the

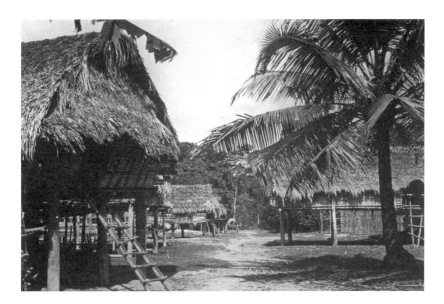

Figure 6.3

Hill-tribe village above Nha Trang in Vietnam. Courtesy of the Institut Pasteur.

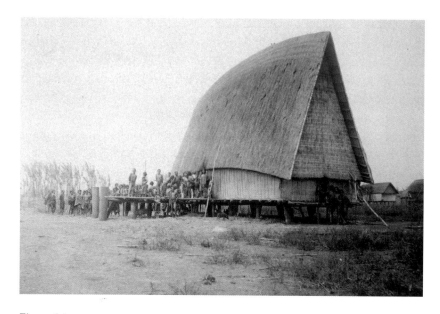

Figure 6.4

Communal 'Banhar' village hut. Photograph taken by Yersin during his travels to the Central Highlands, 1894. Courtesy of the Institut Pasteur.

hagiographical dimension is accentuated by the role played in the matshed's construction by the Italian missionary priest, Father Bernardo Vigano, who negotiated on Yersin's behalf with the authorities and helped him to establish the laboratory.[49]

In more specific ways, Yersin's search for laboratory space was bound up with assumptions about colonial space, race, and social order. At least since the mid-1840s, 'native' matshed dwellings in Hong Kong had been disparaged by the colonial authorities, and their permeability and evanescence associated with the emanation of disease. Thus, government proclamations in the mid-1840s sought to address the anti-social and potentially disruptive influences of native "mat-houses" off Queen's Road.[50] The association of the matshed with disease persisted. One commentator, noting that Europeans sent from Hong Kong to oversee the construction of a paper mill on the mainland in 1890 resided in a matshed, wondered how it was that they did not contract fever "before they were able to put up a brick house."[51] In 1901, matsheds that housed civil staff close to paddy fields at Tai Po in the New Territories were recommended for replacement by permanent buildings on account of the susceptibility of matshed dwellers to malarial fever.[52]

Moreover, matsheds were construed as the abodes of "loitering" and "criminal" indigents who concentrated in insalubrious settlements, such as the nefarious squatters evicted from their matsheds near Kennedy Town in 1886.[53] The 'openness' of the buildings was equated with promiscuity, duplicity, and immorality, even as the structures were deemed to pose a physical threat on account of their combustibility;[54] a subsequent connection between conflagration and disease being intimated by allusions to disease "spread[ing] like wildfire."[55]

Similar assumptions and fears pervaded French colonial perceptions of the *paillotes*—a term that encompassed a miscellany of native wooden, cob, and straw structures—as primitive, fragile, and unhealthy dwellings.[56] In the 1880s, Hanoi consisted overwhelmingly of native housing, prompting a series of colonial edicts from the 1890s aimed at restricting or removing indigenous habitation from the expanding 'modern' city. Such proclamations were known colloquially as the *chasse aux paillotes* and were expressly formulated as countermeasures against the erection of native dwellings in strategic central city locations, reflecting, at the same time, a drive to incorporate the city's 'villages' into the colonial urban fabric, while further reinforcing the divide between spaces of work and living.[57] Under the governor-generalship of Paul Doumer, who later assisted Yersin in establishing the Ecole de Médecine de Hanoi (1902),[58] the capital was moved from Saigon to Hanoi, and an ambitious replanning of the city was undertaken.[59]

In some senses, the *paillotes* became emblematic of French Indochina, which had been represented in the *expositions universelles* since 1878, even before the region's formal absorption into an expanded French empire as the Union Indochinoise in 1887.[60] Characteristically, for example, the *exposition* of 1889 featured an Annamite village with "bamboo *paillotes* covered with straw."[61] Yersin, a keen amateur photographer, recorded his impression of these local matsheds, taking pictures of villages, with their *cabanes paillotes* or *maisons sur pilotis*, on his explorations of the Mekong and the highland plateaux of the Lang Bian, where he 'discovered' Dalat in 1893, a settlement that became the site of French *villeggiatura*, modeled on Simla, Darjeeling, and the British hill stations of the subcontinent (discussed in Chapter 4 by David Pomfret). In Indochina, censorial policies geared to addressing the dangers posed by indigenous habitation coincided in complex ways with anxieties over the pace of industrialization, pollution,[62] and the disappearance of local metropolitan culture, giving rise to a peculiar "congruence" several decades later, in which "beliefs in hierarchy, authenticity, the village, and the soil" conjoined in a conservative "nativism."[63]

Recurrent descriptions of Yersin's matshed laboratory or *paillote* thus take place within a complex contestation over colonial space, and precisely at a time when indigenous, 'unsanitary' housing in Hong Kong (and Indochina) was becoming the object of a repressive colonial state campaign determined on the demolition of unhealthy local structures.[64] Yet the status of the matshed remained equivocal, since colonial authorities in Hong Kong continued to erect temporary accommodation, including the New Alice Memorial Hospital referred to by Lowson simply as "the Matshed"—an 'experiment' that was finally blown away by a typhoon in September 1894.[65] As Sir William Robinson noted, numerous matsheds had been put up to accommodate those dislodged from "infected houses in the Chinese quarter."[66] Similarly, in a lecture on the plague published in *The Lancet*, Cantlie explicitly emphasized the salutary nature of the matshed as opposed to the "reeking [Chinese] hovels":

> Those houses were of the vilest kind of habitation mankind is acquainted with; small, windowless, low-ceilinged, reeking with filth and excretions, they presented infection in its most concentrated form.[67]

The lack of ventilation and the obstructed circulation produce a "concentrated" form of infection, which suggests that the buildings are inverted laboratories concocting "unnatural" cultures of disease. Or, as one newspaper declared, they are "plague breeding properties."[68] In contrast, Cantlie commented on:

> ... [the] newly built, commodious and roomy mat-shed. Freely ventilated by being raised three feet from the ground, and its lofty roof constructed so that air swept across between the side walls and the roof, with large apertures in the roof itself, the chance of contracting the disease from so diluted a form was reduced to a minimum.[69]

The matshed was thus recuperated, becoming an 'organic' habitation in contrast to the corrupted, filthy, and windowless slum tenement dwellings and shacks at the center of the plague epidemic. Similarly, bamboo was exalted for its pliability and strength, with the British official and colonial secretary of Hong Kong, James Stewart Lockhart, proclaiming:

> To start with the bamboo has *seven* virtues of its very own: it is clean and unspotted in itself: a sheath covers the stem as it pierces the dark earth so the bamboo has protection from the world: being hollow it is symbolical ... of a pure heart: it is strong and unyielding: the stem being divided into segments is orderly: the stalk is pure green without blemish: and is lastly eternal and enduring.[70]

The bamboo is identified by Lockhart with cleanliness, strength, resolution, order, and endurance—precisely those characteristics hitherto deemed lacking in the makeshift bamboo mat-houses of the 'natives.' Notions of the 'eternal' and trustworthy qualities of bamboo, and of the 'original' matshed, undoubtedly hark back to the foundational myth of the colony: to the matshed huts of the fishermen on the beaches,[71] to the settler matshed church and clubs, and specifically to William Caine's erection of a mat-hut as his first dwelling on the island.[72]

There is a sense in which the Chinese abandonment of matsheds for tenements, which created the unsanitary conditions so deplored by the civil authorities, prompted a return to the 'original' dwelling. The qualities associated with the matshed, namely its vulnerability to the elements, became benefits in a sanitary and hygienic discourse that placed emphasis on healthy circulations. In colonial Hanoi, locals were not easily convinced to move out of their wood-framed, thatched dwellings, which combined living space with workspace and defined the *ville indigène* in contrast to the 'modern' and 'efficient' colonial brick or stone buildings (with a clear separation of work and living space) of *Hanoi Française*. Although the French condemned the 'crude' native dwellings as offering little protection against natural disasters, such as typhoons, floods, or epidemics, the local population saw the matsheds, which were more quickly and easily rebuilt, as "a strategy for dealing with [such] recurring catastrophes."[73]

Yersin's 'primitive' matshed laboratory might also, perhaps, be linked to late nineteenth-century debates about the nomadic origins of European habitation (Figure 6.5). Anthropological discourse in France, for example, emphasized the migratory nature of Europe's "Aryan" inhabitants, suggesting that "the national home was nothing more than the wagon of the nomad that had come finally to rest, its wheels replaced by a solid foundation."[74] In their comprehensive survey of architecture from prehistoric times to the modern era, *L'habitation humaine* (1892), for example, the French architect Charles Garnier and the anthropologist Auguste Ammann sought to chart the Westward migration of Aryan "tent dwellers" from Asia and their subsequent sedentarization in Europe. For Garnier and Ammann, the "primitive" dwellings of "savage" tribal societies in Africa, North America, Asia and the Pacific, were a link back to the primeval antecedents of European architecture. At the same time, the prehistory of the nation's "nomadic life" furnished a specific context within which scientists such as the biologist and zoologist Henri de Lacaze-Duthiers conceptualized mobile

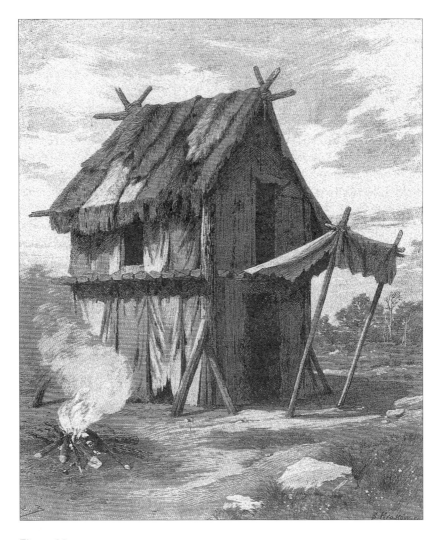

Figure 6.5

"Aryan dwelling in the age of migration," from Charles Garnier and Auguste Ammann, *L'habitation humaine* (Paris: Librairie Hachette, 1892), 401.

laboratories, or "scientific caravans," in relation to permanent research centers, such as the Station Biologique de Roscoff, established in Brittany in 1872.[75]

The sociologist of science Karina Knorr-Cetina has observed that: "The power of the laboratory (but of course also its restrictions) resides precisely in its enculturation of natural objects."[76] Accordingly, "[t]he laboratory subjects natural conditions to social overhaul and derives epistemic effect from the new situation."[77] Yet, Yersin's expeditionary matshed, even while it underscores the complex open-endedness of the field and laboratory, also intimates the reciprocal 'naturalization' of experimental space. If laboratories served to frame natural conditions in the field, by the same token, the field impacted upon the meaning and scope of laboratory space. In short, Yersin's matshed laboratory is a hybrid space, reminding us of colonial architecture's adaptive strategies that strove to indigenize the modern[78] and modernize the indigenous,[79] incorporating local elements and conjoining them with metropolitan values.[80] Indeed, the coupling of the 'primordial' matshed with the laboratory—described by the architectural historian Julien Guadet in his *Eléments et théorie de l'architecture* (1905) as a subject that was "absolutely modern"[81]—into the composite term "matshed laboratory" produces an oxymoron, since, while 'laboratory' suggests modernity, 'matshed' evokes pre-modernity.

Chadwick had called attention to a darker consequence of this indigenization of the modern in his *Report* of 1882, which linked the dismal living conditions of the Chinese to the prevalence of disease in Chinese neighborhoods. He had noted, for example, the way in which, although the Chinese were influenced by Europeans to move into brick houses, they invariably subdivided the interiors of these houses with board partitions, creating separate "cabins about 9 feet long and 10 feet wide," which were tantamount to makeshift shelters within the walls of the dwelling.[82] In other words, disease was understood, in part, as a consequence of the indigenization of colonial planning.

This tension between the permanent and the transitory, the institutionally sanctioned and the peripheral, the modern and the authentic, was echoed in Yersin's own ambiguous position as a naturalized French Pastorian working within a British crown colony. Lacking any knowledge of English and sidelined by Lowson, who favored the Japanese, Yersin was compelled to work both within and outside the colonial establishment. In a literal, as well as a political sense, he moved across borders and between camps. Thus, while the authorities granted him permission to put up his matshed in the grounds of the new makeshift Alice Memorial Hospital, Yersin was initially denied access to specimens for autopsy. He was forced to procure bodies illegally by bribing sailors. As he noted in his diary for June 20, 1894:

> The bodies before they are carried to the cemetery are deposited for one or two hours in a cellar (*une sorte de cave*). They are already in their coffins in a bed of lime. The coffin is opened. I move the lime to clear the crural region. The bubo is exposed, within less than a minute I cut it away and race to my laboratory.[83]

Here, the makeshift morgue and the improvised autopsy by lantern in the *cave* reinforce the connection between space and practice, even as they re-inscribe the difference between field and laboratory: specimens from the world must be hastily ferried for analysis in the sanctuary of the provisional *paillote*.

Sacred Dwellings: The Pastorian Laboratory

Yersin's matshed intimates the permeability of hierarchical boundaries differentiating outside from inside, colonized from colonizers, indigenous from European. It also reflects an impetus, in the midst of an epidemic crisis, to re-affirm the value of specialized spaces: in this case, the sanctuary of the laboratory. To be sure, Yersin was familiar, in a practical sense, with the construction of such specialized spaces. As the first resident of the Institut Pasteur on Rue Dutot in 1889, he had been left to deal with the numerous contractors finishing off the project; he was later to be instrumental in the building of scientific and medical institutions of research and teaching at Nha Trang and Hanoi, drawing upon his firsthand experience of the new Institut Pasteur's construction in Paris. Moreover, the assertion of a 'specialized' space lay at the heart of the so-called laboratory 'revolution' articulated from the 1860s. In *An Introduction to the Study of Experimental Medicine* (1865), the physiologist Claude Bernard had famously visualized the laboratory as the inner sanctum, the place of modern medical research entered through the gateway of clinical experience in the hospital: "The true sanctuary of medical science is a laboratory."[84]

Although Bernard's physiological laboratory in the College de France was very different from Pasteur's experimental laboratory, geared to the manufacture of vaccines and sera, nonetheless, his idea of the laboratory as an inner precinct was promoted by Pasteur and Robert Koch in the context of bacteriological research. The laboratory was construed as a fortress (defending) and a sanctuary (preserving), both of which were defined in relation to the field outside. This opposition of interior and exterior constituted, as Laura Otis contends, part of a new preoccupation with regulating borders.[85] Just as life and disease were increasingly conceptualized "in terms of units with distinct boundaries," so bacteriological laboratories were construed as places where germs were made visible by being constrained.[86]

In the late 1860s, both Pasteur and Bernard had argued for the need to expand existing networks of state-sponsored laboratories.[87] Pasteur had vented his frustration at the scarcity of laboratories in France: while millions of francs were being spent on erecting a new opera house, he had to make do with a dank basement laboratory.[88] As he observed in a projected article in the *Moniteur* in January 1868:

> I implore you, take some interest in those sacred dwellings meaningly described as *laboratories*. Ask that they may be multiplied and completed. They are the temples of the future, of riches and of comfort. There humanity grows greater, better, stronger; there she can learn to read the works of Nature, works of progress and universal harmony, while humanity's own works are too often those of barbarism, of fanaticism and of destruction.[89]

During the Third Republic, the laboratory was exalted as a sanctuary in the cult of science, becoming an "obligatory point of passage" through which new scientific knowledge looped back to medical practice and hygiene.[90] The push for laboratories continued through the 1870s as part of an overhaul of medical education in France that sought to integrate clinical and research components into a unified medical curriculum. Thus, in 1876, the inspector of medical education, Jules Gavarret, called for more extensive research facilities in "an age when the experimental method unquestionably plays a predominant role in the scientific domain."[91] Particularly in the 1890s, there was a discernible shift from laboratories as sites of basic research to the development of clinical laboratories and ward laboratories.[92]

As Pasteur observed in 1871: "Laboratories and discoveries are correlative terms; if you suppress laboratories, Physical Science will become stricken with barrenness and death."[93] Or: "Away from their laboratories, physicists and chemists are but disarmed soldiers on a battlefield."[94] Such mixed metaphors point to more than a lexical confusion: they suggest a latent instability within the biomedical sciences between bacteriology and medicine, laboratory and clinic. The laboratory was at once a sanctuary and a battlefield: a place removed from the field and a place in the midst of the field.[95]

Microbes and Mobility: The Civilizing Mission

From 1889, Roux and Yersin had begun teaching a course in microbiology at the Institut Pasteur in Paris, training students for a laboratory life, but also equipping them for the field. Particularly in France's overseas possessions, distinctions between laboratory and clinic blurred, while it was often difficult to differentiate between the activities of doctor, bacteriologist, and public health official. Invariably, the colonies were construed as extended fields for experimentation and crucial spaces for testing and yielding up new knowledge.

The development of bacteriology became entangled with imperialism, particularly with the surge to acquire colonies and 'protectorates' in the 1880s and 1890s. The French defeat by Prussia in 1870 gave a new impetus to imperial expansion, including ambitions centered on Indochina. During the Third Republic, an 'imperial' outlook began to cut-across party lines, permeating popular culture.[96] By the same token, the laboratory was deemed to be part of a civilizing mission against "barbarism, fanaticism and destruction." From its outset, the 'Pastorian mission' was thus expansionist.[97] As Pasteur had famously proclaimed at the inauguration of the Pasteur Institute on November 14, 1888: "science has no borders" (*la science n'a pas de patrie*).[98] In other words, although science had a global reach, the scientist had an obligation to exploit scientific knowledge for the benefit of the nation.

In contrast to the situation within the British Empire, where there were few research facilities, the Pasteur institutes played an important role in the development of France's colonial possessions.[99] Albeit disastrous, the expedition to investigate the cholera outbreak in Egypt in 1883 set a precedent for the Institute's involvement in colonial scientific research more generally. The establishment of the Paris Institut Pasteur in 1888 was soon followed by the opening of satellite institutes, such as the one established in Saigon in 1891 by Albert Calmette. The Pastorian expansion in the 1890s coincided with the development of a colonial administrative structure and policies geared to rationalizing colonial space with a view to the more systematic extraction of resources.[100]

The Pastorian remit extended from microbiology to epidemiological investigation, immunization strategies, vaccine production, and hygiene concerns.[101] Medical-scientific investigation was integrated into a broader program of activities:

> Such research showed a continuous pendulum movement between laboratory and field observation which narrowed the gap between the

exterior (natural) environment and the interior (artificial) environment of the laboratory.[102]

As Bruno Latour has observed, "the boundaries of hygiene [were] vague," and this open-endedness functioned as a source of power since "it was necessary to be able to act everywhere and on everything at once":[103]

> Only in the colonies was the coordination between those who designed sewers, provided pure water, regulated frontiers and instigated the quarantines, supervised and wiped out epidemics, and the public authorities, usually harmonious.[104]

Far from being a homogeneous field, then, Pastorianism comprised a variety of practices and knowledges, often in tension. In this sense, Pastorian science might be understood as a genre of 'exploration': "a set of cultural practices"— material, social, and literary—that involved "the mobilization of people and resources, especially equipment, publicity and authority."[105] The 'microbe' provided the grounds for this mobilization and the tie between these disparate practices. As Latour has observed, the microbe was a means of action and "locomotion for moving through the networks" of knowledge upon which Pastorianism was predicated. If, on the one hand, the laboratory functioned as an "ideal" space for making "invisible agents visible," on the other hand, the ideal existed in relation to the terrain of the "hastily constructed laboratory" on the frontline, in the field. From this perspective, the 'laboratory' can be seen, not as stationary, monolithic space, but in terms of a "succession of displacements."[106]

Yersin's own career, in this respect, was fundamentally Pastorian. In 1895, he returned from Paris to Nha Trang, where he established a laboratory (later to evolve into the Pasteur Institute), subsequently helping Doumer to found the medical school in Hanoi and embarking on ambitious agronomic projects, including the cultivation of rubber trees imported from Brazil and the acclimatization of quinine trees.[107]

Explorations: Frontiers and Interiors

The fusionist, hygienic approach, which brought together epidemiological investigation and laboratory science within the context of the colonial state's security and welfare, is evident in Yersin's paper on the bubonic plague in Hong Kong. Here, as Latour has noted, the boundaries between laboratory, clinic, and city are blurred to produce a continuous space of knowledge.

Yersin casts himself as the epidemiologist, the sanitarian, and urban planner, as well as the physician and laboratory technician.[108] There is a telescoping throughout between the micro-scale of the laboratory and the macro-scale of colonial planning.

The paper opens by establishing the broad colonial context of the research in Hong Kong:

> The disease raging for a long time, in an endemic state, on the highlands of Yunnan has from time to time made an appearance very close to the frontiers of our possessions in Indochina at Lang-Tcheou and Pakhoi.[109]

Yersin, the bacteriologist, assumes the role of explorer, sketching the geographical trajectory of disease as it connects with colonial frontiers. From the geopolitical setting, Yersin details the building of his *paillote* before following a rhythm of expanding and contracting scales: from macro to micro and back again. While he focuses on the pathology of the disease as the trained clinician, Yersin moves again to consider the epidemiological evidence, including the native Chinese dwellings and defective sewer system.

The arc of Yersin's narrative suggests a complex correlation between the mapping of geographical space and the exploration (and discovery) of the microbe. Mapping had, in fact, been one of the reasons for Yersin's exploratory trips in 1892–94, the years immediately preceding his work in Hong Kong. Visiting the highland regions of central and southern Annam (present-day Vietnam), he had noted in his report: "There is there a vast country, placed under our protection, and which, in the meantime is almost completely unknown."[110] His aim, in part, had been to map the unknown interior with a view to opening up new roads "which would facilitate communications and would allow us to seriously penetrate the interior."[111] In December 1893, Yersin had met the celebrated explorer Auguste Pavie in Saigon, when various missions for the demarcation of frontiers were being organized by the Chinese, French, and British. As the *British Medical Journal* asserted in 1897:

> Dr. Yersin did a good deal of exploring in Indo-China, and especially in a part of the Annamite country which was then almost unknown. In 1895 the Minister of Public Instruction entrusted him with a new scientific mission "to explore the unknown regions of the Black Country from the geographical and ethnological points of view, and to continue in Indo-China the study of various epidemic diseases of men and animals."[112]

Yersin's trips in Indochina were part of a systematic mapping of the peninsula, which entailed the 'invention' of the Highlands (*Hauts Plateaux*), and included

Pavie's mission of 1879–95, an ambitious attempt to map Indochina; indeed, Captain P. Cupet, a member of Pavie's mission, had advised Yersin on the route of his second exploration in 1892.[113] In Yersin's travel accounts, like those of his contemporaries, geography functions as a "geopolitics of conquest" that produces cartographic, economic, scientific, and medical knowledges.[114]

"Boundary anxieties" and concerns about the security of frontiers[115] were connected to fears of microbial invasion[116] and to the dangers posed by the state's penetration and assimilation of the colony's unmapped interior. Indeed, *explorateur* was a noun used of both bacteriological scientists and travelers who were opening up new territories of knowledge. As Calmette observed, microbiologists, as "scientific explorers," had a critical role to play in defending the colonies.[117] Thus, while Yersin autopsied and probed the 'interiors' of diseased animals and human cadavers, his mission was to close off circulations and establish "a really effective quarantine" so that "Indo-China would not be invaded by the epidemic."[118]

Yersin had been trained as a physician, and fieldwork had formed an important part of his experience in Paris, where he arrived from Lausanne in 1885 on "a great voyage of exploration." Taking an interest in tuberculosis and particularly in diphtheria, he worked between the Hôpital des Enfants Malades and Roux's laboratory at the Pasteur Institute—research that led to the identification of the toxin produced by diphtheria bacteria. Yersin's correspondence reflects his interest in the city and suggests the extent to which his urban encounters were inseparable from his laboratory work: Paris ceased "to be simply the chaotic, mysterious antithesis of the laboratory and the clinic, becoming instead a space and object of bacteriological and epidemiological knowledge."[119]

In particular, Yersin's research on diphtheria entailed visits to the hospital, where he took swabs from children's throats. In a perceptive article, Andrew Mendelsohn has sought to read Yersin's bicycle trips through the capital's suburbs, sometimes equipped with a microscope, within the context of the Parisian *flâneur*, a particular, post-1860s genre of mobile 'spectator' theorized by Baudelaire in "The Painter of Modern Life" (1859–60)—Yersin was an avid reader of the 'frontier' novels of James Fenimore Cooper and Victor Hugo's *Les Misérables* (1862). Mendelsohn also suggests reading Yersin's excursions in relation to the artistic practice of *plein air*: the notion that artists ought to move out of their studios to capture the immediacy of life out of doors. Roux was to call this new scientific field of study *bacteriologie en plein air*. Thus, "[t]he studio, the library, the municipal bureau, the writer's *cabinet*, the laboratory and clinic—these were all necessary to artistic and scientific practice, but their walls had to be breached to get at *la verité du plein air*."[120]

The new mobility of knowledge involved the conflation of laboratory techniques with the urban environment. As Mendelsohn remarks, Yersin and Roux sought to verify the hypothesis that infectious disease was caused by activation of attenuated microbes latent in the bodies of humans and animals. The city was thus construed as an aggrandized laboratory, a site in which micro-organisms became pathogenic, while, reciprocally, the laboratory became, "a city of controlled contagions." And yet, as one newspaper remarked in 1897—in an interview conducted with Yersin as he passed through Singapore carrying his plague serum to India—the bacteriologist's decision to site his laboratory in the remoteness of Nha Trang was not fortuitous. The laboratory's very seclusion was an attempt to remove "all chance of blame for infecting large cities" in the event that the "controlled contagion" went wrong and seeped out into the world.[121]

The photographic representations of the bacilli with which Yersin's paper on the bubonic plague concludes have been taken to exemplify a crucial epistemic break.[122] From this perspective, the post-1860s laboratory has been envisaged as an increasingly abstracted space, removed from the field, in which, as the pathologist and cell biologist Rudolf Virchow expressed it, the scientist could "learn to see microscopically."[123] Here was a novel way of discerning disease, which occasioned a shift of emphasis from environment to population. Laboratory space, and the equipment it housed, such as microscopes, test tubes, and animals, were prerequisites for producing 'new' experimental knowledge. Accordingly, the laboratories of Pasteur and Koch constituted "the germ theory put into bricks and mortar."[124]

This predominantly staticist view of laboratory revolution—the laboratory as "bricks and mortar"—however, fails to acknowledge the constantly shifting relationship between laboratory and field, indeed the fundamental 'mobility' of the laboratory as it was (re)-configured within different but overlapping and dynamic contexts. As Thomas Lamarre has written in connection with Mori Ōgai (1862–1922), the Japanese physician, novelist, and poet: "There is a hitch in the laboratory construction of pure culture . . . Bacteria refuse to remain objects. They threaten to exceed their medium and swarm out of their tubes and plates into the world."[125] This seepage—the swarming of laboratory objects out into the world and, conversely, the leakage of the world into the laboratory—is certainly suggested in Yersin's account of the plague in Hong Kong, a fundamental porosity exemplified by his matshed.

The linkage between the laboratory and the field is further underscored by the photographic depictions of the bacterial 'colonies' and Yersin's photographic records of indigenous cultures. As Monnais-Rousselot has noted in relation to the archive of Yersin's photographs, which cover "the heterogeneity of his domains of research," photography was an important medium of observation: "For Yersin photography was an invaluable medium for observing and deducing."[126] In the 1890s, in particular, photography had become closely associated with exploration: of far-off peoples and metropolitan slum-dwellers—and of the exotic flora and fauna represented in the plates of scientific publications. Thus, writing in the foreword to his book *Through China with a Camera* (1898), the celebrated photographer John Thomson declared that his aim was "to show how the explorer may add, not only to the interest, but to the permanent value of his work by the use of photography."[127] As Felix Driver has observed, however: "The business of the scientific explorer was not always, or easily, distinguished from that of the literary flaneur, the missionary, the trader or the imperial pioneer."[128] Consequently, the history of field sciences "is a history of constant efforts to differentiate between, and within, the categories of travel, exploration and discovery."[129]

Conclusion: Hybrid Spaces and Sites of Knowledge

This chapter has sought to demonstrate the fundamental perviousness of the borders that defined the colonial laboratory, while suggesting that the institution of the laboratory, as it took shape from the 1890s, needs to be understood within wider discursive fields. The 'macrocultural' was always a key component of the 'microbiological'; the laboratory existed in a complex interrelationship with the field. New approaches to disease causation, promoted by 'germ theory', did not replace the politics of hygiene and sanitation. On the contrary, as several other chapters in this volume argue, a sanitary discourse overlapped and conflicted with 'new' microbiological science to produce a complex configuration of ideas and assumptions about the meaning and scope of medicine, medical research, and public health.

In 1886, Emile Duclaux, Pasteur's successor as director of the Institut Pasteur, to whom Yersin had imparted the news of his discovery of the plague bacterium in 1894, observed:

> Medicine is a crumbling edifice. While tradition still maintains the general structure, it is more useful that everything crumbles. There is nothing that can be rescued except the building blocks. Were I a doctor, I would be the first to demolish it.[130]

For Duclaux, the laboratory provided a new scientific foundation for medicine, entailing a fundamental re-planning and re-building. This chapter has sought to explore the implications of Yersin's makeshift laboratory in 1890s Hong Kong within a series of overlapping contexts, including the racialized politics of colonial space, and debates about a laboratory 'revolution' in medicine—a process that entailed a de-construction, as Duclaux expressed it, since it involved tearing down the old to make way for a new science-driven medicine: microbiology and bacteriology. Part of the enduring power of the Yersin 'legend' is precisely the way in which the matshed laboratory, as a hybrid space, encapsulated this concept of transition: from edifice to bare foundations. The temporary, improvised, half-open, half-closed laboratory intimated at once the prospect of the new, without fully relegating the authority of the old.

In Hong Kong, it would take time to establish Duclaux's edifice. The secretary of state, Joseph Chamberlain, and officials in the Colonial Office repeatedly questioned the rationale for a bacteriological institute, pointing to the waste of funds in replicating research that was further advanced elsewhere:

> The question is then, if Hong Kong can afford this money, is it to be expended in the most useful manner. What is wanted is investigation into bubonic plague. I submit that in such an enquiry decentralization is simply [a] waste of money. Far better results would be obtained at less expense by contributing to research in India or some other place where elaborate work is already in progress.[131]

At issue in the debate over the establishment of a permanent bacteriological laboratory in Hong Kong were wider concerns about the colony's place in an imperial network of medical science. The Colonial Office's stance on the futility of fostering a research culture in Hong Kong stood in contrast with the vision of Hong Kong's medical destiny articulated by Sir Patrick Manson in his inaugural address as dean of the Hongkong College of Medicine for Chinese in October 1887 at City Hall. There, Manson had envisaged the colony as a hub of medical science spreading out across East Asia, "a centre and distributor, not for merchandise only, but also for science."[132]

As advisor to the Colonial Office in 1901, Manson's influence was critical in securing support for the development of a bacteriological capacity in the colony. However, even when a candidate had finally been identified for the post of bacteriologist, the feasibility of a bacteriological laboratory was still being debated. As Governor Blake wrote to the secretary of state in connection with William Hunter's disinclination to accept the position: "He did not see the aim of going out to Hong Kong as bacteriologist if he was not to be given a laboratory and apparatus."[133] In the event, when Hunter arrived to take up his position in February 1902, he had to make do with a temporary laboratory:

> As there was no Bacteriological Laboratory in the Colony, and no suitable place for the immediate establishment of such, the Principal Civil Medical Officer proposed that I should be allowed to establish, temporarily, a Laboratory in the Kennedy Town Infectious Diseases Hospital.[134]

In 1903, the greater part of bacteriological work was "carried out at the Mortuary owing to the want of a Bacteriological Laboratory."[135]

Temporary, makeshift: these adjectives may seem antithetical to the regulated space of pure, experimental science with which the laboratory 'revolution' is so frequently equated. Yersin's *cabane à paillote*, reflective of the provisional, embodied Duclaux's creative demolition of institutional edifices. In this sense, the field laboratory, no less than the readily reconstructable matsheds of the *ville indigène*, constituted "a strategy for dealing" with "recurring catastrophes."[136] The mobile laboratory functioned as a strategic response to the mobility of vector-borne disease agents. As Edward Eigen has observed: "Having no fixed formal structure apart from evolving methods of experience and practice, this very contingency is what validated the laboratory's claim to being absolutely modern."[137]

The impermanent and the provisional were defining features of colonial laboratories, no less than indigenous dwellings. Although there remains a tendency to essentialize colonialism as an oppositional discourse, re-considering Yersin's extemporized matshed in Hong Kong reminds us, first, that colonial science was never a homogeneous institution, comprising standardized practices: scientific procedures and the scope of laboratory operations varied from context to context. Second, the shift to public health, particularly as it developed from the 1890s, did not entail the uniform dissemination of laboratory-science into the world. On the contrary, as a form of 'exploration,' bacteriology was always 'makeshift,' entailing different kinds of practices, even as it produced different kinds of grounded knowledges.

III

Circulations

7

"Contagion of the Depot": The Government of Indian Emigration

Sunil S. Amrith

Introduction

The second half of the nineteenth century witnessed a vast expansion in Asian migration. In the century between 1840 and 1940, close to 20 million Chinese and 30 million Indians journeyed across the Bay of Bengal and the China Sea to the frontier regions of Southeast Asia.[1] A significant proportion of those migrants who survived eventually returned home. This world of circulation, of bodies in transit, stimulated fears of contagion (both real and imagined); concern about contagion underpinned imperial attempts to govern mobility. Then, as now, contagion served as a metaphor for an accelerating global traffic in people, pathogens, ideas, and objects. Expanding imperial states viewed human mobility as a threat, but also as a necessity: the expansion of capitalism into Asia's frontier zones depended on the supply of migrant labor from the heartlands of India and China. In this context, the containment of contagion related, always, to the management of labor.[2]

In the settler colonies of the 'new world,' fears of contagion fed anxieties about racial purity. The history of immigration exclusion acts in North America, Australasia, and South Africa illustrate the close relationship between the ideology of white supremacy and the fear of contagious aliens.[3] In the mobile waters of South and Southeast Asia, by contrast, the relationship between migration, citizenship, and the threat of contagion was more complex. The restriction of human mobility was more difficult to imagine than in the settler colonies, and even more difficult to enforce.[4]

Contingency and compromise governed the balancing of sanitary concerns with wider political imperatives. The free movement of people was both economically essential to the functioning of European colonialism in Southeast

Asia and part of its ideological edifice, representing freedom of trade and movement. The threat of contagion raised questions about the government of human migration, but so, too, did the fugitive movement of people across imperial boundaries—the boundary, for instance, between the British and Dutch empires across the Straits of Melaka.[5] In the imperial imagination, pilgrimage represented one of the most threatening kinds of mobility—for both political and sanitary reasons—and yet one that was politically difficult to restrain.

Focusing on Indian migration in the age of empire, and on Indian migration to Southeast Asia in particular, this chapter argues that fears of contagion stood within a broader set of anxieties around the government of mobile bodies. Migrants were at once branded as potential vectors of disease and as political subjects whose bodies and capacities had to be cultivated, protected, and enhanced to make them more productive workers and more useful citizens. Emigration camps ('depots'), where so many South Asian migrants began their journeys, served to prevent the contamination of indigenous populations by new arrivals; but were also a starting point in a project to 'improve' the population of migrant workers. Fears of contagion were always situated within the broader development of ways of governing human migration. The juridical and spatial practices that resulted from the imperatives of sanitary control were shaped equally by attempts to govern other kinds of movement across national and imperial frontiers.

Imperial Contagions and Indentured Labor

In his great novel of indentured migration, *Sea of Poppies*, Amitav Ghosh evokes the emigrants' first sight of the emigration camp as their convoy arrives in Calcutta:

> Beyond lay a newly cleared stretch of shore, still littered with the stumps of recently felled trees. Three large, straw-thatched sheds stood in a circle at the centre of the clearing; a short distance away, next to a well, was a modest little shrine, with a red pennant flying aloft on a pole.[6]

The camp is makeshift; it is hastily constructed; it aims, with its "modest little shrine," to provide some sense of continuity to the migrant lives that have been radically disrupted. From the beginnings of Indian indentured emigration to the sugar colonies of the West Indies and the Indian Ocean—in the aftermath of slavery abolition in the British Empire—the emigration camp was essential to the government of migration.

There were many similarities between Indian emigration camps and the process through which West African slaves were inducted into a 'new order' before embarking on slave ships: Markus Rediker has described it as an order designed to "objectify, discipline, and individualize the labouring body through violence, medical inspecting, numbering, chaining."[7] On the account of Hugh Tinker, who held fast to the nineteenth-century humanitarians' critique of indentured labor as a "new system of slavery," the emigration camp was "a place where one's life became submerged in a routine imposed from above." The camp played a strategic role in disciplining bodies and creating pliable emigrants. On arrival at the camp, Tinker writes, "the labourer was ready to begin the process of becoming an indentured coolie"; within, "he was just one of many human parts in a vast assembly process."[8]

The camp, in Giorgio Agamben's terms, stands as "the pure space of exception"—a model and a metaphor for practices of exclusion and segregation, in this case underpinned by colonial fears of contagion.[9] It was from the outset a hybrid space: at once the private preserve of labor recruiters and emigration agents and a site of state sovereignty where imperial magistrates and medical officers intervened directly in migrants' journeys.

The first, and shared, aim of labor recruiters and imperial officials was to ensure the productivity of labor migrants. The camps deployed a regime of medical inspections to try to prevent 'unfit' men, women, and children from departing Indian shores. In practice, these inspections were cursory, and only the visibly disabled failed their inspections. Mortality on the plantations was in any case so great, and the turnover of labor so high, that many planters did not inquire too closely into their recruits' state of fitness. In time, the rigor of the pre-departure examination would animate debates between planters and colonial authorities across the seas: charged with excessively high rates of mortality among indentured laborers, planters and their representatives would argue that recruits had arrived from India in a poor state of health. By contrast, Indian officials argued that "ill usage" and poor conditions turned healthy emigrants into "sickly" returnees. A Nagapattinam port surgeon put it starkly in 1880:

> For the authorities on the other side of the water to pretend that the sickly, starved, ill-used looking wretches who return to this port from Penang after the fulfilment of their contract are returned in the same condition as when they left, or owe their present appearance to the weakly state in which they were when they emigrated, must seem to any one with my experience of the matter . . . a contention far worse than ridiculous.[10]

A second kind of anxiety underpinning the emigration camps was the fear of contagion on board ships, and the related fear of emigrants as sources of contagion at their destinations. These were not idle fears. When epidemics broke out on emigrant ships, they could be devastating. This was particularly the case on the lengthier voyages that took Indian emigrants to the West Indies. To take just one example of many: in 1883, the *Sheila* arrived in Surinam; 49 of the 451 indentured workers on board had died of cholera en route.[11] Paradoxically, the emigration camps were often themselves the site and source of contagion. Only by the early twentieth century did the emigration depot in Calcutta benefit from piped water supplies.

Fears of contagion were at the root of the earliest attempts to regulate the circular movement of people between coastal South India and the ports of Southeast Asia in the middle of the nineteenth century. Until the late 1850s, migration to Southeast Asia was less intensively governed than indentured migration to more distant sugar colonies. Fears of contagion were significant in the institution of emigration camps in the ports of the Coromandel Coast. Initially, these were fears of contagion on board the Indian-owned ships that carried an increasing number of laborers across the Bay of Bengal each year. In 1846, for the first time, regulations were passed to govern the maximum number of passengers permitted to embark on any ship crossing the Bay, specifying certain minimum conditions of space and sanitation on board. Two years later, a British official on Prince of Wales Island (Penang) wrote to the Madras government that it was "notorious the crowded manner in which the vessels arrive at Penang," and "the consequences this year have been very fatal, many passengers having died on the way."[12] Epidemics were frequent, yet regulation seemed pointless: "Asiatics wishing a passage," Penang's governor noted, could simply "embark [or disembark at] the adjacent Malay coast."[13] Nevertheless, the Madras and Penang authorities passed more stringent regulations in 1857, governing conditions on board ship, and intensifying surveillance of departures from the Coromandel Coast.

Emigration from South India to Southeast Asia accelerated from the 1870s. The British India Steam Navigation Company secured a monopoly over passenger routes across the Bay of Bengal. Improved sanitary facilities at the camps, and on board ships, led to a significant reduction of mortality and morbidity on the crossing.

By the turn of the twentieth century, Tamil laborers journeying from South India to Malaya were among the most intensively governed of all Southeast

Asia's migrants. Upon arrival in the ports of Singapore or Penang, new migrants had their first experiences of Malaya in the quarantine stations of St John Island (Singapore) or Pulau Jerejak (Penang), where they remained for at least five days and up to three weeks. Oral histories collected much later in the twentieth century show that the experience of quarantine stations was traumatic for many migrants to the Straits Settlements and Malaya. In the words of the Straits Settlements' Quarantine Act of 1886, the goal was "preventing the introduction into the Colony of infectious and contagious diseases," which would be effected by "placing vessels arriving at any port of the Colony in Quarantine," from which only first-and second-class passengers would be exempt.[14]

Both quarantine campsites later became leper colonies; St John Island eventually became a drug rehabilitation center. This is symbolic of the close relationship in the twentieth century among migration, isolation, and the fear of contagion, all refracted through the logic of quarantine.[15]

Biological Agents and Political Subjects

At every stage, imperial fears about the ungoverned circulation of human beings as 'biological agents' came together with anxieties about the ungoverned circulation of human beings as political subjects. From the outset, Indian indentured migration throughout the British Empire had attracted the attention of humanitarians and anti-slavery campaigners. Many of them suspected that, in the words of Lord John Russell, indentured labor migration would lead to "a dreadful loss of life on the one hand, or, on the other, to a new system of slavery."[16] The earliest emigration depots included a mechanism through which the state (and employers) could demonstrate that the emigrants had signed their contracts of indenture freely and voluntarily. As well as medically inspecting the bodies of migrants, colonial magistrates examined them to determine whether their decisions to emigrate were coerced.

The emigration depot, that is to say, was centrally designed to investigate the agency of 'free' labor. The protector of emigrants, a local magistrate, would "examine every intending immigrant brought before him." He would inquire into each emigrant's "knowledge of the place to which he is to be taken," and his awareness "of the contract and terms on which he is sent to be employed."[17] The process allowed the colonial state to hold each act of migration as the free and willed decision of an individual. The emigration camps for Indian emigrants served a more complex role than simply to prevent contagion. The camps brought together a juridical and a biopolitical discourse on migration; the intersection of the two would generate new ways of governing movement throughout the British Empire.

The attribution of agency to the individual migrant, rather than to the recruiting agent who had brought him to the depot, was crucial in order for the colonial state to attribute responsibility for migration.[18] To take a specific example, the ideological justification for the system of labor recruitment for Malaya after 1870 rested on freedom of contract. The term 'indenture' was never used in relation to Malaya, so far had it already fallen into disrepute because of humanitarian critiques earlier in the century. Determining that each migrant had consented to being transported across the Bay of Bengal was an essential part of holding him responsible for the performance of his contract. Such contracts included punitive sanctions for "desertion," and often the contracts consisted of a "joint and several agreement" that "binds [each migrant] to make good the advances made to any other party to the same agreement, who might abscond, die, or become incapable to work."[19]

Colonial observers could not avoid the question of why Tamil laborers would consent to such onerous conditions, beyond the frequent invocation of the "wretched" or "miserable" state of the South Indian countryside.[20] One British official explained the South Indian propensity to migrate to Southeast Asia in terms of the "*contagion of the depot*."[21] This reference to the 'contagion' of the depot suggests that migration was akin to infection, sweeping through the crowd as a force of nature. Migration emerges on this view as the product of emotion—'discord,' 'discontent'—rather than reasoned choice. Contagion could refer to emotional states and particular kinds of action as much as to infectious disease. Seeing migration as a kind of contagion denied the Tamil emigrant a characteristic that philosopher Charles Taylor defined as fundamental to the exercise of human agency: the ability to evaluate one's own desires qualitatively; in this case, migrants were deemed unable to ask themselves whether they were migrating for the 'right' reasons.[22]

While they subjected migrants to sanitary and bodily discipline and surveillance, the quarantine stations also marked the passage of sovereignty—sovereignty over the migrants' bodies and their lives—from the government of British India to the colonial government of the Straits Settlements or the Federated Malay States. Given the dominance of European planters over the government of the Straits Settlements, it seemed to many that, in fact, sovereignty over the migrants passed from the government of India to the planters themselves, who would exercise almost complete control over their indentured workers for the three-year period of indenture. It was precisely in trying to determine 'consent' that the British government of India aimed to free itself from responsibility for the lives of Tamil migrant workers in Malaya once they passed beyond the sovereignty of the Indian Empire.[23]

Contagion and Containment on the Plantation

The quarantine paradigm assumed that India was invariably the source of contagion: contagion that had to be contained, in transit, by the regime of sanitary inspections and segregation. Testimony from Malaya, however, suggested that conditions on the plantations of Southeast Asia's frontiers could themselves be home to lethal contagions.

The conditions of plantation life were illuminated in testimony that moved back across the Bay of Bengal to the Madras administration from the 1870s. In one of the first accounts in the archives, a government of India official expressed his shock at the conditions that official inspections had exposed in Province Wellesley. He highlighted the "existence of a very deplorable state of things on at least two estates in Penang," where "coolies are habitually flogged; that some of them have died from ill usage, chiefly flogging and neglect while sick; that no proper hospital accommodation is provided." Even in normal times, he noted, the "sanitary condition of the coolies' quarters is as bad as can be; that they are stinted in food, and their wages arbitrarily cut."[24] Only because the government of India wished not to take action that would be "injurious to the general body of planters," he admitted, did they refrain from "ordering at once the immediate cessation of emigration."[25] An investigation following reports of particularly awful conditions at Alma Estate in Penang revealed a picture of numerous Tamil plantation workers suffering from extreme distress and privation. The medical officer reported several cases of dysentery, widespread malnutrition, and a litany of injuries left untreated.[26]

This represents quite a significant reversal in perspective, with the rise of social and environmental explanations for the suffering of Tamil workers that tended to undermine the logic of quarantine. These were to suggest that, far from being the 'source' of contagion, needing containment and sequestration, Tamil laborers arrived in Malaya in a healthy state, to find their bodies ravaged by conditions on the plantation. The plantations themselves—their soil, their insanitation, their work discipline—became the *source* of illness and death, in this view. Because both British and Malayan authorities inevitably stopped short of a direct critique of the planters, they resorted to environmentalist ideas of disease in order to explain the extremely high rates of mortality on the plantation—water supplies, local ecology, the situation of the workers' housing. Inspecting a Malayan estate that suffered from exceptionally high mortality, Malayan officials determined that "this water does not seem to have induced what might be expected from a continued use of it, fever, but it doubtless had some influence in inducing diarrhoea and dysentery."[27]

The space of the camp, the labor lines, became in their own right the object of a program of sanitation and reorganization. Yet, even here, the Tamil estate workers were held at least partly responsible: "the filthy habits of the natives as regards conservancy are too well known to require explanation," one medical officer wrote.[28] This was to suggest that the lethality of the Malayan soil was in part a result of the migration of particular bodily practices and dispositions from India. The main source of contagion, without question, was malaria, which took a huge toll on the lives of fresh recruits from India, many of whom lacked immunity. Only in 1911 did the Malayan government establish a malaria advisory board to focus on anti-malarial campaigns on the estates. Hookworm, too, was a significant cause of debility and illness.[29]

Though it began to decline in the 1910s, the death rate on Malaya's plantations remained very high, as illustrated in Table 7.1. A Malayan government official lamented as late as the 1920s that "the wastage was too rapid; it was not worthwhile to bring coolies over from India, however strictly they were bound to fulfil their term of contract if, in fact, they died before the term was up."[30] The concern about "wastage" on the part of the colonial state and employers stimulated an intensified biopolitics of population management in the early decades of the twentieth century. Moving beyond a focus on contagion and on epidemic disease, the colonial state began to see disease on the plantations as something that—in Michel Foucault's words—"sapped the population's strength, shortened the working week, wasted energy, and cost money, both because they had led to a fall in production and because treating them was expensive." This was "illness as phenomena affecting a population"; death, in this view, "was now something permanent, something that slips into life, perpetually gnaws at it, diminishes it and weakens it."[31]

The colonial state in Malaya held to a conception of multiple, discrete populations rather than a homogeneous national body; it devised carefully targeted interventions to improve particular populations in all their diversity. Given

Table 7.1
Mortality rates on Malaya's rubber estates, 1911–23

Year	Total number of estate labourers	Deaths	Death rate (per 1000)
1911	143,614	9040	62.9
1912	171,968	7054	41.02
1913	182,937	5592	29.6
1914	176,226	4635	26.3
1915	169,100	2839	16.78
1916	187,030	3299	17.61
1917	214,972	3906	18.71
1918	213,425	9081	42.55
1919	216,573	3384	15.16
1920	235,156	4367	18.57
1921	175,649	3195	18.19
1922	159,279	2556	16.05
1923	147,276	1924	13.06

Source: Amarjit Kaur, "Indian Labour, Labour Standards, and Workers' Health in Burma and Malaya, 1900–1940," *Modern Asian Studies* 40, no. 2 (2006): 425–75.

the high death rates on the plantations, medical services were directed entirely towards ensuring the productivity and the reproduction of Indian labor; in the case of the Chinese in Malaya, the colonial state sought to work through Chinese intermediaries and to harness Chinese voluntary associations as a tool of government.[32] While it stimulated an expanded biopolitics (the technologies of managing whole populations), the problem of contagion among Tamil migrant workers on Malaya's plantations also stimulated a new form of what anthropologist Didier Fassin calls a "politics of life." A "politics of life," Fassin argues, in his work on the humanitarian imagination, is a politics that gives "specific value and meaning to human life," in part by producing representations of the human life to be saved or defended (for instance, in depicting the person as wholly a victim, and not an agent).[33]

That is to say, witnessing suffering allowed claims to be made on behalf of plantation workers. By the 1880s, the plantation Tamil population in Malaya emerged as a population to be governed: no longer simply a temporary, floating mass of labor, nor simply vectors of disease. By the 1880s, efforts were underway to 'improve' the population of plantation labor, through halting efforts at education, and limited but growing provision of health facilities. One of the early reports by the protector of Indian immigrants in the Straits made an argument for the government to support Tamil schools, "for most of the Tamil people here are too poor to keep schools unaided by the Government."[34] By the turn of the twentieth century, the question of the gender balance within the Tamil laboring population in Malaya emerged as a key point of debate. In common with officials in the West Indies, Fiji, and Mauritius, administrators overseeing migration to Malaya expressed increasing concern by the early twentieth century that the absence of women in the Straits had a morally deleterious effect on Tamil society.[35] "Married couples make more useful citizens," one official concluded by the end of the century's first decade, "than loose man and loose woman."[36]

These claims to care for the welfare of the plantation labor force came not only from the colonial state but, increasingly, from within the educated elite of Indian 'civil society' in Malaya. A Kuala Lumpur-based journalist, J. D. Samy, wrote in 1911 that "the coolie is literally unrepresented." He described in detail the "sufferings that the poor, illiterate and ignorant coolies daily undergo." He called for Indian nationalists to publicize the "dark side of things" by publishing photographs that would depict the suffering of Tamil plantation workers, "people working during the mid-day sun, men suffering from ankylostomiasis, malaria, beri-beri . . . coolies sentenced, hand-cuffed and publicly paraded."[37]

From the calculus of the planters, the life of Indian indentured labor in Malaya—life as productive power: muscle, bone, and sinew—had a price. They took into account what Marx called "abstract labour," the notion that "all labour is an expenditure of human labour-power, in the physiological sense," a "productive expenditure of human brains, muscles, nerves."[38] Planters, like slave owners before them, had a "direct material interest in the health and survival" of their labor force.[39]

But the interest of Indian social reformers, and even some Indian government officials, in the lives of their subjects overseas was of quite a different order. From the perspective of humanitarian concern with indentured labor migration, it was not only or primarily the laborers' "bare life" at stake—to use Agamben's terms—but also the "qualified," particular lives that they could lead outside India.[40] Discussion in India of the conditions of indentured labor focused on the 'shame' and degradation that indentured migrants experienced, often because of the small number of women who made the journey overseas. The 'loss of caste' and the 'loss of self-respect' was thought to be the most serious consequence of migration. Indian nationalists and British missionaries alike highlighted lurid stories of 'de-moralization,' often focusing on the consequences of the overwhelmingly male populations of Indians abroad; the only Indian women in the colonies, it appeared, were those of 'loose morals.' A powerfully gendered vision of dissolute and defeated Indians overseas—suffering bodies stripped of their dignity, bringing shame upon their motherland—dominated public discussions of the migration of Indian labor overseas.[41]

Conclusion: Contagions, Multiplied

Fears of contagion took their place in a contested field, amid a much broader range of legal and spatial practices governing the circulation of peoples, cultures, particular ways of life, religious performances, rituals, and sacrifices. From this point of view, the space of the plantation became at once a model for "traveling culture" and another form of containment.[42] Creating the plantations as sacred space allowed Tamil estate workers to live "qualified," particular lives in Malaya; it provided a way of transplanting and localizing particular religious practices derived from the South Indian village.

But the plantations and estate temples also served as a means of containment, keeping South Indian religious practices in their place, preventing them from spilling out and over, and 'infecting' other sections of the community. Observing as early as 1834 a performance of the rite of *thaipusam*, popular among Tamil migrants to Malaya, James Low wrote that "when people forsake their own country and voluntarily settle in another, they should be satisfied with the permission to celebrate their religious rites only which do not outrage the proper feelings of the other portions of the community, and which are not injurious to public morals, the decencies of life, and order."[43] The threat of these kinds of popular religiosity spilling over the boundaries created to contain them was also, then, discussed in the language of 'contagion.' Brenda Yeoh's work on the government of space in colonial Singapore argues that sanitary fears were at the root of colonial attempts to control public space; but so, too, were other kinds of fears of contagion.[44]

There were many kinds of 'traffic' that the colonial state and elite Asian reformers alike sought to control and to channel: the traffic between plantations and neighboring Malay villages; between the hinterlands and the port cities; and across the carefully policed boundaries of ethnicity and religion. The logic of 'contagion'—and its counterpart, quarantine—served as a model and a metaphor for thinking about these kinds of flows. By the 1920s, such a model also began to shape imperial thinking about the movement of political ideas, with fears of the 'contagion' of Communist influence within Malaya's Chinese community, or the 'contagion' of pan-Islamic ideas along the routes of pilgrimage between Mecca and Java.[45] But the model was also constantly undermined by flows that exceeded its bounds: epidemics; constant ungoverned migration, outside the purview of the colonial state; the 'traffic' and exchange of popular religious ideas, practices, and even emotional regimes, in the public sphere.

In the context of this volume's concern with contagion and the built environment—rural as well as urban—this chapter has tried to make a case for broadening our conception of the subject beyond some of the traditional concerns of the 'history of medicine' as a field, to encompass studies of migration, circulation, and their imperial regulation. We need to situate fears of contagion within a broader study of imperial mobility as a problem of government in its biological, political, and legal dimensions.

8
Carter and Contagion in India: Anatomy, Geography, Morphology

Ruth Richardson

Introduction: Leprosy and Empire

This chapter explores scientific research on leprosy, tuberculosis, relapsing fever, cholera, and malaria in India between the 1850s and the 1880s, a period when emerging scientific processes of disease investigation were being applied there. In the last decades of the century, novel instrumentation and methods of research associated with 'germ theory' prompted heated debates about whether leprosy could be explained in terms of inheritance or contagion, whether cholera was caused by a waterborne organism, whether malaria could be ascribed to a parasite, and whether famine fever even existed.

Focusing on the Indian Medical Service career of Henry Vandyke Carter, the chapter argues, first, that the production of new scientific knowledge in this period needs to be understood in a transnational setting: in the case of Carter and the diseases on which he worked, within the context of personal and professional networks linking India with Norway and Britain. Indeed, transcolonial and imperial interconnectedness is a key theme of *Imperial Contagions*, which explores how epidemic events and anxieties over 'contagion'—real or imagined—made visible the often invisible "webs of empire"[1] and the various forms of mobility that sustained it.

Although leprosy was a disease with a low level of infection, it underscored latent anxieties especially as the century progressed, in England and India alike, about the dangers of contagion posed by traffic between metropole and colonies. These anxieties about the vulnerabilities of imperial networks provided an often tense political context within which scientific investigation was conducted.[2]

Biomedical research in the nineteenth century was a collaborative process, involving many interlocutors and institutions across the globe. 'Colonial' science and medicine, as other contributors to this volume also suggest, therefore need to be understood as forms of knowledge and practice constituted across and between sites. The international and polycentric dimension of nineteenth-and early twentieth-century science posed significant challenges in relation, for example, to the development and implementation of preventive measures, as Carter acknowledged in his *Report on Leprosy and Leper-Asylums in Norway, with References to India* (1874), in which he sought to draw on and apply the experience of Norway in developing preventive measures against leprosy to the considerably more complicated terrain of the Bombay Presidency.

Second, the chapter traces a relationship between Carter's anatomical and microscopical illustrations, his interest in the morphology of disease, the profile of the fever chart, the mapping of disease prevalence geographically, and epidemiological mapping by the collection and analysis of statistical data. Understanding the interrelationships among these different visualizations of disease offers a way of reflecting on the links between clinic and laboratory in the developing field of public health (including statistics) in the generation before the British parasitologist Sir Patrick Manson defined the field of 'tropical medicine.'[3] Finally, the chapter suggests that, at a time when leprosy provoked widespread revulsion and the existence of famine fever was publicly denied by the medical establishment in India, Carter's approach exemplifies an emergent tradition of humanitarianism, highlighting the heterogeneity of colonial medicine and the complicated, and often conflicted, but little-studied relationship between colonialism and compassion.[4]

The International Dimension: Norway and British India

Professor Edmund Parkes was nearing the end of his life when, in 1873, he addressed a meeting of the British Medical Association (BMA). He looked back over the changes he had seen in his medical lifetime, including recent controversy surrounding what was then known as 'germ theory,' and Joseph Lister's work on antisepsis. Then Parkes looked *forward* with hope. Abreast of scientific change, unlike many of his contemporaries, Parkes had become convinced that contagious diseases had a material basis.[5]

As a way of explaining why discovery had been so slow, Parkes observed that "it was not known how far behind the delicacy of the problem were the instruments of the day."[6] Even the latest microscopes were not quite good enough. Parkes did not live long enough to appreciate just how many improvements would have to occur in microtechnique—not only in the capabilities of lenses, but also in microtomes, dyes, and specimen-fixing processes, as well as in methods of germ cultivation, testing, and interpretation— before 'germ theory' would become accepted as scientific truth. Parkes did, however, have a clear understanding of the difficulty of the process. "The recognition of these agents," he declared, "is evidently a task more difficult than to seize the light of the planets, or the dim luminosity of the nebulae."[7]

Parkes was speaking about the *detection* of germs, but his use of the word *recognition* (both grasping identity *and* acknowledging validity) suggests that he knew the idea would meet with resistance. Understanding the importance of tracking down the causal organisms of contagious diseases, Parkes predicted that, if government were to take the new science seriously, the eradication of diseases might in future be possible:

> . . . if allowed to guide the action of the State it is not too much to say that the diseases which caused so great a mortality in times past, and which even now kill so many persons, will become things gone by, and as little known in England as leprosy and plague.[8]

"At present," he concluded, "inquiry has carried us to the very threshold. How long will it be until someone opens the door and bids us enter?"[9]

The sense of being poised on the brink of an era of discovery is palpable in Parkes's words, which express the buzz of optimism in medical circles in the early 1870s, a period associated with such luminaries as Virchow, Pasteur, Lister, and Tyndall. Within three years of the BMA meeting at which Parkes spoke, Koch was to demonstrate his new technique for isolating and cultivating anthrax bacilli to Ferdinand Cohn in Breslau.[10]

There were also many less prominent figures working in the scientific landscape in 1873. Parkes may have been aware that Otto Obermeier, an assistant of Virchow, had noticed curious mobile filaments in the blood of patients suffering relapsing fever (famine fever or recurrent typhus) in Europe.[11] But Parkes is unlikely to have known that, at the very time he was speaking, two little-known doctors were meeting in Norway. Dr Henry Vandyke Carter, the subject of this chapter, was an Englishman who had crossed half the world from India to visit the other, Dr Armauer Hansen of Bergen.[12]

Hansen was the son-in-law of Dr D.C. Danielssen, co-author with Dr C. W. Boeck of *Traité de la Spédalskhed* (1848), the best-known book on leprosy at that time. In the first half of the nineteenth century, an awareness had grown within Norway that the country was in the grip of a leprosy epidemic, and with royal support, a medical plan had been drawn up whereby the state instituted a national program of leper segregation, in an effort to prevent the further spread of the disease. The first reliable census of lepers in Norway had been completed in 1856.[13]

Today, it is known that leprosy is caused by a mycobacterium, which causes an initial fever, but the typical outward signs of the disease—proliferation of the skin (especially of the face) and areas of numbing (especially in the limbs) appear only after a long incubation period, often of several years duration. Leprosy is a progressively mutilating mortal disease of the entire body, which distorts facial features, maims limbs, and causes pain, blindness, and suppurating stinking sores all over the body. The bacterial organisms are found throughout the body, not only in the skin but also in the viscera and nerves. There is an acute form, but leprosy usually takes years to kill those who suffer from it. Until the twentieth century, the disease was completely incurable. The causal organism of leprosy is highly resistant to artificial cultivation, and it is only recently that it has been discovered how to study the disease in the laboratory on animal models. It is now believed to be spread by exposure to infected mucosal products—by coughs and sneezes. Recent research on the genome of leprosy has shown that, worldwide, the disease derives from a single ancient clone that probably originated in East Africa.[14]

At the time Carter and Hansen met in 1873, the medical orthodoxy was that leprosy was a 'taint' transmitted by heredity. The existence of leper castes in India suggests that a similar belief operated there. Leprosy carried a social stigma, and those afflicted by it were often shunned by communities as if the disease were contagious.[15] No doubt similar anxieties operated among medical men, because almost no work had yet been done on its pathology and post-mortem appearances: when Carter arrived in India in 1858, he had found an open field of study.

The Norwegian effort constituted what would now be termed a nationwide public health campaign, designed to change public opinion in a significant way concerning leprosy. It promoted the idea that affected individuals ought not to have children, so as to prevent passage to future generations.[16] The Norwegian state asylum system provided housing and support for people afflicted with leprosy and unable to support themselves—many in the debilitating final stages of the disease and ostracized by society. Wealthier patients were encouraged to isolate themselves within their own homes.

Carter visited Norway because of his strong interest in this national effort to grapple with leprosy. He was a trained scientist, a microscopist, a London MD working in Bombay, a city with large numbers of beggars afflicted with leprosy on its streets. The general ward for the chronically ill, or 'incurables', in the native hospital in which Carter worked was always full of lepers, many of them in the end-stages of disease. There were never enough beds for those needing care: "This useful refuge for the helpless is now wholly occupied by the leprous," Carter wrote in the 1870s.[17] The city of Bombay, and the region of colonial India in which it stood (known at that time as the Bombay Presidency) had no other provision for them, nor for people suffering other incurable diseases, such as cancer.

What Carter found in Bergen, perhaps, was a kindred spirit. Hansen not only showed him round his institution, and explained the history and rationale behind the Norwegian leprosy initiative, but he eventually also showed Carter the bacillus he had discovered in the brown matter from the fresh tubercles of patients in the Bergen asylum. Hansen had himself doubted his own discovery for a long while, and he had not yet published his findings in any international forum. Not even Danielssen (Hansen's father-in-law) believed in these bacilli, nor did he believe the disease contagious.

Carter was receptive to the idea of a bacterium for at least two reasons: first, he had already discovered the power of an exterior organism—another mycobacterium—in the deep-tissue pathology of mycetoma; and second, because Carter had actually seen, drawn, pondered, and described the brown matter of leprosy in his dissections in Bombay. The lenses on his prized microscope had permitted Carter to discern the mycelia and spores of mycetoma, but not the detailed structure of the mycobacterium of leprosy. Hansen was probably pleased to meet another microscopist supportive of his findings, and it is clear from Carter's references to Hansen that he had great admiration for the Norwegian. The two men remained in touch for many years.[18]

Reporting on Leprosy in India

Carter had trained in medicine at St George's Hospital Medical School, London, and subsequently at one of the foremost scientific institutions in Britain at the time, the Museum of the Royal College of Surgeons. He had won a two-year studentship there, serving under Richard Owen (later the first director of the British Museum of Natural History, at South Kensington) and under the celebrated microscopist John Quekett. Key messages Carter had taken away with him from Owen's lectures were that one has to be *trained* simply to observe, and that "two persons are generally concerned in every fact—one discovers part: the other completes & corrects."[19]

Carter was an introspective man, a religious non-conformist from a provincial background. His father and brother were marine artists. Although young Carter shone academically (winning several scholarships and prizes), he did not fit in well with the prevailing ethos at St George's, and he disliked the bonhomie and social climbing that seemed the norm. He could not pay for entry into the hierarchy and refused to pull strings, preferring to make his own way by merit and hard work. Disaffection with the corrupted promotion process in the London hospital scene was probably why Carter was among the first cohort of medical men to join the Indian Medical Service by examination rather than by influence, as had hitherto been the case. It took a generation for this change to be accepted within the service in India itself: many older doctors recruited under the earlier system were dubious about the new men, and Carter found himself as isolated in India as he would have been in London.[20]

Carter had arrived in Bombay fresh from a two-year stint as a tutor at St George's (1856–57) working alongside Henry Gray, during which time Carter had created all the illustrations for the first edition of *Gray's Anatomy*.[21] It would be true to say that he was a very well-trained observer, and that his close work on normal human anatomy had given him a profound understanding of anatomical perfection. His first impression of the local talent in Bombay was admiring. After attending a prize-giving at the Grant Medical College where he was to work, he commented in his diary, "sharp fellows, these Parsees and Hindus,"[22] demonstrating himself to have been a man ready to respect and appreciate the native peoples of India, untypical of prevailing colonial attitudes at that time, where disease prevalence was linked to the hereditary traits, predispositions, and habits of the local population.[23]

Working initially as professor of anatomy at the medical school, Carter witnessed a wealth of local pathology both among living patients and dead. He was sent many fresh specimens to dissect for the medical school museum from the operating theater next door at the native Jamsetjee Jeejeebhoy Hospital. Among the first cases to catch his interest was a hideously distorted lower limb, amputated from a patient suffering from what was then known as "Madura Foot." Examining the pathology with the new microscope he had purchased from his earnings illustrating *Gray's Anatomy*, Carter became the first person to discern that the destruction of the tissues and bones of the leg had been wrought by an actively spreading fungus. This was the first discovery worldwide of a deep mycosis of human tissue. Carter attempted to cultivate the fungus responsible and named the disease *Mycetoma* (a tumor caused by a fungus), the name it still bears today. In the first few years of his work in Bombay, Carter also became interested in elephantiasis, another disease causing swelling of the foot and lower leg and also often of the scrotum. His interest in leprosy probably developed in parallel with these studies, as their effects are in some respects similar, and neither symptoms nor causation had been worked out. His careful pathological enquiries served to help differentiate these diseases. He began publishing on leprosy in 1862.[24]

In addition to his clinical and teaching load, Carter became devoted to scientific research on the pathology of India. He worked on a wide range of diseases during his 30-year working life in Bombay, and was actively researching and publishing throughout that time. Leprosy was Carter's most consistent area of interest, starting soon after his arrival in India and continuing almost to the year of his retirement. Before his journey to Norway in 1873, Carter had produced four publications on the disease, and he had already made an important finding: the distinctive brown lesions and swelling of the nerve fibers associated with the anesthesia (numbing) of leprosy.

Carter had also produced a major study of a different kind: geographical and epidemiological. His 1871–72 prevalence report contains a careful analysis of the distribution of leprosy in the Bombay Presidency, including an attempt to map the leper castes of that part of India. Carter appears to have been hopeful that mapping the disease geographically might allow a better understanding of its scale and distribution and perhaps its spread, but his report suggests that after a vast amount of labor on not very reliable statistics, he was not much the wiser, although he had a stronger awareness of the great extent of the problem in India and the pressing need for trustworthy data on which to do decent epidemiological work. It is evident from his work on leper castes that, like most of his contemporaries, at this stage Carter still considered leprosy to be a hereditary condition.

The year following his visit to Bergen, 1874, Carter published three major pieces of work. His illustrated text, *Mycetoma, or the Fungus Disease of India*, was published in London by Churchill. It was an impressive volume, giving detailed descriptions and drawings of the malady, demonstrating in detail its fungal derivation. Apart from a single publication much later (in which Carter discussed actinomycetes and mycetoma), this book was his last word on the subject of his original discovery. It remains the most exhaustive work on the malady yet published.[25]

The other two books Carter published that year also demanded considerable effort to see through the press: first, his official report concerning the journey to Bergen, *Report on Leprosy and Leper-Asylums in Norway, with References to India*, published in London under the auspices of the India Office; and second, *On Leprosy and Elephantiasis*, an extensively illustrated work published in London by Her Majesty's Stationery Office, with maps and large colored plates. This latter book was the up-to-date English equivalent of Danielssen and Boeck's great Norwegian text of 1848. It featured some fine images from Carter's hand, and provided a vivid and comprehensive portrait of the disease. Not surprisingly, it became the major text on leprosy in the Anglophone world for the rest of the nineteenth century.

Carter's official *Report* concerning his visit to Norway (1874) made clear his admiration for the Norwegian leprosy initiative, and argued for a similar effort in Bombay. In Norway, he had found those afflicted with leprosy clean, well fed, well housed, and well cared for in the state-run asylums: a vastly different situation from that with which he was familiar in India, where especially those with end-stage disease were shunned and left to starve:

> No greater contrast occurs to my recollection than that between the spacious buildings which I have lately seen in Norway, with their liberal management, and the little mud hut [he had witnessed at Satara, southeast of Bombay city] . . . the abode of a middle-aged leper-man, a cripple and a beggar . . . or the bare shelter of sticks and leaves put up in a hedge-way amongst fields away from the village, where a poor creature lingered for four months before her death.[26]

The parallels and contrasts between the territories of Norway and the Bombay Presidency were the theme of the *Report*. Stylistically, Carter's manner of mapping the distribution of leprosy in both places emphasizes their kinship: his leprosy maps of both territories are closely similar in size and appearance, each features a delicate black outline for coastal detailing and reddish-brown infill highlighting the extent and intensity of the distribution of the disease. The choice of the additional color lends these two maps an appearance of geographical inflammation, and may perhaps have suggested itself by analogy with the brown matter of leprosy Carter had been investigating at a micro level.

But despite their visual affinities, these two key maps reveal an important distinction in their small print. While the Norwegian map charted the extent of leprosy in that kingdom—that is, the surrounding areas shown in white had no known cases—the other demonstrated affected areas only within the Bombay Presidency, beyond the boundaries of which the disease nevertheless prevailed, and to an unknown and perhaps as pervasive extent: it was a map of imperial ignorance. The deeper affinity here was that both maps were addressing genuinely *national* matters: leprosy was not simply a problem in local Bombay, but concerned the entirety of India. Indeed, Carter subsequently visited Southern Europe and the Middle East and published comparative studies of the disease's diffusion in Greece, Syria, Palestine, and Northern Italy (1876).[27] In his 1874 *Report*, Carter was intent to show that the disease was the same disease in both countries (Norway and India), and that the history of the malady in each locale was centuries long, the great contrast being, as he put it, "in Norway practical measures are in full force, while in India, all has yet to be done."[28]

Leprosy was an incurable disease, implacably devastating the lives of people affected by it. But at a population level, the Norwegian initiative gave grounds for real optimism. "Soon after the establishment of asylums," Carter was able to assert, "the number of new cases began to fall." The impact of the asylum policy in Norway was such that, by 1874, the death rate of those afflicted with the disease far exceeded the rate of new diagnoses. "On this calculation," Carter observed, "one might learn to hopefully anticipate the extinction of the malady."[29] Carter presented the case for asylums, based on the medical and social needs of sufferers and of future generations, urging generous care for those afflicted with the disease and arguing that merciful provision would be regarded by sufferers as a blessing. Coercion, he asserted, was needless.

Throughout this *Report*, Carter spoke to the prevailing colonial-medical belief that the disease was hereditary. But he included a significant footnote, in which he described and endorsed Hansen's new discovery:

> Dr GA Hansen of Bergen is engaged in a series of inquiries which cannot but throw much light upon the origin and nature of leprosy. These point to the parasitic origin of the disease . . . By Dr Hansen's kindness I have myself seen the minute organisms (a species of *bacterium*) which are present in living leprous matter taken from the interior of a [leprous] 'tubercle'.[30]

Carter's statement of recognition regarding Hansen's discovery offers more than a contrast with the bad faith of the German researcher Albert Neisser, who later claimed Hansen's finding as his own.[31]

In his larger published volume, *Leprosy and Elephantiasis* (1874), Carter was more informative about what he had witnessed in Norway. In this volume, he reported the significant information that upon his return to Bombay he had been able to confirm Hansen's discovery, having found the bacteria in fresh samples taken from the tubercles of Indian patients. Hansen's description of his discovery of the bacillus was presented in the English translation as the book's *Appendix I*—its first appearance in any language other than Norwegian. The translation was certified by Carter as correct and true to Hansen's original.[32]

This important volume contained a detailed analysis of the character and appearances of leprosy, and carefully differentiated it from other complaints with which it had hitherto often been confused. Carter's efforts here were intended to assist more rigorous diagnosis and so help relieve many sufferers of less serious conditions—such as elephantiasis, eczema, and psoriasis—from the stigma of leprosy. The dates on some of the large-scale images in the book reveal that Carter had been collecting material for the book since 1862, so this great volume was the fruit of at least 12 years' research. The images range from demonstrations of the nerve atrophy of anesthetic leprosy shown in full-scale dissection to portraits of the dermatological appearances of leprous lesions as observed on brown and white skins (from patients seen in Bombay and in Norway), the extensive bone damage caused by leprosy, and the microstructure of the disease.

The book also included the tabulated results of clinical trials on which Carter had worked extensively in Bombay, concerning likely remedies and treatments for leprosy. The trials included a number of indigenous Indian medicines, and showed that while several of the substances tried were of little value, one in particular—a native medicine, chaulmoogra oil—did offer significant help in some, but not all, cases. The disease remained incurable, but there was some hope that the worst effects of the skin lesions could be mitigated or slowed by active topical and oral treatment with this oil. Although Carter knew that the disease was an incurable systemic affliction, his efforts to help sufferers were serious and committed, and he was open-minded towards the value of native remedies.

Famine Fever

There was a hiatus in Carter's leprosy research between 1876 and 1883. His life and work were disrupted in this period by the impact of the Great Indian

Famine of 1876–78. Monsoon failure brought catastrophic crop failure, and large numbers of rural poor converged on Bombay seeking work. The poorer areas of the city rapidly became more than usually overcrowded, and a highly fatal epidemic fever broke out.[33] On investigation, Carter discovered the fever exhibited the characteristic symptoms and double-peak temperature chart of relapsing—or famine—fever, which is now thought to be the same disease prevalent during the Irish potato famine. Carter demonstrated that the spirillar blood organism discovered by Obermeier in a similar epidemic in northern Europe in 1873 was also present among victims of famine fever in Bombay.

But almost as soon as the discovery of the spirillum was made in 1877, Carter's superior officer published a flat denial that famine fever even *existed* in Bombay: statements concerning the destitution among 150,000 migrants, he announced, were "highly exaggerated" and Carter was "*in error*" concerning the diagnosis of relapsing fever.[34] A visiting "expert" from the Sanitary Commission in Calcutta (well known for his hostility to the idea of disease germs), Timothy R. Lewis, was thanked for providing the microscopical confirmation that the spirillum was a "mere epiphenomenon." The ignorance of these men's pronouncements are matched only by that of Bombay's imperial governor, Sir Richard Temple, who is reputed to have joked that what Carter had seen in the microscope were his own eyelashes.[35]

Carter appears to have suffered the public humiliation of their words in silence. He did not directly confront his local superiors at the time. Instead, he resolutely continued with his own researches, and published his findings in London. His clinical and research workload during the epidemic was demanding, and he became seriously ill himself after suffering a needlestick injury during a post-mortem. But while recovering on sick leave in London the following May, he delivered a highly important paper at a meeting of the Royal Medical and Chirurgical Society, proving that what had been found was a fever never previously recorded in India, with a profile identical to European epidemics of relapsing fever. This fever had a very high death rate, almost 18 percent. The spirochete discovered in 1873 by Obermeier was visible in the bloodstream of sufferers at fever-height, and the fever was not checked by quinine (in other words, it was not malarial). Of 900 fever patients whose fever profile and blood he had examined, Carter estimated that approximately 50 percent were cases of relapsing fever, the rest being mostly ague (or malaria). Carter publicly thanked three doctors by name, all of them Indian, who had been working alongside him through the epidemic at the J. J. Hospital, Bombay. The identity of the organism Carter had isolated in Bombay had been confirmed as Obermeier's spirillum by no less a figure than Ferdinand Cohn. This path-breaking communication was reported in the *British Medical Journal* in June 1878.[36]

The sheer quality and weight of Carter's evidence proved that what had been seen was exactly as he had stated, whether or not his superiors admitted the existence either of the organism or indeed of the famine. Returning to Bombay, Carter continued researching the fever, cases of which were still emerging sporadically, and reported in 1879 that he had cultured the organism and moreover that he had successfully transmitted the disease from human to macaque monkey, and from monkey to monkey.[37] In subsequent epidemiological work on relapsing fever, Carter demonstrated the direct correlation between the recent famine, migration, and excess fever mortality.[38] Over five million people had died in the famine.

The book that emerged from all Carter's work on famine fever, *Spirillum Fever* (1882), was publicly celebrated by the award of the British Medical Association's Stewart Prize in Pathology in 1882.[39] The imperial attitude towards the famine fever controversy is demonstrated by the fact that Carter's superior officer was later conferred with the dignity of Knight Commander of the Order of St Michael and George, and made Honorary Surgeon to Queen Victoria.[40]

Tuberculosis, Cholera, Malaria

In the half-dozen years after this final book and before his retirement from the Indian Medical Service, Carter accomplished several extraordinary things. First, in 1883, using new dyeing techniques and better lenses, Carter confirmed Koch's discovery of the bacillus of tuberculosis, and exhibited it to a medical audience in Bombay, alongside Hansen's bacillus of leprosy.[41]

Then, in 1884, Carter confirmed Koch's cholera bacillus from samples obtained from the evacuations of patients suffering from the disease in Bombay. Three microscopes were set up at a meeting of the Bombay Medical Society to show the elusive "comma-bacillus," and congratulations were made both to Koch for the discovery and to Carter for its confirmation in Bombay. Interestingly, Carter is reported as having said that he considered the organism to be "more of the nature of a vibrio than a bacillus." He was correct in this analysis: this is indeed the form the organism is now understood to take.[42]

In 1887, Carter confirmed Alphonse Laveran's discovery of the complex blood organisms in malaria, proving that what had historically been known as 'ague' in India was the same disease as 'malaria' in Algeria. This was a considerable achievement in that Carter was the only first-wave investigator to find the organism without first being shown how to do so by an initiate direct from Laveran himself. Carter had found it on his own, after having seen a description by William Osler in the *British Medical Journal* in 1887.[43] Carter's micrograph drawings of the complex behavior of the malarial parasite reveal the painstaking nature of his observations in exquisite detail.[44]

In those final few years of his working life in India, Carter also published two memoranda concerning the latest figures sent to him by Hansen, showing that since the establishment of asylums in Norway there had been a continued slow but marked decline in the number of new cases of leprosy: "the diminution of new cases . . . goes, pari passu, with the lessening number of home-dwelling sick."[45]

Carter retired in 1888. After 30 years in India, he returned to England and settled in his home town of Scarborough, where he married and started a family. In 1897, he died of tuberculosis at the age of 66.

Conclusion: Empire and Humanitarianism

Despite Hansen's discovery of the causative organism of leprosy, skepticism concerning the germ theory of its causation (and the implications of what such a route of causation might mean) remained strong, especially among the upper reaches of the Indian Medical Service. However, in 1889, the year after Carter retired, the contagion/heredity debate was transformed when a Roman Catholic priest, Father Damien, died of leprosy on Molokai Island, near Hawaii. The leper colony there had been created in response to an epidemic of leprosy on Hawaii itself.

Despite increasing evidence, medical skeptics remained unconvinced about the bacterial spread of the disease. But it was becoming obvious to all unbiased observers that Damien had acquired it not by inheritance, but from his flock.[46] A remarkable, impassioned and eloquent eulogy of Damien written by Robert Louis Stevenson, who had visited the island, increased publicity worldwide.[47] In England and India, public opinion was fundamentally altered, and the doubters of contagion were soon hushed. Pity, revulsion, and fear mobilized funds unavailable before, missionaries organized for India, and Archdeacon

Wright published his angst-ridden book, *Leprosy, an Imperial Danger*.[48] In 1890, the Leprosy Investigation Commission was dispatched to India by the National Leprosy Fund, which had evolved from the Father Damien Memorial Fund.[49] Carter died in 1897, the year of the first International Leprosy Congress.[50]

Preliminary research on Carter's career in India suggests that he had no support for his work from within the Indian medical hierarchy. Whether this was from personal jealousy of his attainments, social distaste concerning his religious and social non-conformity, contempt for his attitudes towards the indigenous population, skepticism about his scientific discoveries, or professional resentment of his international medical links remains unclear. If mutual suspicion characterized the relationship between the Sanitation Department and the Medical Service in India,[51] an article on Carter's work on leprosy that appeared in the London *Times* in 1876 emphasized the government's lack of support for Carter's drive to contain the disease, ostensibly on the grounds of resources.[52]

However, although Carter found no kindred spirits within the medical hierarchy in India, he was largely left alone to pursue his research. Doubtless, in part at least, because he was working in a native hospital with a high clinical and teaching workload. Indeed, Carter seems to have managed to evade the narrow domination of those immediately above him in three ways: first, by publishing outside India (Carter's important works on mycetoma, leprosy, and relapsing fever all appeared in London); second, by using his own periods of leave to undertake researches abroad; third, by his international correspondence and good relations with Hansen, Laveran, Cohn, and Osler.

There is a tendency in histories of colonial medicine and science to focus upon either recognized scientific 'pioneers,' or upon institutional and technological developments and the sociopolitical contexts that shaped scientific practices. In contrast, this chapter has sought to redress the balance by exploring the role played in evolving knowledge about disease by a lone medical scientist whose work challenged existing orthodoxies. Carter's career underscores the complex interaction between society, politics, and elites. This chapter argues for the need to refocus on lesser-known professionals, like Carter, who, while contesting prevailing beliefs in the 'periphery,' remained active in the wider, transcolonial, and global exchange of knowledge that helped construct modern science.

Carter was not a typical instrument of the imperium in India. A social outsider in Britain, he did not become an East India Company insider or a colonial patronage-wallah when he joined the Indian Medical Service, and never became one afterwards. Being appointed by merit on examination, but answerable to a pre-existing colonial medical hierarchy appointed by patronage, he was already at a disadvantage when he arrived. The Indian Medical Service seems to have become a rigidified structure, and until the chronological retirement of those already appointed under the old system, the domination of the older 'patronage' generation remained in place, dominating Carter's cohort throughout their careers in India. Carter's willingness to undertake a demanding placement in a hospital for the poor in Bombay was probably regarded as eccentric by other medical men, whose focus was usually upon the health of the colonial/imperial army and administration, and their families. Carter was indeed unusual in his settled preference for studying the diseases of the local poor, and in having little interest in developing a large private practice among the colonial/imperial elite, which he easily could have done in Bombay.

In one sense, Carter was an old-fashioned figure, having attitudes towards the indigenous culture and peoples of India that share something of the respectful humility of an earlier eighteenth-century generation of colonialists. But he was not at all of that social type. In this and other ways, Carter was significantly ahead of his time in his scientific attainments and in the scope of his researches, which—being essentially humanitarian—escaped the narrow bounds of contemporary imperial medicine in India, and made it supra-national both in scope and impact.

9
Epidemics of Famine and Obesity: China as the Modern World

Sander L. Gilman

Introduction: Epidemics and 'Imperial' Science Today

Scientists at the annual meeting of the American Association for the Advancement of Science in February 2002 warned the American government that obesity had become a "global epidemic"—no longer confined to Western, industrialized societies.[1] This reflected a growing consensus in the 1990s that obesity (not smoking) was going to be the major public health issue of the new millennium.[2] By 2005, the 'war against obesity' had replaced the 'war against tobacco,' even though worldwide tobacco sales continued to increase. While a mass phenomenon of the end of the last century, the phrase "war against obesity, sloth, and addiction" appeared in the United Kingdom in *The Times* as early as 1981.[3] By the twenty-first century it was this 'war against obesity' that had come to be seen as an 'epidemic' by public health authorities in the West.

The People's Republic of China (PRC) today has also come to see obesity as its primary health concern. But does 'epidemic of obesity' have the same nuances in China as it does in the West? The 'obesity epidemic' seems to be the next great fear of Chinese public health officers, eclipsed only by smoking. According to recent surveys, "an obesity epidemic is imminent, with more than 20% of children aged 7–17 years in big cities now overweight or obese."[4] While the official Chinese journal of preventive medicine (*Zhonghua Yufang Yixue Zazhi*), acknowledged that the prevalence and increment of this problem varied in rural versus urban areas, it estimated that "70 million overweight and 30 million obese Chinese people emerged in China from 1992 to 2002" and that the number affected had increased rapidly in the past decade to 260 million Chinese people, and would continue to increase unless effective intervention was undertaken.[5]

179

The shift seems to be marked. According to the Chinese public health literature, a Body Mass Index of greater than 25 is to be found in 18.7 percent of the
population in urban areas as opposed to 13.7 percent in rural areas. (We should
note that a BMI of 30 is conventionally held to be a marker of obesity.) But the
increase over the past decades is also striking. These figures are for 1997. They
mark a fourfold increase over 1982, when only 3.7 percent of Chinese adults
had a BMI of over 25.[6] Chinese medical and epidemiological studies argue that
"obesity has become a global epidemic" though there seems to be little knowledge of the state of affairs in the People's Republic of China. Looking at "a group
of 2,776 randomly selected adults (20–94 years of age) living in the Huayang
Community in Shanghai, China," a 2002 study argued that, while "the prevalence of obesity" [using Western standards] was lower in China than in the
West, the "overall fat mass-related metabolic disorders were also common."[7]

Obesity is the problem of the twenty-first century, but is it truly a 'Chinese'
problem? Or is obesity, which is clearly seen as a problem in China, a Western
problem read through a Chinese lens? Is this apparent epidemic in China
merely the importation of a Western model of health and illness or a reconfiguration in Chinese terms? This chapter examines the epidemic of obesity
in China in relation to the historical background provided by nineteenth-and
twentieth-century engagements between China and the West. Though never
entirely colonized by Western powers and Japan, much of mainland China was,
in the early twentieth century, part of Europe's 'informal empire,' and relations
with these intruding nation-states were marked by the stark power imbalance
that was a characteristic of formal colonial rule elsewhere. Allopathic medicine
was one of the major tools from the beginning of the nineteenth century of the
establishment of a Western cultural hegemony in China. This chapter addresses
the question of how the circulation of Western medical and health discourses
helped shape Chinese self-awareness during the period leading to the present
acceptance of discourses of public health in the PRC. It builds upon recent
studies foregrounding the importance of Western medicine to the formation
of Chinese ideas about the body, the self, and the nation-state.[8] It considers
how constructions of obesity that drew upon medical discourses circulating in
modern China were informed by cultural anxieties surrounding the import of
Western commodities associated with the public's health, such as tinned milk,
into China.

The 'Fat' Body in China

On the surface, the fear of an epidemic of obesity seems to be a contemporary Western importation. Concern in China's immediate past, as well as in the nineteenth century, had centered not upon an epidemic of obesity but rather on recurring epidemics of famine. James L. Watson notes that the dominant sense of fear concerning the body in modern China is the result of the experience of the great famine under Mao Zedong.[9] This famine, which lasted from 1958 to 1961 and resulted from the collectivization of peasants, killed millions in China and evoked the horrors of the earlier famines of the 1940s during the war against the Japanese, the civil war, as well as the policies of the nationalist government. For adults in today's China, 'famine' recalls their own experiences under Mao and the tales of starvation during the war handed down by their parents and grandparents. Mao's great famine, too, had its echoes of the famine culture attributed to and experienced in China in the nineteenth century. In such circumstances, how did obesity come to be understood?

In early twentieth-century China, there was a medical obsession with the epidemic of famine as the 'famine' that had marked Western views of the pathological body in nineteenth-century China. When the standard 'Western' medical journal published in China, the *China Medical Journal*, is read systematically from the beginning of the twentieth century to the Japanese invasion of China, the central medical discourse concerning 'diet' and the body is that of famine and starvation. In such texts, China is truly the 'sick man of Asia,' as Larissa N. Heinrich discusses in her book, *The Afterlife of Images: Translating the Pathological Body between China and the West*.[10] Heinrich's book is actually an answer, in part, to Shigehisa Kuriyama's central thesis in his *The Expressiveness of the Body and the Divergence of Greek and Chinese Medicine* (1999), which argues for an inherent antithesis between 'Western' (Greek) and 'Eastern' (Chinese) images of the body and therefore its very nature. Heinrich illustrates how the rhetorical commonplace of 'China as the sick man of Asia' is historically structured through the tension between Chinese high culture (including medicine) and Western claims on the inherent inferiority of that culture and Western superiority in all media of expression and representation. It is the re-reading of a 'sick' China through Western medicine and its illustrations that preoccupies Heinrich and, as such, she provides an important corrective to Kuriyama's view.

For Kuriyama, the 'model' body type in classical Chinese medical literature and culture is described as rotund, as opposed to the muscular, svelte bodies of Greek art and medicine. Heinrich shows how Western models of the 'sick' Chinese body came to be accepted within China as an adequate representation of the very nature of what it meant to be Chinese, despite evidence to the contrary (according to Heinrich). The difference between Kuriyama and Heinrich, of course, lies in the historical periods examined by both—Kuriyama examines the ancient roots of both the West and the East, in contexts where contact between the two was extremely limited; Heinrich's book examines the post-Enlightenment world at the height of massive colonial expansion into Asia. The 'sick man of Asia' is the result of experiences of famine and malnourishment in a world reshaped by colonial expansion.

Thus, famine in China takes on two quite different meanings as an epidemic: in the classical world of Chinese medicine, it is caused by an imbalance in nature and in the body; in the modern world, it is—if the food tickets circulated by the Chinese Communist Party in Shanghai in 1927, stating that the British were responsible for the famine, are correct—the result of colonial oppression and its impact on the world of food. In nineteenth-and early twentieth-century China, epidemic and famine were widely seen as interlinked, no matter how they were defined.[11]

The Western medicine of the new age of bacteriology also sees widespread famine and infectious epidemics as linked. According to William Hamilton Jefferys and James L. Maxwell, "in the summer of 1906 there was a frightfully fatal and widespread epidemic of subtertian malaria all over Hupeh and Hunan, owing, it is believed, to a famine in Honan the previous winter which drove southward a hundred thousand or more starving Honanese, whose depressed vitality it is supposed afforded the fertile soil necessary to light up the epidemic. At least this is the theory held by those who report from these provinces."[12] Here, we see not famine as an epidemic but famine as tied to models of epidemic.

Famine and Cure

In nineteenth-and early twentieth-century China, the physicians of the Chinese Medical Missionary Association were concerned with the outcome of such epidemics. They needed to develop models for the treatment of the sequelae of famine and they turned, not surprisingly, to those advocated by allopathic

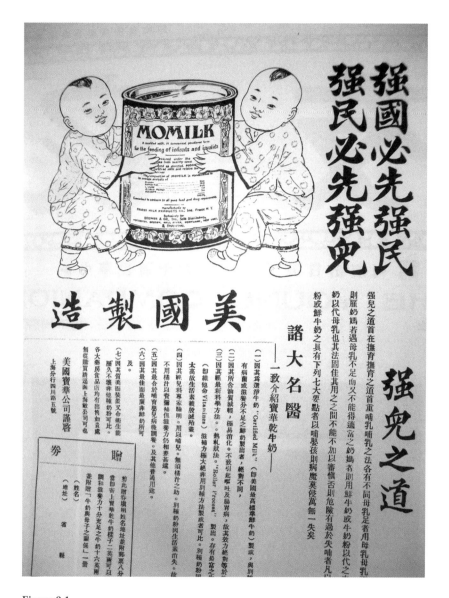

Figure 9.1

Happy Chinese babies on condensed milk. An advertisement from Shanghai in the 1920s.

medicine. They were concerned with ensuring that the food made available in their hospitals had sufficient protein and fat, to the extent that they advocated "crossing foreign and native cows," or introducing canned milk to improve the local diet.[13] Modern treatment advocated for an ancient and endemic problem. Canned, condensed milk, Frank Dikötter notes, was 'modern' in China in the nineteenth century and became a sign of the adaptation of China to the modern world.[14] But it was also a sign of an early attempt to remedy a Chinese 'problem' with a Western solution. Condensed milk presented what was considered by some to be the 'perfect' food in the light of the claims of nineteenth-century science, that cows' milk had a therapeutic influence upon a range of illnesses.[15] In this way, the American neurologist S. Weir Mitchell noted in his 1877 *Fat and Blood*: "Milk is the best and most easily managed addition to a general diet."[16] Certainly in 1877, raw milk, unpasteurized and a source of infectious diseases, was anything but a real 'health food.' (While Louis Pasteur and Claude Bernard developed 'pasteurization' for wine in 1864, its broad use for milk was introduced much later. Indeed, Robert Koch saw pasteurization as unnecessary, as he believed well into the twentieth century that bovine tuberculosis could not be transmitted by milk to human beings.)

Condensed milk is, however, a very poor substitute for mother's milk, given the extremely high percentage of sugar to be found in it. "Preserved condensed milk is simply a combination of sugar and condensed milk, in which the value of the sugar is greater than the value of the condensed milk," noted the son of its inventor Gail Borden, John G. Borden, in 1885.[17] Condensed milk, like boiled water, was not only concentrated but was inadvertently pasteurized (as the process for condensing milk was developed in 1856 well before Pasteur) and was therefore perceived as a healthy alternative food. Yet cows' milk was not the 'perfect food' for the treatment of famine-related diseases in China. Given the "frequency of decreased lactase activity ranges [of] 95% for Han Chinese,"[18] one would imagine that canned milk might actually have had deleterious effects for the infants so fed.

But why was a substitute for mother's milk sought in this world of epidemic famine? Were physicians dealing with the epidemic of famine concerned only with the failure of infants to thrive? According to William Hamilton Jefferys and James L. Maxwell in 1911:

> The Chinese child is devotedly cared for, but after that period of absolute dependence its parental attentions undergo marked deterioration and it does a lot of shifting for itself. One gets the impression that most Chinese

> babies are born with excellent health and are particularly round and fat and chubby; and though congenital deformities are not uncommonly met with, congenital disease is comparatively rarely so.[19]

For:

> . . . the Chinese mother knows nothing of modified milk mixtures and artificial feeding rarely, if ever, crosses the horizon of her thought. In the case of the well-to-do if the mother's milk is insufficient, she readily acquires the cooperation of a wet nurse. In the case of the poor, there is the aunt or the sister-in-law living in the same house with a baby or two of her own, ready to supply the deficiency. We have not infrequently seen the grandmother turned to in such straits—possibly the great grandmother occasionally takes a turn![20]

And thus condensed milk emerged as the answer. Plump babies were understood as healthy babies. Yet concerns remained that the seeming health of the Chinese infant might merely be a sham, quickly giving way to further diseases.

Debates about famine reflect often on the 'peculiarities' of the Chinese. Sometimes the differences were seen in terms of geography and class. Thus, the Chinese diet came to be regionally differentiated and appeared to compensate for levels of wealth. One physician noted that the "rich have rice, vegetables, and meats. The poor have rice, vegetables, and substitutes for meat." It was only "when floods overtake the people year in and year out that so many are driven to our doors for charity."[21] China was from this perspective not a 'famine' culture at all. Rather, from the standpoint of the physicians, it was the distribution of food by the Chinese, especially in times of turmoil or disaster, that seemed to lie at the heart of episodes of famine. In this view, the failure of the local Chinese distribution network caused famine.[22] But the suspicion remained that indigenous foods might not be 'suitable' enough to maintain a healthy diet.[23] The soybean was advocated over and over again as a substitute for other forms of protein, as if by virtue of repetition Western physicians might be convinced that this was true.[24]

Yet when the concern was true starvation, the sense that 'Western' cures, such as a rich, milk-based diet, were most appropriate re-appeared among members of the medical community.[25] It was the child who was seen as most at risk from the effects of famine, both in terms of the deleterious effects of hunger and the pernicious actions of its intransigent parents. The selling of children was closely connected with, and seen as a major consequence of, the famine culture in China.[26] "Cannot the famine relief associations . . . take this matter into consideration and put an end to it?" wrote one irate physician in

1920.[27] Among the myriad concerns expressed about the pathological effects of diet, not a single word was spent on the dangers or effects of our modern concern about the epidemic of obesity.[28]

Western Views of Obesity in the Land of Famine

Yet, from the mid-nineteenth century, China, the 'sick man of Asia,' was imagined by Westerners as a land of obesity and the Chinese as an obese people. In 1849, Jean-Pierre Beaude stated that the Chinese hold "a man . . . in dignity regards embonpoint and even obesity as one of the requirements of his rank." This was because obesity was believed to be the result of a wealthy and pampered status, bringing with it access to an excess and variety of foodstuffs.[29] The Chinese, it was claimed, held a belief that the prosperous and powerful man must be "one who really fills up a chair."[30] From the mid-nineteenth century, however, obesity began to be re-read as a symptom of decadence and degeneracy. Frederic W. Farrar stated that obesity was a mark of Chinese developmental inferiority: "The unmarked features, the serene, blandly-smiling face, the tendency to physical obesity and mental apathy, the feeble, tranquil, childish, gluttonous sensuality, mark the race."[31] Unlike the healthy and hardy European, Arthur de Gobineau claimed, the Chinese were fat and indolent, the people most often likely to be obese.[32]

Chinese obesity thus emerged as a marker of the quality of race as well as a social practice. According to one Western source:

> In China there is every variety of climate, food and social condition . . .
> The whole race displays a remarkable tendency to obesity. The nutritious juices of the body are directed towards the surface, distending and overloading the cellular tissues with inordinate quantity of fat. This general tendency of the whole people can only be attributed to the hereditary diathesis, unchecked by intermarriage with others differently constituted. It is an evil which exclusiveness of that singular people has entailed upon them.[33]

According to J. Richardson Parke, the Chinese were fascinated with obesity as part of their ideals of sexuality:

> In almost all Oriental countries the 'stout lady' is in demand. In fact there are portions of our own where the supply sometimes runs short; but in Turkey and China, where the highest social and matrimonial ambitions are not realized so much through the spirituelle type of feminine loveliness as by the number of fingers of fat over the ribs, the ladies are shut up and stall-fed, like Strasbourg geese, before their prudent parents think of

putting them upon the market. Indeed the pashas and mandarins, who are the chief patrons of this nourishing domestic industry, buying their wives in carload lots, and always on trial, are not as a rule highly spirituelle themselves, running to stomach rather than soul, and paying far greater heed to quantity than to quality.[34]

If marriage traditions were not to blame, then corrupt governance was. For Jefferys and Maxwell:

Apoplexy among the aged officials in Peking, properly disposed to it by their obesity and their having to perform the nine obeisances before the emperor so frequently, is not very uncommon.[35]

While they were obese—unlike the Jews ('a diabetic people'), who have also been represented as suffering from diseases of excess because of their race and marriage practices—the Chinese were less often seen to suffer from diseases attendant to obesity, such as diabetes. Hence, for Thomas B. Futcher:

All authorities agree that the Hebrew race is particularly susceptible. Frerichs states that of his 400 cases 102 were Jews. Wallach clearly demonstrated its greater frequency among the Hebrews of Frankfurt. From 1872 to 1890 there were 171 deaths from diabetes in that city. The proportion 674 of deaths from diabetes to the deaths from all causes was six times greater among the Jews than among the rest of the inhabitants. The factors occasioning this greater susceptibility in Hebrews are not well understood. It has been variously ascribed to greater instability of the nervous system, fondness for sweets, and overeating and sedentary habits particularly among the better classes. Diabetes is very common among the educated and commercial classes in India, and Rose and Sen have shown that it is the Hindoos who chiefly suffer. The disease is said to be very uncommon in China and Japan.[36]

This is somewhat odd given that the Chinese diet was seen as encouraging such pathological developments. Futcher added:

We might suppose that the prolonged excessive use of carbohydrate food would favor the development of diabetes. There seems no satisfactory evidence favoring this view, however. Cantani stated that the majority of his Italian patients subsisted largely on farinaceous food. He believed the diet was an important etiological factor. In Ceylon, also, where diabetes is common, large quantities of saccharine food are taken. The Chinese, on the other hand, rarely suffer from diabetes, although their diet consists chiefly of carbohydrates.[37]

In the argument over whether 'fat' or 'carbohydrates' were most at fault for obesity and the diseases attendant to obesity, carbohydrates were blamed after the great popular success of William Banting's dieting practices at mid-century.

This obsession of China-based Western medical professionals with the obesity of the Chinese reappears in the popular Chinese press of the late Qing and the Republican period as China becomes 'modern.' Though the concern with obesity also appeared in Chinese-language periodicals wherein it may be seen as a response to the past and contemporary, allopathic medicine view of China as a famine culture, it did so in the form of articles by foreigners freely adapted and purveyed for consumption in these journals and magazines. While a minority voice in the perspectives on China of Western allopathic medicine, the concern with the fat Chinese body was consistently voiced as a sign of the inherent disparities of indigenous society.

Obesity in China: Traditional and Revolutionary Views

Obesity seems not to have been a major problem in the various theories of the ill body in Chinese medicine. There was, however, a constant and intense concern with the 'immoderate body' in the medical and dietetic literature of traditional Chinese medicine. In the sixteenth century, Li Shizhen (1518–93) wrote in his *Bencai Gangmu* (Systematic Materia Medica) that the consumption of fresh crabs was healthy "in small quantities" but:

> Gluttons will consume a dozen or more at a sitting together with various kinds of meat and other foods. They eat and drink twice as much as they need . . . then blame [their upset stomachs on] the crabs. But why blame the crabs?[38]

In the world of traditional Chinese medicine, the culture of excess became a hallmark of the degenerate Chinese body in need of regeneration by the early twentieth century. This was quite in contrast to the cultural anxiety about emaciation, which drove thin people to undertake 'special bulking diets' in order to find marriage partners. Such emaciation was often seen as the curse of ancestors who were:

> . . . 'eating' the health and vitality of a descendant in retaliation for neglect or mistreatment. Plumpness, by contrast, was perceived as a clear indication that the person so blessed was in harmony with the supernatural world.[39]

In the writings of Western commentators in early twentieth-century China, the dominant image of China as a starvation culture thus had its answer in the counter-example of the degenerate obese body.

Immediately before the revolution that overthrew the Qing dynasty on October 10, 1911, 'reform' was everywhere. As a new fantasy of the 'reformed' body began to emerge in China, obesity came to be viewed as one of the signs of the degenerate Chinese body, a body clearly in need of reform. Following the model of 'regeneration' that captured most of the ideologies of the day (from Zionism to Marxism to Social Darwinism to Colonialism), obesity defined the ability of the society to reform the individual. In one of the most widely read columns, "Ziyoutan," (unfettered talk) in the renowned newspaper *Shenbao*, the author Wang Dungen, a well-known writer and a key figure in the "Mandarin Ducks and Butterflies School," explored the reform of the body. In the late 1910s and early 1920s, Wang Dungen was under attack by the progressive writers of the May Fourth movement, and in 1914 he created the comic journal *Saturday*, in which he responded to his critics. In a comic essay entitled "Reforming the Human Body," Wang Dungen envisioned a grotesque ideal of the "new" body comprising a newly configured mouth, tongue, ear, eyes, nose, skin, eyebrows, hair, teeth, neck, shoulders, arms, hands, fingers, and feet. The new body possessed hundreds of mouths so that its owner could eat more and yet still be able to talk.[40] This was an ironic response to the starved body, a body desiring reform so that it might consume ever more, and it emerged at a moment when calls were being advanced for the adoption of 'Western' models of regeneration, such as structured physical exercise, as a means of reforming the too-fat body. Chen Duxiu, the leader of the New Cultural Movement, advocated exercise to make the Chinese physically, as well as morally fit, and Mao Zedong in 1917 published a full-scale essay on physical education as a means to reform the body.[41]

By 1913, the classical Chinese medical literature on obesity was beginning to be summarized for an intellectual readership in China. The essay "On Obesity," by Shu Hui and Wei Seng, written in classical Chinese, was published in a leading women's magazine. Such magazines shaped and were shaped by the images of the so-called New Woman (*xin nuxing*) and Westernized Modern Girl (*modeng nulang*), which came into prominence in the first decade of the twentieth century in China as well as in the West. These images were defined in many ways, but to no small extent by their 'thin' body form. As James L. Watson has noted, thinness, even after the establishment of the People's Republic, continued to be a mark of "bad luck, illness, and early death."[42] Thinness was the "stigma of emaciation" that scarred the psyche of the Chinese at both the beginning and the close of the twentieth century. But it was associated not with 'modern' thought, but with village superstition and backwardness among the intellectuals of the early twentieth century.

The "On Obesity" essay of 1913 presented the argument that obesity was an illness that women should not take lightly.[43] The authors referred to figures from ancient China, including as a man named Zilong, who lived in the Warring States period. Considering himself to be too fat, Zilong took *Phragmites communis Trin* (a plant used in traditional medicine) to lose weight. The authors offered this example to prove that obesity had been an illness treatable by medical intervention even in the pre-modern period. One of their sources was *Hanshu* (A History of the Former Han Dynasty), written by the historian Bangu. They argued that, according to *Hanshu*, too much body fat is the cause of obesity. But there are two kinds of obesity; one associated with surfeit and the other with a deficit of blood cells. The causes of the former were, not eating appropriately (too many unhealthy foods such as flour, sugar, and alcohol), not having a balanced lifestyle, and not having enough sex. Obesity of the second type was caused by external injury, overworking, or stress, and sometimes occurred after giving birth.

As with the Western medical literature of the late nineteenth century, in these free adaptations of articles in the Western press, the idea that there are stages of obesity was advanced.[44] For the authors of the 1913 essay, for example, obesity had three phases. In the initial phase, the person would look acceptably plump, which, since it was taken as a sign of prosperity, would mean that others would admire him; in the next phase, he would begin to look overtly obese and would thus take on a comical appearance; and finally, in the last phase, his life would be in danger and others would take pity on him. This final stage of obesity would present with symptoms including sweating, fatigue, backache, heart disease, sexual incompetence, and so forth. The 'cure' for obesity was a balanced diet and lifestyle: avoid eating things that contain too much fat, do not sleep for more than eight hours, take a warm bath two or three times a week, walk for two or three hours everyday, and be persistent. The condition could be medicated with either a traditional cure, such as *wodu* or, better yet, thyroid tablets. The latter offered the classical pharmaceutical intervention and certainly could reduce weight—by making the individual hyperthyroidal and increasing their basal metabolism. While this would lead to weight loss, it could also lead to a wide range of other pathologies, such as Graves' disease.

The treatment of obesity as an endocrinological deficiency, one of the most up-to-date views of early twentieth-century medicine, is suggestive of the way that modern ideas were creeping into classical Chinese views on obesity. The obese body was held by Western observers to be the antithesis of a beautiful and healthy body. And it therefore presented a special problem for contemporary women. In an essay "Keep the Body Slim," adapted and published in a women's magazine in 1922, the author, Dai Zuo, stressed that people with obesity were not beautiful, especially women:

> A person who is too fat looks very ugly. Women especially can't be fat. If a woman gains too much weight and becomes fat, where can one find her beauty?[45]

In addition, obesity was coming to be seen as an important medical problem. Obesity was the result of faulty metabolism, or of a hormone imbalance. Yet obesity was not a random occurrence. Certain people were more at risk than others, specifically people who ate rich food in abundance, were not physically active, had a family inheritance of obesity, and who were, of course, alcoholics. The essay made clear that obesity was dangerous as it led to heart disease. People with obesity had shortness of breath and rapid heartbeats even after walking a few steps. They were more likely to have a stroke. People with obesity had urinary and kidney problems. Dieting offered the solution. The essay advised that one should not overeat and that one should avoid food containing too much fat and eat less meat. Other suggestions for weight loss were physical exercise, the use of laxatives, and electric steam therapy to reduce body fat, which according to the essay was very popular abroad. Electrotherapy certainly was a standard late nineteenth-century Western treatment for the "failure or perversion of nutrition," including diabetes.[46]

Women were clearly the targets of the growing anti-obesity anxiety of Republican China. Chinese intellectuals, as with intellectuals and politicians in Western national states in this period, were focused on what was perceived as a decline in the birth rate among the elites. Women's bodies were the focus of a range of concerns, from the impact of intellectual life on reproduction to the growing sense that obese elites could not reproduce healthy children. In one essay, the author, Zhou Zhenyu, stated that he was a doctor who often had female patients who needed help to lose weight.[47] Zhou Zhenyu commented, "when I was a doctor in Beiping, I often had women patients come asking for the method of losing weight. I would tell them the method, some of them went home and practiced following my suggestions, others would come visit again and want medication. The effects differ because the causes of their obesity vary." "The cause and danger of female obesity" (as Zhou Zhenyu labeled it) was seen either in terms of over-indulgence and the absence of exercise or of an imbalance of the hormones.

This is the classic argument about obesity that dominated the late nineteenth-century discussion of its causes. In the United States, the home of most of the medical missionaries based in China, the editors of the *Journal of the American Medical Association* had published a 1924 editorial entitled "What Causes Obesity?" In it they argued, following a powerful anti-psychological strand in obesity research that began in the late nineteenth century, for an etiology of obesity rooted in malfunctions of normal metabolic processes. See obesity as a "scientific problem," they wrote, and that will free the "fat woman" from the stigma for which she "has the remedy in her own hands—or rather between her own teeth." The new object of scientific interest was the fat woman, who had been charged with carrying "that extra weight about with her unless she so wills."[48] Women, not 'men' or 'people,' were considered to be most at risk from obesity, a far cry from the evocation of Falstaff as the exemplary sufferer from obesity in the mid-nineteenth century. According to this article, although fat people usually ate less than thin people, they did not burn enough calories. There were still large amounts of fat accumulated and stored in their bodies. While the obese did not eat much at every meal, they often ate between meals. Women specifically could suffer from hypothyroidism, hypopituitarism, or a loss of estrogen. Pregnant women were especially at risk. One woman, after giving birth, had to get up and eat every night. She quickly gained weight and became obese.

The danger of female obesity is the collapse of one's health and thus one's ability to bear children, which is the classic definition of women's health. Obese women have compromised immune systems and are likely to catch colds and coughs, which leads to tuberculosis. They have heart disease. Their nervous systems are endangered. The obese are usually slow and lazy, but often they laugh and appear jovial. A disease that can be triggered by pregnancy ends up preventing conception, causing sexual problems, and heightening the possibility of miscarriage.

By 1941, as war raged and famine haunted China, a public discourse on obesity articulated by Western medical professionals was woven into the new 'reformed' Chinese attitude towards the body. These attitudes came to be labeled as a "tragedy at the dinner table."[49] It is always difficult to judge how widespread such views were among urban elites, but the indication that such concerns were read in the 'popular' press may be seen as an indication of the acceptance of such ideas about the fat body, at least among this readership. An essay, "Tragedy at the Dinner Table"—another free adaptation among a number of foreign medical and popular articles, especially those authored by American experts—appeared in the Chinese popular review, *Liangyou*, presenting the pathological consequences of overeating. The author identified middle-aged people as being most at risk, because they seemed to be more easily attracted to fine dining. The essay defined pathology by quoting a saying attributed to an American congressman: "fifty, fifty, fifty," which means if a 50-year-old person is 50 pounds overweight, his life span will be reduced by 50 percent. The author also quoted statistics provided by an American doctor suggesting that out of 2,000 cases of sudden death, 90 percent of those involved had died of heart disease: "Most of them eat too much, are overweight, which causes heart disease."[50] While other foreign cases of overeating were mentioned in the article, such as among the ancient Romans, American Thanksgiving was given special mention as a moment of extreme public gluttony:

> Around Thanksgiving time, there are often cases of death caused by overeating to be found in the mortuary. People in charge of the postmortem examinations are often too busy rushing to luxurious banquets to do their work. It's also quite dangerous to eat too much after fasting. One should definitely divide all the nice dishes into several meals, and never eat everything at once. It is nice to be able to enjoy a full table of luxurious food, but one should remember not to gamble with one's own life. Otherwise tragedy would take place in the holiday season, and one would sadly fall onto the bosom of death.[51]

The result of such gluttony was sudden death, chronic heart disease, or diabetes. A litany of diseases was the result of obesity: high blood pressure, lung disease, cancer, even suicide and accidental death. For, according to the author, people with obesity often had psychological problems and were very slow in reacting to what was going on around them—and thus were prone to accidents. The overweight individual was advised to consult qualified doctors to monitor his or her individual diet. Yet the 'cure' proposed in the essay of 1941 was to pay minute attention to what and how much one ate. The formula did not have much to do with any specific type of food, rather the idea that, as one grew older, one should eat less. By the time one was very old, one should eat only light and simple food, returning in effect to the kind of diet prescribed for infants.

China, like America, seems to be suffering from a new epidemic of obesity but one that now documents its modernity—no model of Oriental, primitive infectious diseases is evident here. Rather, there is a claim of the 'invasion from the West.' Earlier, negative depictions of obesity as a reflection of inherent Chinese problems, whether social or racial, as seen through the eyes of Western observers and consumed by readers of Chinese magazines, become a model for this undesirable circulation. The consumption of modern Western products such as condensed milk, seen initially as a potential 'cure' for the diseases resulting from famine, come to be read as the cause of this new urban, Western phenomenon of obesity. However, the negative aspects of the new economy imported from the West could be addressed and confronted through the importation of models of obesity derived from Western public health. Obesity and its treatment can thus be understood as part of a system of modernization wherein all of the pitfalls of modern living are apparent, just as the 'cure' is apparent and available for consumption. Like concepts such as famine, obesity too is rooted in nineteenth- and early twentieth-century Chinese understandings of health and illness. Evoking the 'Western' causes of obesity, Chinese public health officials today echo this older, Chinese model of an obesity epidemic—for all that is bad in Chinese health must still have its roots in the West.

10
'Rails, Roads, and Mosquito Foes': The State Quinine Service in French Indochina

Laurence Monnais

Introduction

In Daniel Headrick's seminal work *The Tools of Empire*, quinine is presented as a key tool of nineteenth-century Western imperial expansion. This emphasis upon the important role played by quinine in facilitating colonial conquest and administration has been criticized by historians of medicine, notably William Cohen, David Arnold, and Mark Harrison. These historians argue that quinine was not as widely consumed in the nineteenth century as Headrick supposed, that its mode of administration (form and dosage) was probably of limited efficacy and therefore is unlikely to have had such an impact on the health of colonial troops and administrators.[1] Quinine may still have played a role in protecting the health of European troops, enabling them to 'pacify' some territories in Asia or Africa, but we still know very little about how quinine was actually distributed, utilized, and consumed in tropical colonies. Moreover, we need to evaluate its effects on the health of colonized people. Thus, it seems important to ask in what ways and to what extent quinine served not only the conquest, but also the subsequent exploitation and socio-economic development of the territories placed under colonial rule; in other words, to consider whether and how quinine was used, not only as a tool of imperialism but also as a tool of colonization.

To explore these questions, this chapter analyzes how the Service de Quinine d'Etat, or the State Quinine Service (SQS), functioned in French Indochina during the first half of the twentieth century. Established in 1909, the purpose of the SQS was to manage the distribution of subsidized quinine for the prevention of malaria in Indochina, which was constituted by what is now Vietnam (in the colonial period the protectorates of Tonkin and Annam and the formal colony of Cochinchina) and the protectorates of Cambodia and Laos. Quinine was to be provided free of charge in areas where malaria prevalence was highest, and to groups identified as contributing to the development of the colony: soldiers, 'coolies,' migrant farmers, and those employed on public works projects. It is essential that the SQS in Indochina be considered in relation to the larger context of the *mise en valeur*—translated as "rational development" by colonial historian Alice Conklin—which was both a key objective and important justification for colonial rule.[2] At the same time, malaria was the most prevalent infectious disease in the Vietnamese peninsula, accounting for at least 15 to 20 percent of total morbidity. It thus presented a major obstacle to colonization, particularly given that it severely affected the indigenous workforce (especially in some of the areas most likely to form the focus of managed economic exploitation).

Examining the history of the SQS and considering its effectiveness as a means of implementing the mass distribution of 'colonial quinine' as part of a thoroughgoing public health program, this chapter highlights the difficulties that the colonial administration encountered in relation to the distribution and consumption of quinine during the first half of the twentieth century. Did the circulation of quinine adequately follow the circulation of capital, goods, and people created by the *mise en valeur* of colonial administrators? The evidence suggests that the colonial state's efforts to provide quinine to indigenous populations ultimately failed to stem the risk of rising contagion. And it reveals that this risk arose from the economic transformations and the social mobilities produced by the experience of colonialism itself.

Malaria and the *Mise en Valeur*: Creating the State Quinine Service

As early as the 1860s, the first French military physicians who arrived in Cochinchina, in the south of Vietnam, pointed out the devastating effects of "malarial miasmas" in reports to their superiors.[3] This widespread scourge weakened troops and was a constant threat to the Vietnamese population. The novelist and colonial civil servant Jules Boissière described malaria as evil personified, a scourge that made no distinction between Europeans and indigenous people.[4] In 1892, in one of the first large-scale reports on health in Tonkin, an area in the north of Vietnam that was being 'pacified' by the French at the time, it was claimed that malaria was responsible for at least one-third of local morbidity and for one-half of all deaths.[5] Further reports would confirm the magnitude of the problem; in 1904, Dr Edouard Jeanselme declared at the colonial congress in Paris that "malaria is the principal affliction disrupting the development of the indigenous population."[6]

From the late 1880s, the high river valleys and the Dong Trieu massif in the north were mapped and assigned the status of "hyperendemic malaria zones." Only the provinces of the Red River delta appeared to have been spared. As for the Annamitic chain, the mountain range extending from the coast of central Vietnam to Laos, the rate of prevalence was estimated to lie between 80 and 100 percent. In Cochinchina, the wooded areas of the eastern and western provinces were believed to be the worst affected. In 1907, the Pastorian Paul-Louis Simond, a physician and medical geographer, wrote: "Indochina should be considered as divided into two regions: one where malaria is sparse and one where malaria is widespread. The first encompasses the densely populated and cultivated lowlands, with wide river valleys, deltas and coastal plains. The other is made up of all mountainous territories, wooded and uncultivated, and of forested plains."[7] Several Pastorian physicians and scientists would later refine Simond's portrait of malaria distribution in Vietnam. The parasitologists, Constant Mathis and Maurice Léger, for instance, drew a detailed map of the endemic index for malaria in the Tonkin area on the basis of blood tests. Their study showed that the disease prevalence was low in the delta and the middle region, and substantial in the high region, especially towards the northwest in the Black River area.[8] Notwithstanding such variation, Mathis and Léger's general conclusion was that the whole country was badly affected.

During the first decades of French domination, from 1860 to 1880, interventions targeting malaria were sporadic and disorganized. They were deployed in times of crisis resulting from disease epidemics or the threat thereof. Regular distribution of prophylactic quinine took place almost exclusively among the French and Vietnamese military and the European minority. Quinine, an alkaloid obtained from the bark of cinchona, was isolated in 1820 by two French pharmacists: Pierre-Joseph Pelletier and Joseph-Bienaimé Caventou. From at least the 1850s, quinine sulphate was used as a specific treatment for malarial fevers. It was also used to prevent the disease, even though its etiology was still relatively unknown. In 1880, while he was posted in Constantine, Algeria, the Pastorian doctor Alphonse Laveran discovered the hematozoan parasite that caused malaria, the *Plasmodium*.[9] Its mode of transmission by the mosquito vector, the female *Anopheles*, would be discovered by British scientists Patrick

Manson and Ronald Ross in 1897–98. Together, these discoveries prompted the international medical community to consider quinine a valuable preventive medicine, which could be put to collective use. Through large-scale public health interventions, the human parasite reservoir could be reduced.

The time seemed ripe for the launch of precisely such a policy in Vietnam, where the pacification of the northern territory was almost complete by the turn of the twentieth century. Several foreign models for anti-malarial campaigns were examined by sanitary officials and medical doctors in the metropole. The first major road and railway infrastructure works were accompanied by local initiatives to reduce the prevalence of malaria.[10] Indeed, malaria morbidity among 'coolies' working on these construction sites was staggering: from 40 to 70 percent of the workers, depending on the site, were reportedly affected. In 1902, in response to a survey on the health of public workers mandated by Governor-General Paul Doumer, Dr Charles Grall, the chief of the Colonial Health Care Services, called for the immediate introduction of several measures.[11] Intended, in particular, for the workers of the Nha Trang–Dalat road construction site in Annam, these measures included bush clearing around workers' camps, the limitation of working hours, the distribution of healthy and nutritious food rations, as well as the systematic and controlled distribution of prophylactic quinine.

Two years later, in 1904–05, the Pastorian Noël Bernard reported on the malaria situation in work-sites along the railway between Yen Bay and Lao Kay in Tonkin.[12] In his report, Bernard explained that he had applied the measures proposed by Grall, but focused especially on prophylactic quininization. This strategy was not as effective as he had expected. In response to a surge in malaria cases in May 1905, he had increased the daily doses of quinine, and ordered the repatriation of all 'coolies' displaying signs of infection to their 'native' villages. Despite this, the number of cases continued to increase in June. When a third contingent of workers arrived, Bernard requested that his supervisors reduce working days to eight hours, distribute alum to purify water supplies, and increase weekly doses of quinine. In August, 1,264 out of 2,200 workers were ill (approximately 57 percent) and 1,126 were apparently ill with malaria. Bernard concluded that quinine, which had been distributed regularly from February to September, had an impact on morbidity from March to June, but failed to prevent a rise in cases from the beginning of the warm season.

Within military circles, however, more encouraging results were reported. From 1902–03, Dr Montel, head of the army medical service in the marshy and malarial Ha Tien province in Cochinchina, had each of his men take one tablespoon of quinine wine daily. This produced good results: "in February, the number of exemption days due to the fever decreased [from 59 in January 1903] to 14 . . . in March . . . there were only two exemption days . . ."[13] As early as 1908, 313 kilos of quinine sulphate and chlorhydrate in tablet form were supplied to military posts in Indochina. This resulted in a decline in morbidity among European and native military populations by half on average, while the death rate dropped by 20 percent.[14] During the same period, in Tonkin, several trials of prophylactic quinine treatment for civilian communities also seemed to produce good results. Counters for the distribution of low-cost quinine, or *dépôts de quinine*, were set up in the most highly affected zones in the provinces of Ha Dong, Hai Duong, and Thai Binh.[15]

In all of the reports on these trials, however, it was noted that quinine distribution failed to prevent seasonal outbreaks of the disease. If, at the time, ideas concerning climate, and particularly heat, had become unpopular in etiological explanations of tropical diseases, it is no less true that the observations of doctors in service abroad emphasized that, in the case of malaria, the hot season—in other words, the rainy season—was an important factor in the proliferation of *Anopheles* in regions where they were already well represented. Moreover, given that the important infrastructure projects required sending workers into regions known to be unhealthy, it is clear that it was impractical to stop work for several months out of the year. The best that authorities could do was to reduce the number of working hours per day and to distribute more quinine.

Selling Protection: The Quinine Service between Plan and Reality

In 1907 and 1908, high-ranking representatives of the colonial government declared that the time had come to consolidate these efforts in a comprehensive anti-malarial policy for Indochina.[16] Two years earlier, in 1905, Governor-General Paul Beau had officially established a public healthcare system aimed at responding to the needs of the population of Indochina, the *assistance médicale indigène*, or Indigenous Medical Assistance (AMI). The AMI was also promoted as having a key role to play in the 'civilization' of the colony. Its priority was preventive public health; it focused on collective interventions targeting the most prevalent epidemic and endemic diseases, as well as health education.

It also provided for the development of a relatively extensive network of medical facilities. Collective, prophylactic intervention nevertheless remained its primary role throughout the whole colonial period. Through this emphasis, vaccines and (preventive) quinine were the sole medications assigned a prominent role in the system by colonial health authorities.[17]

On December 4, 1909 the Governor-General created the State Quinine Service by decree as "an action of social prophylaxis" (article 2) intended to organize, rationalize, and control the distribution of quinine to the populations of Indochina. The distribution of quinine was to be operated through a system of central and secondary quinine stores, which would be managed by agents authorized by the colonial administration and supervised by representatives of the five Local Directions of Health (*directions locales de la santé*) (article 6). The 1909 text insisted on the quality and the purity of the quinine to be distributed (article 4). Its price was to be determined annually (article 5) and rules for its purchase and use stressed freedom from inconvenience (such as "useless formalities and of the need to travel far"). Access to quinine was to be made as easy and widespread as possible (article 11).

However, the 1909 text also specified that not all regions and segments of the population would be treated equally in terms of distribution. The only groups provided with quinine free of charge were those judged to be "indigents," i.e., the destitute, and groups considered to be most at risk, such as soldiers, 'coolies,' those employed on public works projects, and migrant peasant families (articles 7/9). The beneficiaries also had to prove that they resided within one of the endemic malarial zones appearing on a list that was to be periodically revised. Finally, only in cases of severe epidemics within recognized endemic areas would the SQS distribute quinine for both preventive *and* curative purposes (article 8). Though later directives from the governor-general or his local representatives would modify some aspects of the SQS system, they did not introduce any major changes in the way the service functioned, in spite of the setbacks that the service soon encountered. These included recurrent problems with the definition of malarial zones, the provision of adequate supplies of quinine, distributors' practices, and of course, the actual quantity of quinine consumed by the population.

The provinces of Tonkin were the first to be defined and listed as malarial zones by a decree issued in January 1912. The underlying objective was to set the SQS in motion as quickly as possible in the region with the highest economic potential at the time, both in terms of agricultural and mining exploitation as well as infrastructure development that would facilitate the circulation of people and goods in the interior of the country and towards China or the port of Haiphong. The 'highly malarial' provinces of the protectorate (Son La, Lai Chau, Ha Giang, Hoa Binh, Tuyen Quang) and the provinces with a more moderate risk of malaria transmission (Lao Kay, Yen Bay, Thai Nguyen, Quang Yen, Bac Kan, Phu Tho, Lang Son) were to be supplied different amounts of quinine on a year-round basis. Subsequent studies added to and altered the classification of malarial provinces in Tonkin and elsewhere. The definition of these different zones was made on the basis of the endemic malarial index, which also changed in response to new knowledge about local epidemiology or alerts from local physicians. The complexity of procedures for determining the classification of provinces in these lists is striking. Moreover, the lists do not seem to reflect the real-life situations encountered by inhabitants. For instance, several physicians mentioned disparities within provinces. Non-malarial zones in provinces classified as high-risk were not accounted for, even by refined mapping, and of course the inverse was also possible. The SQS was, therefore, an inequitable system of distribution.

There were also problems with supply. The text of 1909 had emphasized the importance of a regular supply of good quality quinine products but this goal was not achieved. These products were sourced directly from France by the colonial healthcare services, but also sometimes locally from French pharmacists. The choice between these two channels seems to have changed over time, depending on cost.[18] For example, when the SQS was launched in Annam in 1912, quinine was imported by a private pharmacy on the basis of an agreement between the owner of the pharmacy and the local director of health. According to this agreement, 1,000 conditioned tubes of quinine cost the health service 192 francs, which was considered a very good price.[19] During the 1920s and 1930s, however, the central pharmacies of AMI (*pharmacies centrales de l'assistance*) seem to have been the main suppliers of quinine sulphate—in powder form, that is, in bulk. These central pharmacies were set up in three cities, Hanoi, Hué, and Saigon, to optimize the distribution of medicines and pharmaceuticals throughout the country. Through the personnel, equipment, and techniques at their disposal (techniques that included adding talcum powder to quinine salts) they were able to provide better quality control and, most importantly, lower production costs than alternative suppliers.[20]

Money—or the lack of it—regularly caused problems at other levels of the organization and operation of the service. The SQS, according to the 1909 text, was to be paid for by local budgets through direct taxes levied in each region; as was also the case for most healthcare expenditure. This in itself was potentially problematic, since the wealth and the malarial status of each province did not necessarily match. Each province was to allocate a sum in its annual budget for the purchase of quinine on the understanding that this expenditure would eventually be recouped through the sale of state quinine to those Vietnamese who did not have free access to it. In 1911, for instance, one Dr Hermant declared that he had included a credit of 150 piastres for state quinine in the provincial budget of Nghe An, where he was in charge of the AMI. This would allow for the purchase of about 1,500 quinine tubes to be distributed among the province's 11 stores. The budget reportedly reached 1,000 piastres a year later, which was sufficient to provide supplies for 20 stores.

According to Dr Allain, the local director of health in Annam, no fewer than 100,000 tubes of state quinine were sold at the level of the protectorate in 1913. But, of that total, 66,000, or 66 percent, were sent to the wealthy coastal province of Binh Dinh alone.[21] By contrast, in 1917, Dr Havet wrote in his report on the densely populated province of Tay Ninh, in southern Vietnam bordering Cambodia, "the fight against malaria has not even been begun [here] . . . 7 kilos of quinine annually are set against . . . the malarial disease that is spread among the population (80,000 inhabitants), that is, fewer than 9 centigrams per head annually . . ."[22] Disparities were evident, then, and budget shortages were usually blamed for the uneven distribution of the medicine.

Other glaring inequalities appeared in the absence or ineffectiveness of quinine stores in numerous malarial provinces. In Cochinchina, the number of stores increased rapidly, but not necessarily in provinces where they were needed most. For instance, the province of Gia Dinh, near Saigon and relatively protected from the disease, was reported to have no fewer than 36 stores on the eve of World War I. By contrast, further south, in the province of Phan Thiet, Dr Pic explained how, for lack of alternatives, he oversaw the preparation of 0.25g quinine sulphate pills in the small pharmacy of his clinic in a bid to provide sufficient supplies to meet his patients' demands.[23] In some regions, the SQS simply did not exist until the 1920s; the war had delayed its introduction. This was the case for the Tonkin provinces of Ninh Binh, Vinh Yen, Kien An, and Phuc Yen. In any case, in Vietnam as a whole the number of stores was clearly insufficient and would remain so.

Further concerns about the timing and adequacy of the supply system soon emerged, and were set down in a report published by Dr Havet in 1917.

Distributors were meant to inform provincial colonial authorities when they were running short of supplies, and at the same time to send the money acquired from the sale of quinine. Only after this information (and the money) made its way up the chain of command could the central stores, under the authority of the local offices of health, re-order quinine and renew distributors' supplies—provided there was enough money left in the budget. On top of this potentially lengthy procedure, Havet revealed that there were often difficulties in the transportation of quinine, especially in remote regions and at certain times of the year, such as the rainy summer months when malaria was on the increase.[24] Given these issues, many reports mention that distributors in the provinces either failed to receive or obtained inadequate supplies of quinine, even in the late 1930s.

The 1909 decree had emphasized the need for flexibility in channels of access to preventive quinine. Here, again, a substantial gap emerged between planning and reality. Initially, the authorities thought of appointing mainly colonial agents as distributors. These included customs officers and postal office employees, who were considered easy to control and unlikely to refuse this extra task, members of the *gardes indigènes*, and the managers of state-run alcohol and opium stores (*dépôts de la régie de l'alcool et de l'opium*).[25] As early as 1910, the governor of Cochinchina decreed that private pharmacists should be allowed, upon making a formal request, to sell state quinine. While some may indeed have done so, it should be noted that there were only a few private pharmacies at this time, and these were concentrated in the Saigon–Cholon urban area, where malaria was not as prevalent as in other parts of the region. The functioning of the SQS was becoming increasingly unwieldy, especially since responsibility for its operation was spread across several different departments. Navigating the ever-growing administrative hierarchy of the SQS required patience and diligence, as each of these departments had its own codes and regulations to be observed.

From 1921–22, the department of customs and state monopolies (*douanes et régies*) was the only body entrusted by the colonial government with the distribution of state quinine supplies, as well as the supervision of its sales and restocking. It is hard to imagine how this decision could have been unproblematic (*douanes et régies* was also responsible for the distribution of opium and alcohol, both products being state monopolies that were on occasion forcibly sold to certain villages), although the administration seems to have considered the notion of recruiting distributors from communities in the malarial zone.

As early as 1923, the general inspector for healthcare services in Indochina, Dr Audibert, remarked that the distribution of state quinine in Cochinchina had decreased noticeably since the quinine stores had come under the control of the customs department. According to several colonial doctors under Audibert's supervision, this decrease was a direct result of a lack of trust in the intermediaries responsible for quinine distribution among the target demographic. On top of negative perceptions of them as 'tax collectors', agents of the *douanes et régies* were denounced as either too rigid or too lazy. Some were seen as limiting distribution to a circle of family and close friends. Others were accused by some Vietnamese newspapers of selling quinine at a high price or refusing to accept free quinine coupons held by indigent Vietnamese.[26] It was for this reason, the chief medical officer for the province of Binh Dinh explained in 1921, that in the past three years, 14 out of 17 stores had failed to distribute a single tube of quinine.[27]

Medicine and Mobility: Consuming and Distributing Quinine in Vietnam

The colonial government had become aware, and concerned, that an inadequate amount of quinine was being consumed to facilitate the flows of laborers, goods, and resources that were essential to the *mise en valeur*. While the reliability of the AMI statistics can be questioned, these show that the distribution of state quinine varied over time. The lowest rates of distribution occurred during the years 1914–18, which can be explained by the impact of the war on quinine supplies, and which may have had quite serious repercussions for the health of Vietnamese population. Mapping all of these fluctuations and regional disparities would be a formidable task, but it is possible to analyze in more detail several statistical series from the late 1930s in order to illustrate this point.

According to data compiled for January to June 1939, quinine distributions in Tonkin reached 69.4 kg during this six-month period.[28] From this total, 24.9 kg were sold by customs services and 17.7 by other colonial agents; only 26.8, or 39 percent, were distributed free of charge, which does not seem like a considerable amount. Yet, the analysis of healthcare reports from the 1930s indicates that the proportion of paid distributions dropped significantly during the interwar period. Global figures are, however, misleading: while the percentage of free state quinine was only 35 percent in Annam in 1930, it reached 95 percent in Cochinchina (it must be noted that Cochinchina was the only region in Indochina to have a system of indigent identity cards to identify individuals living in poverty).[29] These figures also hide provincial disparities: in Lang Son, Tonkin, 6.5 out of the nearly 7.5 kg, or 87 percent, were handed out for free during the first half of 1939; in contrast, in Phu Ly, not a single state quinine tablet was recorded as having been dispensed free of charge. For the same time period, Lao Kay recorded a distribution of 15.6 kg and Quang Yen, of zero. These differences did not necessarily correspond to the official malarial status of the provinces: Quang Yen, Lao Kay, and Lang Son were all listed as areas of 'moderate' infestation. By contrast, more seriously affected provinces, such as Ha Giang, did not distribute the largest supplies. During the first months of 1939, it seems that the Ha Giang population 'consumed' 9.4 kg of quinine, Hoa Binh 1.8 kg, and Son La, only 87 g.

The sale price of state quinine (that is, for customers other than indigents, colonial agents, and those employed on public works projects) was determined by the colonial authorities. It was the representatives of the governor-general in the colony of Cochinchina and in the protectorates of Annam and Tonkin who set the price; in theory, they were to adapt it to the needs and means of each region. As a result of this decentralized approach, prices fluctuated not only over time but also from one region to another. In 1912, the price for a tube of 10 0.25 g tablets of quinine was 0.10 piastre in both Tonkin and Annam; in 1930, the price per tube in Cochinchina was 0.18 piastres, and 0.15 in Tonkin and Annam. A closer look at prices in Tonkin shows only that they were modified from 0.10 in 1921 to 0.08 in 1922, then to 0.12 in 1934. These prices seem relatively low; yet, a supply of preventive state quinine was probably still too expensive for a large part of the population. When the SQS was created in 1909, the daily preventive dose recommended for an adult varied from 0.50 to 0.60 g, that is, two tablets (one for children). The recommended number of days of treatment per month and the number of months over the year varied according to the prevalence of malaria in the region and the intensity of the symptoms of the disease.[30] In the highlands of Tonkin, a province which was particularly affected by malaria, the following regimen was prescribed: two tablets for 10 days during the first month, and eight days during the second and third months. In the 1930s, malariologists considered that in high-risk regions, such as the Tonkin highlands, adults should take 1 g per day (four tablets) continuously over at least one month.[31]

Complying with these instructions was therefore difficult for the inhabitants of these zones; they required 12 tubes per year in the 1930s—compared to only five in 1909. If a tube cost 0.15 piastre on average, this amounted to 1.80 piastres per month per person, much more for a whole family. The total sum could easily reach 10 piastres, which was a large amount for Vietnamese families, particularly during the economic depression of the 1930s. (The annual tax at this time for a peasant family of five was estimated between 25 and 30 piastres, which accounted for 15 to 30 percent of the annual income per head. Indeed, several AMI doctors complained about the cost of state quinine.)[32] Numerous stores were unable to clear supplies of state quinine for this reason. Such was the case of Lang Son between 1921 and 1926, despite its status as a high-risk malarial zone.[33] In 1924, the local director of health in Cochinchina, Dr Lecomte, wrote in his report on the functioning of the AMI in the colony that "the only provinces to obtain results are those in which administrators and physicians have dared to take the initiative and modify standard departmental procedures . . . In the province of Ba Ria, each village [thus] allocates a sum for the purchase of quinine. It then resells this to its inhabitants at half the sale price, and the rest is covered by the commune's budget . . ."[34]

Yet when the question of how quinine circulated from the colonial state to subjects is considered, the picture remains highly varied. In some regions, for example, stores quickly disposed of state quinine supplies; so quickly, indeed, that they could not re-order in time to meet demand.[35] While some unscrupulous distributors charged customers for quinine intended to be issued free of charge, in other cases unsold supplies might sometimes be distributed free of charge. Other state quinine agents facilitated sales by selling quinine by the tablet, and on demand, instead of by the whole tube, because it was more affordable that way.[36] As for the consumers, they negotiated access to state quinine and did not always comply with the regimen advocated by medical authorities. From the inception of the SQS, the issue of user compliance was regularly brought up by AMI doctors and public health personnel. The AMI administration had insisted from the outset that the goal of the SQS was to persuade rather than coerce the population into adopting preventative quinine treatment. From the first years of the Service, quinine tubes were accompanied by instructions for the proper use of tablets, written in *quoc ngu* (romanized Vietnamese) and in Chinese, as a substitute for medical supervision.[37] In addition, advertising tools were used to diffuse information about the benefits of quinine, as well as how to obtain and use it: notices and posters were hung adjacent to retail distribution points, while leaflets were handed out in busy public places. The following notice, for instance, was in use in 1912:

Notice to quinine buyers.

Quinine is the best known medication to reduce fever . . .

Those who want to reduce fever must use the medicine in the following way:

Take 2 tablets daily for 4 days; no quinine for 3 days

Take 1 tablet daily for 4 days

For children, administer only one tablet daily.

The medicine will work better if it is crushed and dissolved in a *cai-chen* [teacup] before swallowing. It will take more than one day for the fever to disappear; quinine must be taken for a long period of time.[38]

This kind of text was meant to be didactic, yet, in the end, it was probably rather confusing. Most importantly, it failed to emphasize the preventive dimension of quinine, and instead described its curative use, probably in an effort to better 'sell' the product. Other attention-grabbing tactics were used. For example, colorful posters depicted people who had fallen ill because they had not taken quinine, or featured frightening, bloodthirsty mosquitoes.[39]

These posters, however, were put on view mostly in urban centers or in work spaces, both public and private. Up until 1940, distributors were often criticized in medical circles for their lack of effort in promoting the sale of state quinine beyond a very limited geographic perimeter. The issue was even raised in an open letter written by some colonial civil servants that appeared in one of the most widely distributed Saigon newspapers, *L'Echo Annamite*, in 1927. They called for ". . . the intensification of the malaria prophylaxis program with lectures given by assistant physicians, explanatory notices in *quoc ngu* posted in the schools, communal houses, and markets . . ."[40] Quinine distribution was to become an object of mass education through a "mobile promotion" that would reach the most distant regions. The governor of the colony answered the letter by promising improvements to the system. Yet, no significant re-orientation in the administration's approach followed.[41]

Aside from potential problems arising from an inadequate consumption of state quinine, issues also arose in relation to the preventive efficacy of state quinine tablets. One problem related to the issue of dosage. Two hematozoan parasites coexisted in Vietnam; the most harmful, *Falciparum* (discovered by Laveran), and *Vivax*. Yet, the capacity of colonial authorities to identify the two parasites and establish their local prevalence was extremely limited; entomological studies, splenic index evaluations,[42] and blood tests—the most reliable methods—were extremely costly in terms of budget, personnel, and technical support. The failure to address the issue of dosage placed an additional limitation upon the effectiveness of the colonial authorities in preventing these undesirable circulations.

Other problems relating to the form in which the medicine was to be administered threatened the efficacy of state quinine. In the 1920s, a debate emerged among colonial doctors about the advantages of the tablet, which was obviously more practical, versus those of powder, which was said to guarantee maximal efficacy. The latter was also preferred on the grounds of the effect of humid tropical climates on the solubility of tablets. 'Low-quality' tablets were particularly liable to decreased solubility, and therefore reduced efficacy.[43] During the same period, the cheaper quinine sulphate was replaced by quinine chlorhydrate, which was said to be less liable to induce gastric intolerance and to allow for a better identification of the symptoms of 'quinine-induced delirium' (nervous reactions). Chlorhydrate had also a higher solubility and quinine content than sulphate, and was therefore more effective. Indeed, several physicians blamed the prior use of sulphate—thought to be not only inefficient but responsible for severe cases of biliary hemoglobinuric fever—for some of the failures in the anti-malarial campaign.[44] In any case, it took 15 years for the SQS to attend to problems of standardization, inefficiency, and unsafe products. The complaints about low-quality tablets nevertheless hint at the continued circulation of counterfeit products (which sometimes contained no active ingredients) alongside authentic state quinine—an additional threat to the outcome of mass preventive quinine treatment.[45] At the same time, the existence of these counterfeit tablets indicates the attraction of the Vietnamese population to the product and suggests that its supply was facilitated by illegal distributors, most often small-scale Vietnamese and Chinese merchants, with more flexible and efficient distribution practices.

Mass Prophylactics: The Pitfalls of Preventive Quininization in the 1930s

It became clear by the late 1920s that prophylactic quinine treatment was not, on its own, sufficient to realize the planned mass protection of the Vietnamese population. In 1936, malaria was still the primary cause of morbidity in AMI facilities; it accounted for 52,196 hospitalizations in Indochina (or 15 percent of total hospitalizations) and was associated with a death rate oscillating between 10 and 13 percent.[46] Yet, these figures do not even express the full extent of the problem, since they are based on the number of individuals consulted and admitted to colonial hospitals. Entomological studies, blood tests, and splenic index evaluations would have provided a better picture of the malaria situation, but they were only applied in a few target communities due to their high cost. The results of these more detailed experiments and studies are nonetheless revealing. Blood tests performed in Cochinchina and southern Annam under the supervision of Joseph-Emile Borel in 1926 confirmed that in some communities 50 to 70 percent of the population was affected. *Falciparum* malaria in particular was on the rise; it was identified as the main cause of infant mortality as well as of a decrease in birth rates, especially in the so-called new economic zone of the Terres Rouges, where rubber plantations were being established.[47]

By the beginning of the twentieth century, it was already well known among public health specialists and advisors that malaria prevalence rates were increasing in Vietnam in tandem with colonial efforts towards *mise en valeur*. As early as 1904, Dr Jeanselme mentioned that malaria had depopulated "once prosperous" Vietnamese provinces. In 1930–31, an investigation conducted by the local branches of the Pasteur Institute would confirm that all provinces in central Vietnam were malarial—not all to the same extent, but epidemic peaks had now spread to several coastal regions—while the east of Cochinchina was among the most affected areas. The extension of terraced ricefields is likely to have created new breeding grounds for *Anopheles* in many regions. Land clearing in the Terres Rouges and to the north of Saigon had created a serious health hazard for 'coolies' working on plantations and for immigrant farmers settling on the lands. Indeed, many administrative reports mention that, in the early 1930s, resettled peasant communities had deserted the lands they had been provided with after only a few months in order to escape malaria.[48] Moreover, in regions in which malaria had been seasonal, irrigation extended the transmission season throughout the year. The increased movement of people, especially workers traveling between places of work and villages, had also influenced the distribution of the disease. For example, when the Son Tay province in Tonkin was added to the list of the highly malarial provinces in the late 1910s, this was accounted for by workers' increasing mobility.[49]

Advances in knowledge about malaria and increasingly refined maps of disease prevalence in Vietnam should have made non-pharmaceutical preventive measures a priority, particularly measures to control mosquito vectors and protect populations from their bites. In fact, clear and insistent calls for greater vector control came from several Pastorians working in Indochina during the interwar period. These scientists were aware of the huge challenges facing colonial projects of rational development; challenges arising both from attempts to develop previously uninhabited malarial regions, and from the more recent proliferation of anopheles populations as a result of ecological disruptions. In 1931, the Pastorian Léon Bordes spoke of the spread of malaria as a global trend and warned of serious consequences for the inhabitants of Vietnam.[50] Randall Packard's recent history of malaria is similarly critical of the priority given to interventions targeting the parasite and its human reservoir until the 1950s. By neglecting the important socio-economic dimensions of malaria epidemiology, he argues, vertical strategies dominated by a biomedical logic had a limited impact on malaria in tropical territories.[51]

This was certainly the case in colonial Vietnam.[52] Not only did the colonial administration still lack precise knowledge of local malaria epidemiology at the time, it also lacked the means of stemming the global trend Bordes described, and of implementing a comprehensive malaria control policy. Such a strategy would have included country-wide blood tests to provide detailed information about regional distributions, as well as anti-larval and vector control measures ranging from marsh filling to the promotion of mosquito nets and glass windows. Yet these measures were, time and again, pushed aside by the colonial administration; they were deemed unrealistic, unmanageable, and too costly. Only in small groups of workers, seen as easy to control and economically worthwhile, were such measures implemented as part of pilot projects. From the late 1920s, for example, Pastorian malaria control strategies were applied in several rubber plantations. These were openly described in 1938 by the General Inspector of Healthcare Services of Indochina, Dr Pierre Hermant, who had been very active in preventive quinine treatment campaigns in Annam in the 1910s, as a "plan for the rich and only for the rich."[53]

In 1923, a formal agreement was reached between the general government and the Indochinese branches of the Pasteur Institute to coordinate research on malaria in Vietnam. Under Borel's direction, several rubber plantations soon became laboratories for an integrated malaria control endeavor, of which the Suzannah plantations (société des plantations An Loc), situated 100 kilometres from Saigon, was one. The method used there combined aggressive education campaigns on how to prevent malaria, anti-larval measures (spreading fuel on bodies of water or larvicide powder on breeding grounds, and rearing larvae-eating fishes), as well as both preventive and curative treatments targeting the parasite. These measures are believed to have contributed to a reduction of as much as 50 percent in the number of children harboring the parasite on the plantation.[54] They also cost the rubber-producing private firm that sponsored them a fortune; this cost could not have been borne by the colonial government or most other private companies.

At the same time, the monopoly held by Dutch Indonesia over cinchona cultivation resulted in frequent increases in the price of the alkaloid.[55] The introduction of the first synthetic anti-malarial drugs in the late 1930s did not solve the problem for the colonial administration. Not only were most of these new pharmaceuticals expensive, they were also no more effective than traditional quinine salts, and were considered to be more useful for treating episodes of malaria than for their prevention.[56] In addition, they had to be taken for fairly long time periods and preferably under strict medical supervision, given their experimental and toxic nature.[57] Thus, while trials of Quinacrine, Plasmochine, Rhodoquine, and Premaline took place in Vietnam in the late 1930s, the use of these medicines remained restricted to small, well-defined, and, again, often privileged communities: a few groups of 'coolies' working on private sites (where private companies paid for the experimental medicines), a few prisons, in which therapeutic experiments took place, and some small agricultural settlements.

At that time, Indochina's anti-malaria policy was considered to be backward compared with that of its neighbors, namely British Malaya and Dutch Indonesia, or Taiwan under Japanese rule. In Indonesia and Taiwan, prophylactic and curative quinine treatment had already been relegated to a limited ancillary measure in the late 1920s, in accordance with the guidelines published by the Malaria Commission of the League of Nations.[58] Moreover, at the Conference on Rural Hygiene in Eastern Countries (held in Bandung in August 1937), several public health specialists, some of whom were fighting against malaria for the American Rockefeller Foundation, denounced the limits of what was then called the 'French method.' The French method relied more on quinine prophylaxis and treatment and less on a policy of mosquito eradication using pesticides in *Anopheles* breeding sites (the 'Anglo-American method') and was a process deemed to be costly and difficult to control, as well as requiring an elaborate relationship between well-trained personnel—doctors, nurses, distributors of quinine—and the ill or potentially ill.[59]

In addition, the Vietnamese population never had full access to state quinine, despite the priority given in texts and discourses to flexible and widespread accessibility, and to the preventive and collective dimensions of the program. This is indicated in various obvious problems described in reports: inefficient and insufficient supplies, problems with the management of distribution points, the high price of quinine, etc. Indeed, the report of a study mandated by the League of Nations in 1932 exposed the absence of quinine consumption on a mass basis in Vietnam. According to the report, it was calculated that the Indochinese would have to consume at least 30,000 kg of quinine on the basis of estimated rates of prevalence in the territory. That year, less than 3,000 kg of quinine was officially reported to be available in the Union.[60] World War II was to severely affect the supply of anti-malarial drugs: state quinine distribution was restricted from 1941, and by 1942 synthetic drugs were no longer available in Vietnam.

Conclusion

The distribution of quinine remained the cornerstone of the fight against malaria in Vietnam from the creation of the AMI in 1905 to World War II. How is this emphasis to be explained, given that its basis was largely theoretical? Medicines and pharmaceuticals played only a minor role within the state-run healthcare system in Indochina except for preventive medicines, including vaccines and quinine. This faith in prophylactic medication remains difficult to explain, even when we take into consideration its links, in France, to Pastorism and the pharmaceutical industry, in particular to the Rhône Poulenc company, which was at the time in competition with the German pharmaceutical industry, two industries that were soon to focus on the market for synthetic anti-malarial products.

In Indochina, a yawning gulf appeared between plans to tackle a disease that was officially declared a public health priority, and the actual malaria control measures that resulted, which revolved around a very limited and unpopular therapeutic intervention, an intervention regularly denounced by many of those involved—doctors, Pastorians, journalists, consumers of healthcare, residents of malarial regions. This analysis of the Vietnamese SQS from 1909 to 1945 has suggested that malaria control was never really a priority of French sanitary policy in Vietnam.[61] This conclusion is supported by the numerous and recurring problems encountered by the SQS and its relatively weak impact, which was a result not only of apparently low rates of quinine consumption, but also the system's incapacity to respond to the rapidly evolving geographical distribution of the disease; or, in other words, its inability to circulate quinine within the populations of the peninsula. Quinine was never, in this context, a tool of colonialism, except perhaps in playing a limited role alongside other (more effective) preventive measures in reducing malaria morbidity in a few restricted areas and in small and relatively privileged communities of workers.

This conclusion leads to further questions concerning the *mise en valeur* and its limitations. As Conklin writes in her *Mission to Civilize*, "confronted with the economic poverty of the indigenous populations [of their empire], the French believed that civilization required that they improve their subjects' standard of living through . . . the *mise en valeur* of the colonies' natural and human resources. This objective, they thought, could best be achieved by building railroads . . . and by improving hygiene to eliminate the parasites."[62] If one focuses on malaria, the most prevalent disease in Vietnam throughout the colonial period, it is evident that the development of natural resources was prioritized over the development of human resources. Worse still, mosquitoes and malaria became more mobile because of colonization, while quinine never circulated as it should have, given its inability to 'follow' the increasingly mobile insects and people who carried the parasite.

The SQS did not facilitate or support the flows of laborers, goods and resources that were essential to the *mise en valeur*. Both in its goals and its achievements, the service slowed the development of the country, revealing in so doing the inefficiency and unresponsiveness of the French colonial administration, or at least its inertia and excessive bureaucracy, which were no match for a disease diffused through a complex and evolving relationship with the environment. Malaria was perhaps a 'colonial disease' more than a tropical one—and it was certainly an imperial contagion.

Afterword: 'Global Health' and the Persistence of History

Priscilla Wald

The essays collected in *Imperial Contagions* investigate the complex relationships among disease, politics, economic interest, and the development of medical research and public health in colonial Asia. Drawing on evidence from different case studies, each of the essays engages with a number of critical issues concerning the conceptualization and management of communicable disease as evident in colonial state health policies and institutions. These essays make clear that there were no stable categories through which to define, much less determine, the health of an individual or to understand and predict the course of a devastating communicable disease, as there are not today. The emergence of new technologies and discoveries and the fashioning of new practices and policies invariably occur within the context of social and political negotiations. Changing ideas about health and medicine are always highly charged socially and politically, and they illustrate the intricate entanglements of the conceptual and the material that find particular and often poignant expression in the experience of devastating communicable disease outbreaks.

Although the focus of the volume is primarily on the period between 1880 and the foundation of the People's Republic of China in 1949—with a particular emphasis on the 1890s and the first decades of the twentieth century—these questions remain critical today in the (re)formulation of 'Global Health.' In a 2008 article in *The Lancet*, for example, Margaret Chan, director-general of the World Health Organization (WHO), issued a call to return to the bold vision articulated in the 1978 Declaration of Alma-Ata, in which 134 member nations of the WHO and 67 international organizations affirmed the UN's definition of 'health,' broadly defined, as a "fundamental human right" and pledged to work for the goal of universal access to "primary health care" by 2000.[1]

Publishing "Return to Alma-Ata" in anticipation of the release of the WHO's World Health Report in 2008, entitled "Primary Health Care (Now More Than

Ever)," Chan reiterated the basic principles of the Declaration as she contemplated the many challenges that had prevented the realization of its goals. The intervening decades, she explained, had witnessed "an oil crisis, a global recession, and the introduction, by development banks, of structural adjustment programmes that shifted national budgets away from the social services, including health." Additionally, "the emergence of HIV/AIDS, the associated resurgence of tuberculosis, and an increase in malaria cases moved the focus of international public health away from broad-based programmes and towards the urgent management of high-mortality emergencies." [2]

Although the events that Chan enumerates drew both attention and resources away from the goals of the Declaration, their doing so is in fact symptomatic of deeper structural problems that Chan did not address in her (widely circulated) *Lancet* piece. These are, however, precisely the problems addressed in *Imperial Contagions*, where, from different perspectives, contributors consider conceptualizations of health and healthcare within the context of European global expansion, consolidation, and retrenchment. In so doing, they provide an important historical framework for reflecting on contemporary challenges, helping to elucidate deep-rooted assumptions that have, at least in part, contributed to the "stalled progress" of global health. [3]

It was during the late colonial period that health, conceived as a basic right of citizenship, began to lead to the articulation and subsequent espousal of an ambitious pan-Asian, and global, program of disease eradication and prevention, culminating, in April 1948, in the metamorphosis of the Health Organization of the League of Nations into the WHO. [4] *Imperial Contagions* provides a prehistory of this 'decolonizing' of international health in Asia, exploring the shifting boundaries that demarcated state power, welfare, disease, and development in different colonial settings from colonial India to Singapore, Indochina, and Hong Kong. If war was a stimulus to the development of disease control and, indeed, to the internationalization of health in the mid-twentieth century, the emphasis here is on colonial systems under stress and the ways in which colonial 'public health' was articulated and shaped in relation to upheavals and conflated crises: social, economic, political, and biological.

The essays chronicle the consequences of the inter-articulation of medicine, geopolitics, and socioeconomics, showing how policies in each of these areas were informed by anxieties raised by the others. The particular medical focus of the volume is communicable disease, because it is the medical issue that most explicitly affected the social and economic interactions within Europe's empires, although, as the contributors to this volume explain, the impact of such diseases was as much conceptual as material. As Peckham and Pomfret contend in the Introduction, "contagion worked as metaphor and practice through the development, planning, and segregation of colonial-era East and South Asian cities."

Central to that insight is an understanding of the importance of the spatialization of communicable disease. Disease, as these essays show, confounded the spatial expression of social distances that distinguished between a colonial 'us' and a colonized 'them.' That idea found common expression at the turn of the twentieth century, as the discoveries of bacteriology made it increasingly possible to chronicle microbial routes. In the words of Cyrus Edson, New York City's commissioner of health in 1895:

> We cannot separate the tenement-house district from the portion of the city where the residences of the wealthy stand, and treat this as a separate locality. The disease we find in the tenement-house threatens all alike, for a hundred avenues afford a way by which the contagion may be carried from the tenement to the palace.[5]

Concern about communicable disease in particular intertwined with, and dramatized, anxieties about social distance, as imperialism and urbanization brought populations into unprecedented contact. Microbes mapped the many interactions—unwitting and illicit—that had previously remained obscured. Communicable disease brought into view the fact and consequences of the promiscuous spaces of a shrinking globe. From their earliest identification, it was clear that microbes notoriously knew no boundaries, and their spaces were the spaces of networks rather than nations, of social interactions rather than distinct spatial hierarchies. *Contagion*, from the Latin *contagio*, meaning 'to touch,' gave material expression to largely unspoken concerns about the new possibilities for social contact afforded by the radical geopolitical transformations at the turn of the twentieth century.

If communicable disease gave expression to this dangerous social promiscuity, however, boundaries—national and social—were simultaneously reinforced by an emerging geography of disease. Warwick Anderson and others have documented how Europeans' encounter with the diseases of the tropics troubled colonial settlement and gave rise to the specialty of tropical medicine.[6] The essays in *Imperial Contagions* illustrate the resulting pathologization of places by the colonial state and the spatial responses instigated to curtail the diffusion of disease. At the same time, they suggest how this pathologization of the places and spaces of the global South—invariably construed as 'breeding grounds' of infection—crystallized anxieties about an increasingly interconnected world and continue to inform contemporary constructions of disease emergence. Indeed, *Imperial Contagions* offers insight into the constitutive processes through which the past shapes contemporary approaches to health, including the understanding and management of communicable disease.[7]

Among the most pressing circumstances that deflected attention from the goals of the Declaration of Alma-Ata, Chan lists communicable diseases such as HIV/AIDS and tuberculosis, diseases that shifted the focus from comprehensive healthcare reform to that of crisis management and expediency. Indeed, medical professionals first began to notice the surge in unusual opportunistic infections that eventually led to the identification of the HIV virus just two years after the Alma-Ata conference. The conference came at the end of a decade in which the countries of the global North had witnessed a marked decline in the severity of the problem of communicable disease and an increasing sanguinity about the ability of the medical establishment to minimize the threat of communicable disease worldwide. The eradication of naturally occurring smallpox in the late 1970s, in an initiative led by D. A. Henderson at the Centers for Disease Control, seemed to the medical establishment proof that any serious threat from communicable disease would soon be a distant memory. While the concept of primary healthcare came from health programs in the southern hemisphere in such nations as China (which was notably absent from the Conference at Alma Ata), Tanzania, and Venezuela, and arose from revolutionary ideas about social organization, as well as medical care, the confidence of the Euro-American medical establishment that medical science would soon have rendered medical catastrophes largely obsolete facilitated the broad acquiescence in the stated goals of the Declaration.

The sanguinity, of course, was short-lived. HIV/AIDS was one among many new and resurfacing devastating communicable diseases, albeit the most visible among them. Ebola, Marburg, Hantavirus, and many others had already begun to surface in relative isolation, even while the medical establishment was declaring victory in their war on communicable disease, and, by the end of the decade, what Chan calls "the urgent management of high-mortality emergencies" had become a priority. In 1989, epidemiologists, medical researchers, and tropical and infectious disease specialists came together in a well-publicized conference in Washington, DC, to discuss a problem that they named "disease emergence."[8] The problem and accompanying analysis that emerged from this conference quickly seeped not only into the medical literature, but also into the mainstream media and popular culture and has shaped ideas about contagion, especially pandemics, and global health generally, since that time.

"Disease emergence" refers to disease-producing microbes that have come newly into contact with human hosts for a variety of reasons, most of all because of human encroachment in previously uninhabited environments as a result of population explosions and increased development. This analysis shared one important feature with the Declaration of Alma-Ata: both insisted on the social as well as medical dimensions of human health. But in other ways, the analyses are almost antithetical. The concept of Health For All includes an analysis of global poverty as a problem of the inequitable circulation of resources largely originating in the developed nations of the North and disproportionally affecting the developing nations of the South. Conversely, the geography of disease that emerged from the 1989 conference depicted the threat of catastrophic communicable disease as emanating from the ostensibly mismanaged and pathologized spaces of the South and threatening the metropolises of the North.[9] This geography of disease is clearly a legacy of the re-ordering of colonial space explored in *Imperial Contagions*. In particular, this geography of disease, a function of the pathologizing of the colonial (and, subsequently, postcolonial) spaces of the South, reinforces the boundaries that were troubled by the spatial challenges to social hierarchies posed by contagion, real or imagined.

The geography of disease that has become associated with devastating communicable disease in the North registers a sense of danger that becomes indelibly associated with the spaces of the South. The journalist and novelist Richard Preston, who has mastered the art of blending his media in sensational accounts of communicable disease as national threat, exemplifies this geography when he explains, in *The Hot Zone*, that "a hot virus in the rain forest lives within a twenty-four-hour plane flight from every city on earth. All of the earth's cities are connected by a web of airline routes. The web is a network. Once a virus hits the net, it can shoot anywhere in a day—Paris, Tokyo, NY, LA, wherever planes fly."[10] The sensational style of Preston's account of an airborne strain of Ebola discovered in primates in a Reston, Virginia, primate quarantine facility reads like a novel, and it is accordingly widely read and taught. *The Hot Zone* both exemplified and helped to shape and disseminate conventional ways of thinking about disease emergence in the North, including the preconditions for emerging infections, their routes and means of travel, and the means with which to address the problem. These conventions appear in the mainstream media and popular fiction and film and constitute what I have elsewhere referred to as "the outbreak narrative."[11]

The geography of disease is among the most evident of these conventions, finding expression in fiction, film, and the mainstream media with the appearance—or anticipated appearance—of each new outbreak of a devastating communicable disease. An account of the SARs outbreak in a May 2003 issue of *Newsweek*, for example, described Guangdong, which it identified as the Ground Zero of SARS, as:

> . . . the same Chinese province that delivers new flu viruses to the world most years. Pigs, ducks, chickens and people live cheek-by-jowl on the district's primitive farms, exchanging flu and cold germs so rapidly that a single pig can easily incubate human and avian viruses simultaneously . . . The clincher is that these farms sit just a few miles from Guangzhou, a teeming city that mixes people, animals and microbes from the countryside with travelers from around the world. You could hardly design a better system for turning small outbreaks into big ones.[12]

Concerns about avian flu have found characteristic expression in such phrases as "The Flimsy Wall of China" and the Asian "hot zone"; "Asia today" is "the perfect incubator" for such a disease. And avian flu is itself "Nature's Bioterrorist."[13]

The last phrase in particular exemplifies how global threats begin to converge. Here communicable disease meets another threat that allegedly emerges from the formerly colonized world: 'terrorism.' The connection is evident in the familiar metaphors that describe microbial danger. Microbes, for Madeline Drexler, are "secret agents [that] shadow ecological change everywhere"; they are "nature's undercover operatives," capable of "hijacking the cell's metabolic machinery," and they even have their own mode of transmitting information: a "wireless communication system, called 'quorum sensing,' enables microbes to coordinate their activities . . . the most menacing bioterrorist is Mother Nature herself."[14] For Joshua Lederberg, one of the two primary organizers of the 1989 conference, the communicable diseases that are produced by our "ever-evolving adversary," the microbe, are "'Nature's revenge,' for our intrusion into forest, irrigation projects, and climate change."[15] And Richard Preston calls them "molecular sharks, a motive without a mind . . . Compact, hard, logical, totally selfish . . ."[16]

These metaphors logically extend the apparently irresistible tendency for scientists and science writers to attribute cognition and intentionality to microbes. Microbes, insists Richard Krause in a conventional formulation:

> . . . are not idle bystanders, waiting for new opportunities offered by human mobility, ignorance, or neglect. Microbes possess remarkable genetic versatility that enables them to develop new pathogenic vigor, to escape population immunity by acquiring new antigens, and to develop antibiotic resistance. [They are] more than simple opportunists. They have also been great innovators.[17]

A Darwinian instinct for survival becomes a will to survive. Motivated by that will, microbes manifest, according to science writer Laurie Garrett, the "ability to outwit or manipulate the one microbial sensing system *Homo sapiens* possess: our immune systems."[18] In medical thrillers about outbreaks, which have proliferated since the early 1990s, microbes that turn hosts into walking viruses have become stock characters. Many of these hosts begin deliberately to seed new outbreaks to avenge what they perceive as a desecrated Earth; they become, that is, ecologically motivated bioterrorists.

The twinning of the threats of devastating communicable disease outbreaks and terrorism find their clearest expression in these figures. The geography of disease applies as well to the geography of terror, with both threats typically viewed as emanating from the South—and, in particular, from formerly colonized locales. They represent the legacy of what the editors refer to in their introduction as "the re-ordering of colonial space" that *Imperial Contagions* addresses: the geopolitical return, in effect, of a colonial repressed.

These narratives have consequences similar to those explored in the essays contained in this volume. Communicable disease and non-state-sponsored violence constitute genuine threats to public health and wellbeing, but the geo-political logic of these narratives shapes the analysis of the threats and, conse-quently, the proposed solutions. The geographies of disease and terror, which suggest that these threats move from South to North, constitute the problems as originating in those locales. Asia is "the perfect incubator"; Africa, as Garrett writes in her widely hailed *The Coming Plague*, is a place in which:

> . . . the Andromeda strain nearly surfaced . . . in the form of Ebola virus; megacities were arising in the developing world, creating niches from which 'virtually anything might arise'; rain forests were being destroyed, forcing disease-carrying animals and insects into areas of human habita-tion and raising the very real possibility that lethal, mysterious microbes

would, for the first time, infect humanity on a large scale and imperil the
survival of the human race.[19]

The May 2003 issue of *Newsweek* that featured articles on the SARS outbreak
reported the "good news" that the material global networks that enabled the
virus to spread around the world had information counterparts that enabled
its containment. If the geography of disease moves from South to North, the
geography of techno-medical expertise, according to accounts such as the
Newsweek articles, moves in the opposite direction.

The concept of primary healthcare that motivated the Declaration of Alma
Ata emerges from an alternative geography of disease. As the healthcare
activist Paul Farmer puts it, "diseases themselves make a preferential option
for the poor," and the conditions of poverty in formerly colonized locations
certainly promote the emergence and spread of communicable disease.[20] But
the Declaration of Alma Ata came out of a global analysis of poverty, which
emphasized the inequitable distribution of resources that produced those conditions of poverty. According to that analysis, the origins of the conditions of
global poverty are complex and multifactorial, and they include the policies
and regulations of global capital that emerge from the alliances of governments and corporations in the North. The idea of primary healthcare is that a
local population is in the best position to determine its own healthcare needs
and terms and that national governments and global healthcare organizations
should work to ensure that populations have access to the resources that would
enable them to address the concerns that they determine to be most relevant
to them.

The nature of the link between poverty and 'terrorism' is less clear than
its shared geography, but, historically, prohibition of self-determination has
yielded large-scale violence, which has been variously interpreted; the labels
attributed to such violence may include *revolution, uprising, terrorism* or any
number of other possibilities that are as likely to reflect the perspective of the
narrator as the nature of the violence. Each term, that is, reflects the standpoint—the figurative and literal location—of the viewer. 'Terrorism' registers a
view from without—typically, at present, like the outbreak narrative, from the
North to the South. The rhetorical link between microbes (and human carriers) and terrorists in the accounts described above illustrates the way geopolitical threats mutually inform each other and distort the nature of both threats as
well as the underlying conditions that give rise to them.

Farmer offers an alternative mapping of disease in which a global align-ment of corporate interests amplifies the conditions of impoverishment that in turn fuel epidemics in *Aids and Accusation: Haiti and the Geography of Blame*. From oral histories, he constructs an account of how an alliance of U.S. cor-porate interests and Haitian elites resulted in the building of the Peligré Dam, which displaced farm communities from arable to non-arable land. The dam thereby helped to create one of Haiti's most impoverished regions. While acts of violence that get labeled 'terrorism' cannot be so directly linked to poverty, a more global analysis, such as the example of the Peligré Dam provides, would similarly offer a more geopolitically distributed analysis of causality. Such an analysis can change the way problems such as disease and violence are con-ceptualized, anticipated, and addressed. While media accounts anticipating an avian flu pandemic typically stress vaccine and drug research and plans for quarantine as the chief means of anticipating that threat, for example, a shift in the understanding of the geopolitics of disease could result in an addi-tional—or alternative—focus, such as the return to the goals of the Declaration of Alma-Ata for which Margaret Chan called in 2008.

Imperial Contagions contributes to that alternative conceptualization by making visible the spatialization of contagion. As cultural geographers have argued, building on the work of Henri Lefebvre, space serves as a grounding term that naturalizes power relations and social hierarchies. Those hierarchies are, however, always evolving, and challenges to them produce anxieties that find expression in a variety of forms, such as fears about contagion. Those fears only work when there is some basis for them. There is genuine reason for concern about impending pandemics of devastating communicable disease, such as avian flu. Indeed, the call to return to the goals of the Declaration of Alma-Ata is in part motivated by the conviction both that such events are inevitable and that a restructured healthcare system would significantly mel-iorate its catastrophic effects. But, as the essays in this volume make clear, the health concerns are inextricably informed by anxieties that attend the desta-bilizing effects of social and geopolitical transformations. With mobility both a threat and a necessity, as the contributions here have shown, anxieties about the management of labor and the preservation of familiar social relations and forms have found and continue to find expression in fears about contagion. Turn-of-the-century concerns about racial purity informed fears about con-tagion—how, that is, space is racialized—and they continue to do so, if not always as explicitly.

Both the Declaration and the concept of primary healthcare that informs it face challenges that are intrinsically spatial. Both work against the assumptions of the geography of disease that maps both the routes of contagion and the idea of expertise in ways that ignore the deeper causes of those routes and the important contribution of local knowledge to the management of health. The spatial logic of the Declaration is, moreover, local in its goals and global in its conceptualization of the problem of healthcare, but nonetheless has to work through nations to achieve those goals. National boundaries are intrinsically at odds with movements of microbes, people, and expertise, and organizations such as the WHO are designed specifically to address those flows. However, global regulation and governance typically lack the means to enforce policies that still belong to national governments. The spatial imaginary of contagion manifests an intrinsic tension between networks and nations, yet, as the essays in *Imperial Contagion* demonstrate, the management of contagion becomes an important logic through which national boundaries and their social relations and hierarchies are reinforced against alternative spatialities.

Understanding these spatial contradictions can help epidemiologists and medical professionals to manage the problem of communicable disease outbreaks more effectively, while making visible the terms that have naturalized geopolitical tensions. Investigating these relations will therefore offer greater insight into the nature and consequences of political anxieties, and the anticipation and management of communicable disease outbreaks. Such investigations can also help to reduce the stigmatizing of individuals, groups, places, and behaviors associated with communicable disease. They might also facilitate a rethinking of the management of communicable disease pandemics. In place of the almost exclusive focus on quarantine and the production of vaccines and pharmaceuticals, for example, the ideas of primary healthcare and health for all arguably offer not only a more humanitarian system of healthcare, but also a more economically sound anticipation of and long-term solution to crises such as pandemics. Nothing is a better vector for a devastating communicable disease than an impoverished population without sufficient access to healthcare. A more just distribution of access to healthcare and an improved standard of living worldwide could create the conditions through which such an emergency would be more easily and effectively addressed.[21]

The study of contagion thus has important lessons to offer about contemporary geopolitics. While poverty correlates more obviously and directly with communicable disease than with terrorism, the metaphorical association between microbes and terror is not incidental. The goals to which the Declaration returns stress self-governance and global cooperation, and they raise the issue of the spatialization of contagion. At the heart of these goals, and of the concepts that they articulate, is a conceptualization of human beings and of human communities that foreground precisely the priorities to which the authors of this volume call our attention. The question that motivates this volume is what we can learn from our inquiry into the spatial imaginary of contagion, not about whether or how we might survive the coming plague, but how we do—and ought—to live together in the networks of the contemporary world.

Notes

Introduction

1. Diarmid A. Finnegan, "The Spatial Turn: Geographical Approaches in the History of Science," *Journal of the History of Biology* 41, no. 2 (2008): 369. See also Simon Naylor, "Introduction: Historical Geographies of Science—Places, Contexts, Cartographies," *British Journal for the History of Science* 38, no. 1 (2005): 1–12; Veronica della Dora, "Making Mobile Knowledges: The Educational Cruises of the *Revue Générale des Sciences Pures et Appliquées, 1897–1914,*" *Isis* 101, no. 3 (2010): 467–500; Peter Meusburger, David N. Livingstone, and Heike Jöns, eds., *Geographies of Science* (Dordrecht and New York: Springer, 2010).

2. Nancy Leys Stepan, *Picturing Tropical Nature* (Ithaca, NY: Cornell University Press, 2001).

3. See Charlotte Furth, "Introduction: Hygienic Modernity in Chinese East Asia," in *Health and Hygiene in Chinese East Asia: Policies and Publics in the Long Twentieth Century*, ed. Angela Ki Che Leung and Charlotte Furth (Durham, NC: Duke University Press, 2010), 2. The volume focuses, for the most part, on towns and villages in Taiwan, Manchuria, Hong Kong, and the Yangzi River delta during the 'long' twentieth century from the late Qing reforms in the 1860s.

4. Ibid.

5. Nicholas Thomas, *Colonialism's Culture: Anthropology, Travel and Government* (Cambridge: Polity, 1994), 2.

6. Anna Lowenhaupt Tsing, *Friction: An Ethnography of Global Connection* (Princeton, NJ: Princeton University Press, 2005).

7. Aldo Castellani, *Climate and Acclimatization: Some Notes and Observations* (London: John Bale, 1931), vii.

8. Ibid.

9. Michael Worboys, *Spreading Germs: Disease Theories and Medical Practice in Britain, 1865–1900* (Cambridge: Cambridge University Press, 2000); "Was There a Bacteriological Revolution in Late Nineteenth-Century Medicine?", *Studies in History and Philosophy of Biological and Biomedical Sciences* 38, no. 1 (2007): 20–42.

10. Daniel R. Headrick, *The Tools of Empire: Technology and European Imperialism in the Nineteenth Century* (New York and Oxford: Oxford University Press, 1981); *The Tentacles of Progress: Technology Transfer in the Age of Imperialism, 1850–1940* (New York: Oxford University Press, 1988); Teresa Meade and Mark Walker, eds., *Science, Medicine and Cultural Imperialism* (New York: St Martin's Press, 1991); Roy MacLeod and Milton Lewis, eds., *Disease, Medicine and Empire: Perspectives on Western Medicine and the Experience of European Expansion* (New York: Routledge, 1988); David Arnold, *Colonizing the Body: State Medicine and Epidemic Disease in Nineteenth-Century India* (Berkeley: University of California Press, 1993).

11. Biswamoy Pati and Mark Harrison, eds., *Health, Medicine and Empire: Perspectives on Colonial India* (Hyderabad: Orient Longman 2001); Sokhieng Au, *Mixed Medicines: Health and Culture in French Colonial Cambodia* (Chicago: University of Chicago Press, 2011).

12. Bruno Latour, *We Have Never Been Modern*, trans. Catherine Porter (Cambridge, MA: Harvard University Press, 1993). Latour borrows the concept of "quasi-object" from Michel Serres. In relation to Latour, bacteria, and colonial agency, Thomas Lamarre observes: "The hybridity of bacterial and national colonies begins with the agency of bacteria and peoples in the colonial network" ; see "Bacterial Cultures and Linguistic Colonies: Mori Rintarō's Experiments with History, Science, and Language," *Positions* 6, no. 3 (1998): 620.

13. Fa-ti Fan, *British Naturalists in Qing China: Science, Empire, and Cultural Encounter* (Cambridge, MA: Harvard University Press, 2004), 64–65.

14. D. A. Griffiths and S. P. Lau, "The Hong Kong Botanical Gardens: A Historical Overview," *Journal of the Royal Asiatic Society Hong Kong Branch* 26 (1986): 58.

15. Ibid., 60.

16. Fan, *British Naturalists in Qing China*, 65.

17. On Ford's annual reports, see Grifftiths and Lau, "The Hong Kong Botanical Gardens," 64–71.

18. Christopher A. Bayly, *Empire and Information: Intelligence Gathering and Social Communication in India, 1780–1870* (Cambridge: Cambridge University Press, 1996).

19. Dwayne R. Winseck and Robert M. Pike, *Communication and Empire: Media, Markets, and Globalization, 1860–1930* (Durham, NC: Duke University Press, 2007); see also Deep Kanta Lahiri Choudhury, *Telegraphic Imperialism: Crisis and Panic in the Indian Empire, c.1830–1920* (Basingstoke: Palgrave Macmillan, 2010).

20. Tony Ballantyne, *Orientalism and Race: Aryanism in the British Empire* (Basingstoke: Palgrave, 2002), 13–17.

21. Alan Lester, *Imperial Networks: Creating Identities in Nineteenth-Century South Africa and Britain* (London and New York: Routledge, 2001); Gary B. Magee and Andrew S. Thompson, *Empire and Globalisation: Networks of People, Goods and Capital in the British World, c.1850–1914* (Cambridge: Cambridge University Press, 2010).

22. Deborah J. Neill, *Networks in Tropical Medicine: Internationalism, Colonialism, and the Rise of a Medical Specialty, 1890–1930* (Stanford: Stanford University Press, 2012).

23. Michael Hardt and Antonio Negri, *Empire* (Cambridge, MA: Harvard University Press, 2000), 135–36.

24. "News in Brief," *Times* [London], June 13, 1894, 5.

25. Heinz-Gerhard Haupt and Jürgen Kocka, eds., *Comparative and Transnational History: Central European Approaches and New Perspectives* (New York: Berghahn, 2009), 53–57; and Ryan Johnson and Amna Khalid, eds. *Public Health in the British Empire: Intermediaries, Subordinates and Public Health Practice, 1850–1960* (London: Routledge, 2011).

26. Larissa N. Heinrich, *The Afterlife of Images: Translating the Pathological Body between China and the West* (Durham, NC: Duke University Press, 2008).

27. Ken De Bevoise, *Agents of Apocalypse: Epidemic Disease in the Colonial Philippines* (Princeton, NJ: Princeton University Press, 1995).

28. See, for example, Miriam R. Levin, Sophie Forgan, Martina Hessler, Robert H. Kargon, and Morris Low, *Urban Modernity: Cultural Innovation in the Second Industrial Revolution* (Cambridge, MA: MIT Press, 2010).

29. Carl Nightingale, *Segregation: A Global History of Divided Cities* (Chicago: University of Chicago Press, 2012).

30. Michael R. Bristow, "Early Town Planning in British South East Asia, 1910–1939," *Planning Perspectives* 15, no. 2 (2000): 139–60.

31. Eric Jennings, "Urban Planning, Architecture, and Zoning at Dalat, Indochina, 1900–1944," *Historical Reflections/Reflexions Historiques* 33, no. 2 (2007): 346; Robert K. Home, *Of Planting and Planning: The Making of British Colonial Cities* (London: E&FN Spon, 1997); Ambe J. Njoh, "Urban Planning as a Tool of Power and Social Control in Colonial Africa," *Planning Perspectives* 24, no. 3 (July 2009): 301–17; Zeynep Celik, *Empire, Architecture and the City: French-Ottoman Encounters, 1830–1914* (Seattle: University of Washington Press, 2008).

32. Ilana Löwy, "Making Plagues Visible: Yellow Fever, Hookworm, and Chagas' Disease, 1900–1950," in *Plagues and Epidemics: Infected Spaces Past and Present*, ed. D. Ann Herring and Alan C. Swedlung (Oxford and New York: Berg, 2010), 270.

33. Ed Cohen, *A Body Worth Defending: Immunity, Biopolitics and the Apotheosis of the Modern Body* (Durham, NC: Duke University Press, 2009).

34. Lamarre, "Bacterial Cultures and Linguistic Colonies," 620. On the relation between bacteriological and colonial cultures, see Heinrich, *The Afterlife of Images*, 155–56. On Korea and Taiwan as 'laboratories,' see Ping-hui Liao and David Der-wei Wang, *Taiwan under Japanese Colonial Rule, 1895–1945: History, Culture, Memory* (New York: Columbia University Press, 2006), 98, 203; and Ramon H. Myers and Mark R. Peattie, *The Japanese Colonial Empire, 1895–1945* (Princeton, NJ: Princeton University Press, 1987), 16, 84, 85.

35. Warwick Anderson, *Colonial Pathologies: American Tropical Medicine, Race, and Hygiene in the Philippines* (Durham, NC: Duke University Press, 2006), 111–14;

"Excremental Colonialism: Public Health and the Poetics of Pollution," in *Contagion: Historical and Cultural Studies*, ed. Alison Bashford and Claire Hooker (London and New York: Routledge, 2001), 85.

36. Ruth Rogaski, *Hygienic Modernity: Meanings of Health and Disease in Treaty-Port China* (Berkeley: University of California Press, 2004), 260.

37. Lenore Manderson, *Sickness and the State: Health and Illness in Colonial Malaya, 1870–1940* (Cambridge: Cambridge University Press, 1996); G. M. van Heteren, M. J. D. Poulissen, A. de Knecht-van Eekelen, and A. M. Luyendijk-Elshout, eds., *Dutch Medicine in the Malay Archipelago, 1816–1942* (Amsterdam: Rodopi, 1989).

38. Laurence Monnais-Rousselot, "'Modern Medicine' in French Colonial Vietnam: From the Importation of a Model to its Nativisation," in *The Development of Modern Medicine in Non-Western Countries*, ed. Hormoz Ebrahimnejad (London: Routledge, 2008), 130–32; *Médecine et colonisation. L'aventure Indochinoise, 1860–1939* (Paris: CRNS Editions, 1999).

39. Peter Zinoman, *The Colonial Bastille: A History of Imprisonment in Vietnam, 1862–1940* (Berkeley: University of California Press, 2001), 4–7.

40. Gwendolyn Wright, *The Politics of Design in French Colonial Urbanism* (Chicago: University of Chicago Press, 1991).

41. Roy MacLeod, "Scientific Advice for British India: Imperial Perceptions and Administrative Goals, 1898–1923," *Modern Asian Studies* 9, no. 3 (1975): 343–84. See also Thomas R. Metcalf, *The New Cambridge History of India, Vol. 4: Ideologies of the Raj* (Cambridge: Cambridge University Press, 1995). As Paul Rabinow has remarked, the colonies are a "laboratory of experimentation for new arts of government capable of bringing a modern and healthy society into being" (Paul Rabinow, *French Modern: Norms and Forms of the Social Environment* [Cambridge, MA: MIT, 1989], 289).

42. Frederick Cooper and Ann Laura Stoler, eds., *Tensions of Empire: Colonial Cultures in the Bourgeois World* (Berkeley: University of California Press, 1997), 5.

43. Patricia A. Morton, *Hybrid Modernities: Architecture and Representation at the 1931 Colonial Exposition, Paris* (Cambridge, MA: MIT Press, 2000), 5.

44. William S. Logan, *Hanoi: Biography of a City* (Seattle: University of Washington Press, 2000), 99–110.

45. Anthony D. King, "Colonial Cities: Global Pivots of Change," in *Colonial Cities: Essays on Urbanism in a Colonial Context*, ed. R.J. Ross and G.J. Telkamp (Dordrecht: Martinus Nijhoff, 1985), 12.

46. Wright, *The Politics of Design in French Colonial Urbanism*, 306–7.

47. Although, as James Clifford has argued, travel and "intercultural connection" are not the exception, but the norm; see *Routes: Travel and Translation in the Late Twentieth Century* (Cambridge, MA: Harvard University Press, 1997), 5.

48. See, however, the arguments made for reconsidering scientific practices in relation to both the local and the global in Leung and Furth, eds., *Health and Hygiene in Chinese East Asia*.

49. On colonial medicine and transnational themes, see Anne Digby, Waltrud Ernst and Projit B. Mukharji, eds., *Crossing Colonial Historiographies: Histories of Colonial and Indigenous Medicine in Transnational Perspective* (Newcastle: Cambridge Scholars, 2010).

50. Bashford and Hooker, *Contagion: Historical and Cultural Studies*; Priscilla Wald, *Contagious: Cultures, Carriers, and the Outbreak Narrative* (Durham, NC: Duke University Press, 2008).

51. Nightingale, *Segregation Is Everywhere.*

52. Jennings, "Urban Planning"; Michael G. Vann, "Of Rats, Rice and Race: The Great Hanoi Rat Massacre, an Episode in French Colonial History," *French Colonial History* 4 (2003): 191–203; Michael R. Bristow, "Early Town Planning in British South East Asia: 1910–1939," *Planning Perspectives* 15, no. 2 (2000): 139–60.

Chapter 1   Combating Nuisance

*   The author would like to thank Mishko Hansen and Marilyn Novell for their support and critical comments on this chapter.

1.   Philippa Levine, "Modernity, Medicine, and Colonialism: The Contagious Diseases Ordinances in Hong Kong and the Straits Settlements," *Positions* 6, no. 3 (Winter 1998): 681–682.

2.   For an overview of the history of racial segregation in British colonial cities, see Robert Home, "'The Inconvenience Felt by Europeans': Racial Segregation, its Rise and Fall," in *Of Planting and Planning: The Making of British Colonial Cities* (London: E & FN Spon, 1997), 117–40.

3.   For just a few examples, see Jyoti Hosagraher, *Indigenous Modernities: Negotiating Architecture and Urbanism* (London and New York: Routledge, 2005); Brenda Yeoh, *Contesting Space in Colonial Singapore: Power and Space in the Urban Built Environment* (Singapore: Singapore University Press, 2003); William Glover, *Making Lahore Modern: Constructing and Imagining a Colonial City* (Minneapolis: University of Minnesota Press, 2008); and McFarlane, "Governing the Contaminated City: Infrastructure and the Sanitation in Colonial and Post-Colonial Bombay," *International Journal of Urban and Regional Research* 32, no. 2 (June 2008): 413–35.

4.   Hosagrahar, *Indigenous Modernities*, 6–7.

5.   See Frederick Cooper's critique on this subject, in *Colonialism in Question: Theory, Knowledge, History* (Berkeley: University of California Press, 2005), 3–32.

6.   Christopher Hamlin, *Public Health and Social Justice in the Age of Chadwick: Britain, 1800–1854* (Cambridge: Cambridge University Press, 1998), 2–15.

7.   For a discussion of the reception of Western medicine in colonial territories, see Roy Macleod and Milton Lewis, *Diseases, Medicine, and Empire: Perspectives on Western Medicine and the Experience of European Expansion* (London and New York: Routledge, 1988); and Myron Echenberg, *Plague Ports: The Global Urban Impact of Bubonic Plague, 1894–1901* (New York and London: New York University Press, 2007).

8. David Scott, "Colonial Governmentality," in *Anthropologies of Modernity: Foucault, Governmentality and Life Politics*, ed. Jonathan Zavier Inda (Oxford: Blackwell, 2005), 39.

9. Here I am referring to communities with shared sets of beliefs and knowledge that have established themselves as power blocs, seeking to influence policy-making. For a formal definition of the term, see Peter Haas and Emanuel Adler, "Do Regimes Matter? Epistemic Communities and Mediterranean Pollution Control," *International Organization* 43, no. 3 (1992): 377–403.

10. Emery Evans, "The Foundation of Hong Kong: A Chapter of Accidents" in *Hong Kong: The Interaction of Traditions and Life in the Towns*, ed. Marjorie Topley (Hong Kong: Hong Kong Branch of the Royal Asiatic Society, 1975), 1–41.

11. For an explanation of Hong Kong's early land policies and the leasehold system, see Robert Nissim, *Land Administration and Practice in Hong Kong* (Hong Kong: Hong Kong University Press, 2008), 3–15; and Christopher Munn, *Anglo-China: Chinese People and British Rule in Hong Kong, 1841–1880* (Richmond, Surrey: Curzon, 2001), 89–98.

12. E. G. Pryor, *Housing in Hong Kong* (Oxford and New York: Oxford University Press, 1983), 8–13; Frank Leeming, *Street Studies in Hong Kong: Localities in a Chinese City* (Hong Kong and New York: Oxford University Press, 1977), 20–27.

13. For a discussion of urban development in early Hong Kong and the patterns of Chinese property ownership, see Carl Smith, *A Sense of History: Studies in the Social and Urban History of Hong Kong* (Hong Kong: Hong Kong Educational Publishing, 1995), 38–49.

14. Successive waves of refugees were driven to Hong Kong during the Taiping Rebellion, which lasted from 1851 to 1864.

15. For an overview of the 'invasion' of Chinese houses in this period, see Pope Hennessy to Earl of Carnarvon, September 27, 1877; and Surveyor General to Colonial Secretary, May 8, 1877, Enclosure 1 in No. 1, *China. British Parliamentary Papers: Correspondence, Dispatches, Reports, Returns, Memorials and other Papers Respecting the Affairs of Hong Kong 1862–81*, vol. 25 (Shannon: Irish University Press, 1971), 647–51.

16. "Report of the Colonial Surgeon on His Inspection of the Town of Victoria, and on the Pig-Licensing System," April 1874, Enclosure in No. 29, *British Parliamentary Papers*, 701.

17. "Statement of His Excellency Governor Sir John Pope Hennessy, K.C.M.G., on the Census Returns and the Progress of the Colony," Enclosure 2 in No. 42, Legislative Council, Hong Kong, 1881, *House of Common Papers* LXV, 42, Public Record Office, Kew, London (hereafter PRO).

18. For Pope Hennessy's policy agenda, see Kate Lowe and Eugene McLaughlin, "Sir John Pope Hennessy and the 'Native Race Craze': Colonial Government in Hong Kong, 1877–1882," *Journal of Imperial and Commonwealth History* 20, no. 2 (May 1992): 223–47.

19. "Insanitary Houses in Hong Kong," surveyor general to colonial secretary, March 23, 1878, Enclosure D in No. 45, *British Parliamentary Papers*, 750–51.

20. Ibid.

21. Ibid.

22. "Chinese Houses," *Hongkong Government Gazette*, July 27, 1878, 370–72.

23. Ibid., 371.

24. Ibid.

25. For a discussion of the problems associated with drainage and water supply in this period, see Martin V. Melosi, *The Sanitary City: Environmental Services in Urban America from Colonial Times to the Present* (Pittsburgh, PA: University of Pittsburgh Press, 2008); and Patrick Joyce, "The Water and the Blood of the City: Naturalising the Governed," in *The Rule of Freedom: Liberalism and the Modern City* (London and New York: Verso, 2003), 62–97.

26. Chadwick, *Report on the Sanitary Condition of Hong Kong*, CO882/4; and "Report on the Sanitary Condition of Hongkong," *Papers Laid Before the Legislative Council of Hongkong*, April 10, 1902, 3–5.

27. Osbert Chadwick, "Part II, Section 5: Water Supply," *Report on the Sanitary Condition of Hong Kong*, 1882, Great Britain, Colonial Office, Series 882, CO882/4, 76–8, PRO; Francis A. Cooper, "Water and Drainage Department Report for the Year 1891," *Papers Laid Before the Legislative Council of Hongkong*, January 13, 1892, 119–124.

28. Chadwick, "Part II, Section 5: Water Supply," *Report of the Sanitary Condition of Hong Kong*, 1882, PRO; "Report on the Sanitary Condition of Hongkong," April 10, 1902, 3.

29. Ibid.

30. Ibid.

31. "Report of the Meeting of the Legislative Council," *Papers Laid Before the Legislative Council of Hongkong*, June 23, 1902, 28–29.

32. Joyce, *Rule of Freedom*, 70.

33. Lord Kimberley to Hennessy, August 20, 1881, *British Parliamentary Papers*, vol. 25, 759–60.

34. Chadwick, *Report of the Sanitary Condition of Hongkong*.

35. Chadwick, *Preliminary Report on the Sanitary Condition of Hongkong*, April 10, 1902, 2–18.

36. "Ordinance 29 of 1902, Waterworks Consolidation," Gascoigne to Chamberlain, August 29, 1902, CO129/312, 280–89.

37. "The Humble Petition of the undersigned Chinese Inhabitants and Firms of Hong Kong on behalf of themselves and their fellow Countrymen residing Thereat," August 29, 1902, Enclosure 3, CO129/312, 291–93, PRO.

38. Ibid., 293.

39. Ibid., 292.

40. "Water Ordinance," October 2, 1902, CO129/312, 347, PRO.

41. The term "resumption" refers to the exercise of eminent domain, where the government takes possession of a private property with due monetary compensation to the owner, but without the latter's consent.

42. For an overview of plague outbreaks and responses to them in non-European territories, see Echenberg, *Plague Ports*. For a primary account of the bubonic plague in Hong Kong, see report by Governor William Robinson, *Annual Report for 1894*, No. 148, Hong Kong, 3–10. For secondary sources, see Echenberg, "An Unexampled Calamity: Hong Kong, 1894," in *Plague Ports*, 16–46; Mary Sutphen, "Not What, but Where: Bubonic Plague and the Reception of Germ Theories in Hong Kong and Calcutta, 1894–1897," *Journal of the History of Medicine* 52 (January 1977): 81–113; E.G. Pryor, "The Great Plague of Hong Kong," *Journal of the Royal Asiatic Society* 15 (1975): 61–70; Arthur E. Starling et al., eds., *Plague, SARS and the Story of Medicine in Hong Kong* (Hong Kong: Hong Kong University Press, 2006), 26–37.

43. Robinson to Chamberlain, July 10, 1895, *British Parliamentary Papers*, vol. 26, 437.

44. Sutphen, "Not What, but Where," 94–103.

45. "Sanitary Improvement of Taipingshan," October 1, 1894, CO 129/263, 741–42, PRO.

46. See the frequent editorials on this subject in the *Hongkong Telegraph* and the *Hongkong Daily Press* between May 1894 to May 1895.

47. Granville Sharp, "Plague and Prevention," Nos. 1 to 13, *Hongkong Daily Press*, July 30–August 17, 1894.

48. Ibid., August 17, 1894.

49. Ibid., August 13, 1894.

50. "Report of the Meeting of the Legislative Council," September 17, 1894, *Papers Laid before the Legislative Council of Hongkong*, 60–68.

51. The unofficial members of the Legislative Council have always been drawn from the largest commercial enterprises in Hong Kong. For a discussion on the organization of the council, see Norman Miner, *Hong Kong Under Imperial Rule: 1912–1941* (Hong Kong: Oxford University Press, 1987).

52. A full list of Taipingshan property owners was published in the *Hongkong Daily Press*, March 11, 1895.

53. For a discussion of Ho Kai's life and career, see G. H. Choa, *The Life and Times of Sir Kai Ho Kai* (Hong Kong: Chinese University Press, 1981).

54. "Report on the Meeting of the Legislative Council," September 17, 1894, *Papers Laid before the Legislative Council of Hongkong*, 66–68.

55. "Taipingshan Resumption Ordinance," October 1, 1894, CO 129/263, 729–42, PRO; "Taipingshan Resumption Ordinance," October 22, 1894, CO 129/264, 127–34, PRO; and "Taipingshan Resumed Area," CO 129/266, 588–99, PRO.

56. "Rents Memorial from Certain Persons," April 1, 1895, CO129/266, 373–98, PRO.

57. Ibid., 376.

58. Ibid., 377–78.

59. Ibid.

Chapter 2   'Tropicalizing' Planning

1. "Insanitary Singapore," *Straits Times*, September 13, 1910.
2. I am following in this chapter the British colonial administrators' use of "native" to refer to not just the indigenous Malay population but also the Chinese and Indian immigrant population.
3. See "Insanitary Singapore."
4. Martin V. Melosi, *The Sanitary City: Urban Infrastructure in America from Colonial Times to the Present* (Baltimore, MD: Johns Hopkins University Press, 2000), 28–39.
5. Jiat-Hwee Chang, "Tropicalising Technologies of Environment and Government: The Singapore General Hospital and the Circulation of the Pavilion Plan Hospital in the British Empire, 1860–1930," in *Re-Shaping Cities: How Global Mobility Transforms Architecture and Urban Form*, ed. Michael Guggenheim and Ola Söderström (London: Routledge, 2009), 123–42; Mark Harrison, *Public Health in British India: Anglo-Indian Preventive Medicine 1859–1914* (Cambridge: Cambridge University Press, 1994), 60–98.
6. Douglas Melvin Haynes, "The Social Production of Metropolitan Expertise in Tropical Diseases: The Imperial State, Colonial Service and Tropical Diseases Research Fund," *Science, Technology & Society* 4, no. 2 (1999): 205–38.
7. Ronald Ross, *Report of the Malaria Expedition to West Coast of Africa 1899* (Liverpool: Liverpool School of Tropical Medicine, 1900); W. J. Simpson, *Report on Sanitary Matters in Various West African Colonies and the Outbreak of Plague in the Gold Coast, Presented to Parliament by Command of His Majesty* (London: His Majesty's Stationery Office, 1909); Mary Sutphen, "Not What, but Where: Bubonic Plague and the Reception of Germ Theories in Hong Kong and Calcutta, 1894–1897," *Journal of the History of Medicine* 52 (1997): 81–113.
8. See, for example, Birendra Nath Ghosh and Jahar Lal Das, *A Treatise on Hygiene and Public Health, with Special Reference to the Tropics*, 2nd ed. (Calcutta: Hilton and Co., 1914); W. J. Simpson, *The Principles of Hygiene as Applied to Tropical and Sub-Tropical Climates* (London: John Bale, Sons & Danielsson, 1908).
9. Anderson to Lyttelton, September 12, 1905, Great Britain, Colonial Office, Series 273, CO 273/310, Public Record Office, Kew, London (hereafter PRO); "Improving Singapore: Measures for Compulsory Resumption," *Straits Times*, July 13, 1907.
10. "The Calcutta Improvement Trust," *Garden Cities & Town Planning, incorporating the Housing Reformer* 6, no. 5 (1921): 113; Prashant Kidambi, "Housing the Poor in a Colonial City: The Bombay Improvement Trust, 1898–1918," *Studies in History* 17, no. 1 (2001): 58.
11. This phrase was used to describe the notion of colonial mimicry in Homi K. Bhabha, *The Location of Culture* (London: Routledge, 2004 [1994]).
12. See, for example, Jyoti Hosagrahar, *Indigenous Modernities: Negotiating Architecture and Urbanism* (London and New York: Routledge, 2005); Abidin Kusno, *Behind the Postcolonial: Architecture, Urban Space, and Political Cultures in Indonesia* (New

York: Routledge, 2000); Joe Nasr and Mercedes Volait, eds., *Urbanism Imported or Exported? Native Aspirations and Foreign Plans* (Chichester: Wiley-Academy, 2003). See also Dipesh Chakrabarty, *Provincializing Europe: Postcolonial Thought and Historical Difference* (Princeton: Princeton University Press, 2000).

13. See, for example, Richard Harris, "Development and Hybridity Made Concrete in the Colonies," *Environment and Planning A* 40 (2008): 15–36; Felipe Hernández, "Introduction: Transcultural Architectures in Latin America," in *Transculturation: Cities, Spaces and Architectures in Latin America*, ed. Felipe Hernández, Mark Millington, and Iain Borden (New York: Rodopi, 2005), ix–xxv.

14. Duanfang Lu, "Travelling Urban Form: The Neighbourhood Unit in China," *Planning Perspectives* 21, no. 4 (2006): 369–92.

15. Stephen J. Collier and Aihwa Ong, "Global Assemblages, Anthropological Problems," in *Global Assemblages: Technology, Politics, and Ethics as Anthropological Problems*, ed. Aihwa Ong and Stephen J. Collier (Malden, MA: Blackwell Publishing, 2005), 11.

16. Ibid., 10.

17. Michel Foucault, "Governmentality," in *The Foucault Effect: Studies in Governmentality*, ed. Michel Foucault et al. (Chicago: University of Chicago Press, 1991), 100.

18. Michel Foucault, *Society Must Be Defended: Lectures at the College De France, 1975–76*, trans. David Macey (New York: Picador, 2003), 241. It is also translated as "*foster* life or *disallow* it" in Michel Foucault, *The History of Sexuality: An Introduction, Volume 1*, trans. Robert Hurley (New York: Vintage, 1990 [1978]), 138.

19. Paul Rabinow and Nikolas S. Rose, "Introduction," in *The Essential Foucault: Selections from Essential Works of Foucault, 1954-1984*, ed. Paul Rabinow and Nikolas S. Rose (New York: New Press, 2003), xv–xvii.

20. Ibid.; and Paul Rabinow, *Anthropos Today: Reflections on Equipment* (Princeton: Princeton University Press, 2003), 49–54.

21. Ibid., xvi.

22. Gyan Prakash, *Another Reason: Science and the Imagination of Modern India* (Princeton: Princeton University Press, 1999), 125.

23. David Arnold, *The Problem of Nature: Environment, Culture and European Expansion* (Oxford: Blackwell, 1996), 141–68.

24. The seminal study on Simpson's report in relation to sanitary improvement and town planning in colonial Singapore is Brenda S. A. Yeoh, *Contesting Space: Power Relations and the Urban Built Environment in Colonial Singapore* (Kuala Lumpur: Oxford University Press, 1996). My chapter is of course indebted to Professor Yeoh's study although my focus is different and I deploy different theoretical frameworks.

25. Sutphen, "Not What, but Where"; Malcolm Watson and Mary Sutphen, "Simpson, Sir William John Ritchie," in *Oxford Dictionary of National Biography* (Oxford: Oxford University Press, 2004); R. A. Baker and R. A. Bayliss, "William John Ritchie Simpson (1855–1931): Public Health and Tropical Medicine," *Medical History* (1987) 31: 450–465.

26. Patrick Joyce, *The Rule of Freedom: Liberalism and the Modern City* (London: Verso, 2003).

27. W. J. Simpson, *The Sanitary Conditions of Singapore* (London: Waterlow, 1907), 7.

28. Nikolas S. Rose, *Powers of Freedom: Reframing Political Thought* (Cambridge: Cambridge University Press, 1999), 203.

29. Yeoh, *Contesting Space*, 104.

30. For maps, see Joyce, *Rule of Freedom*, 35–56; Rose, *Powers of Freedom*, 36–40.

31. Simpson, *Sanitary Conditions of Singapore*, 29.

32. Robert Bruegmann, "Architecture of the Hospital: 1770–1870" (unpublished Ph.D. dissertation, University of Pennsylvania, 1976); Anthony D. King, "Hospital Planning: Revised Thoughts on the Origin of the Pavilion Principle in England," *Medical History* 10, no. 6 (1966): 360–73.

33. Jiat-Hwee Chang and Anthony D. King, "Towards a Genealogy of 'Tropical Architecture': Historical Fragments of Power-Knowledge, Built Environment, and Climate in the British Colonial Territories," *Singapore Journal of Tropical Geography* 32, no. 3 (2011): 283–300.

34. See, for example, Ronald Ross, *Report on the Prevention of Malaria in Mauritius* (London: J & A Churchill, 1908).

35. Simpson, *Principles of Hygiene*, 305.

36. Cited in William Atkinson, *The Orientation of Buildings or Planning for Sunlight* (New York: John Wiley & Sons, 1912), 1.

37. Felix Driver, "Moral Geographies: Social Science and the Urban Environment in Mid-Nineteenth Century England," *Transactions of the Institute of British Geographers* 13, no. 3 (1988): 275–87.

38. The RIBA Joint Committee on the Orientation of Buildings, *The Orientation of Buildings, Being the Report with Appendices of the Riba Joint Committee on the Orientation of Buildings* (London: RIBA, 1933), 3.

39. Atkinson, *Orientation of Buildings*.

40. Raymond Unwin, *Town Planning in Practice: An Introduction to the Art of Designing City* (New York: Benjamin Blom, 1971[1909]), 310–13.

41. Bruno Latour, *Science in Action: How to Follow Scientists and Engineers through Society* (Cambridge, MA: Harvard University Press, 1987).

42. Singapore Housing Commission, *Proceedings and Report of the Commission Appointed to Inquire into the Cause of the Present Housing Difficulties in Singapore and the Steps Which Should Be Taken to Remedy Such Difficulties*, vol. 1 (Singapore: Government Printing Office, 1918), A9.

43. E. P. Richards, "Appendix H, Improvement Trust for Singapore: Report by Deputy Chairman, May to December 1920," in *Administration Report of the Singapore Municipality for the Year 1920* (Singapore: Straits Times Press, 1921), 125–27.

44. Robert K. Home, *Of Planting and Planning: The Making of British Colonial Cities* (London: E&FN Spon, 1997), 81.

45. H. V. Lanchester, "Calcutta Improvement Trust: Précis of Mr. E. P. Richards' Report on the City of Calcutta, Part I," *Town Planning Review* 5, no. 2 (1914): 115–30; H.V.

Lanchester, "Calcutta Improvement Trust: Précis of Mr. E. P. Richards' Report on the City of Calcutta, Part II," *Town Planning Review* 5, no. 3 (1914): 214–24; H.V. Lanchester, "Notes on the Calcutta Report of Mr E. P. Richards, Summarised in Nos. 2 and 3 of Vol. V," *Town Planning Review* 6, no. 1 (1915): 27–40.

46. Patrick Abercombie, "Town Planning Literature: A Brief Summary of Its Present Extent," *Town Planning Review* 6, no. 2 (1915): 93.

47. E. P. Richards, "Appendix E, Improvement Trust for Singapore: Report for 1921 by Deputy Chairman," in *Administration Report of the Singapore Municipality for the Year 1921* (Singapore: Straits Times Press, 1922), 101.

48. There were different accounts of why Richards resigned. One held that he was in the bad books of the president of the municipal commissioners. See Han Hoe Tan, "A Study of Singapore Slum Problem, 1907–41: With Special Reference to the Singapore Improvement Trust" (unpublished academic exercise, University of Malaya, 1959), 24. Another noted that Richards was "[l]ike all planning pioneers . . . regarded as an unrealistic dreamer and . . . gave up the unequal struggle." J.M. Fraser cited in Home, *Of Planting and Planning*, 84.

49. See, for example, Joyce, *Rule of Freedom*; Latour, *Science in Action*.

50. Richards, "Appendix H, Improvement Trust for Singapore: Report by Deputy Chairman, May to December 1920," 126.

51. Ibid.

52. W. H. Collyer, "Appendix B, Improvement Trust for Singapore: Report for 1924 by Deputy Chairman," in *Administration Report of the Singapore Municipality for the Year 1924* (Singapore: Straits Times Press, 1925), 1–12; W. H. Collyer, "Appendix B, Singapore Improvement Trust," in *Administration Report of the Singapore Municipality for the Year 1925* (Singapore: Straits Times Press, 1926), 1–35.

53. The 1918 Report describes the data from the colonial decennial censuses as "estimating in a very high form." Commission, *Report of the Commission on Housing Difficulties*, A3.

54. Collyer, "Singapore Improvement Trust 1925," 28.

55. Ibid., 3.

56. See the ordinance "Town Planning in Malaya" in PRO CO273/539, 1.

57. J. M. Fraser, *The Work of the Singapore Improvement Trust 1927–1947* (Singapore: Singapore Improvement Trust, 1948), 4.

58. *Report of the Housing Committee Singapore, 1947* (Singapore: Government Printing Office, 1947), 48.

59. Fraser, *Work of the Singapore Improvement Trust 1927–1947*, 6.

60. See, for example, the Health Officer's reports on Victoria Street, Nos. 256, 258, 260, 262, 264, National Archives of Singapore (NAS), Housing Development Board (HDB), Singapore Improvement Trust (SIT), HDB1079 SIT29/8, 27.

61. Fraser, *Work of the Singapore Improvement Trust 1927–1947*, 6.

62. Tan, "Study of Singapore Slum Problem, 1907–41," 35–36.

63. "Clearing Singapore Slums: Report on Home Policy," *Straits Times*, April 29, 1936.

64. "Rehousing Slum Tenants," *Straits Times*, May 18, 1936.

65. "Eastern Slums and Western Cities," *Straits Times*, May 4, 1936.
66. "Weisburg Building Policy Report," NAS HDB1061 SIT70/41, 3.
67. Ibid., 6.
68. "Singapore's Housing Problem: Mr. W.H. Collyer's Lecture," *Straits Times*, July 12, 1930.
69. "History and Development of Tiong Bahru Estate," NAS HDB1080 SIT744, 50
70. "Steel Windows for Tiong Bahru," NAS HDB1079 SIT242, 35.
71. "Bomb-Proof Shelters for New Blocks of Flats," *Straits Times*, June 28, 1939; "Tiong Bahru Flats Will House 1000 by End of 1938," *Straits Times*, October 13, 1937.
72. James M. Fraser and Lincoln Page, "Singapore Improvement Trust, 1950 Programme: Two Blocks of Flats and Shops Tiong Bahru Road, Singapore," *The Quarterly Journal of the Institute of Architects of Malaya* 1, no. 2 (1951): 37–42.
73. Collyer, "Singapore Improvement Trust 1925"; "Housing Scheme at Henderson Road," NAS HDB1003 SIT148/25.
74. "Bad Housing and Disease," *Straits Times*, October 4, 1932; "Improvement Trust Housing Off Lavender Street," NAS HDB1079 SIT582/25.
75. Home, *Of Planting and Planning*, 113.
76. "Amended Layout of Lavender Street Housing Scheme," NAS HDB1080 SIT28/26.
77. "Trust to Build Detached Two-Storey Houses," *Straits Times*, November 13, 1940.
78. Fraser, *Work of the Singapore Improvement Trust 1927–1947*, 10.
79. "A Healthier Singapore," *The Malayan Architect* 5, no. 5 (1933): 107.
80. Ibid.
81. *Attap* is the Malay word for the palm leaves used for the roofing of these houses. These are traditional houses commonly found throughout the Malay Peninsula, especially in the Malay villages or *kampongs*.
82. *Report of the Housing Committee Singapore, 1947*, 7.
83. For the Victorian origin of such an argument, see Robin Evans, "Rookeries and Moral Dwellings: English Housing Reform and the Moralities of Private Space," in *Translations from Drawing to Building and Other Essays* (London: Architectural Associations, 1997), 93–118.
84. See, for example, "Housing Position Has Reached a Dangerous Point," *Straits Times*, November 6, 1937; "Just Another Report?" *Straits Times*, August 18, 1948.
85. Matthew Gandy, "Planning, Anti-Planning and the Infrastructure Crisis Facing Metropolitan Lagos," *Urban Studies* 43 (2006): 371–96; Colin McFarlane, "Governing the Contaminated City: Infrastructure and Sanitation in Colonial and Post-Colonial Bombay," *International Journal of Urban and Regional Research* 32, no. 2 (2008): 415–35; Vijay Prashad, "The Technology of Sanitation in Colonial Delhi," *Modern Asian Studies* 35, no. 1 (2001): 113–55; Awadhendra Sharan, "In the City, Out of Place: Environment and Modernity, Delhi 1860s to 1960s," *Economic and Political Weekly* 41, no. 25 (2006): 4905–11.
86. "A Beneficial Epidemic," *Eastern Daily Mail and Straits Morning Advertiser*, May 3, 1906.
87. "Editorial," *Straits Times*, July 4, 1907.

88. For the case of colonial Singapore, see Jiat-Hwee Chang, *No Boundaries: The Lien Villas Collective* (Singapore: Pesaro, 2010), 33–34; Henry Probert, *The History of Changi* (Singapore: Changi University Press, 2006 [1965]).

89. See, for example, Swati Chattopadhyay, *Representing Calcutta: Modernity, Nationalism, and the Colonial Uncanny* (London: Routledge, 2005); William Glover, *Making Lahore Modern: Constructing and Imagining a Colonial City* (Minneapolis: University of Minnesota Press, 2008).

90. Anthony D. King, *Colonial Urban Development: Culture, Social Power, and Environment* (London: Routledge & Kegan Paul, 1976). For the idea of a medical and sanitary enclave in a colonial city, see also Chang, "Tropicalising Technologies of Environment and Government."

91. Cited in McFarlane, "Governing the Contaminated City," 419. On a related note, David Arnold has argued that the medicalization of the population in British India during the nineteenth century was initially restricted to specific socio-spatial enclaves, where grids of intelligibility through medically knowing, evaluating, and intervening in the lives of the inhabitants could be attained. David Arnold, *Colonizing the Body: State Medicine and Epidemic Disease in Nineteenth-Century India* (Berkeley: University of California Press, 1993), 28.

92. Home, *Of Planting and Planning*.

93. "Report of the Gillman Commission," CO273/538, 3, PRO; J. F. F., "Changi Cantonment 1933–1937," *Royal Engineers Journal* 51 (1937): 355–62; L. N. Malan, "Singapore: The Founding of the New Defences," *Royal Engineers Journal* 52 (1938): 213–35; "Correspondence Relating to the Provision of Barrack Accommodation at the Straits Settlements," 1896, WO33/56, PRO.

94. "Military Contribution," PRO CO273/546, 6; Walter Makepeace, "The Military Contribution," in *One Hundred Years of Singapore*, ed. Walter Makepeace, Gilbert E. Brooke, and Roland St. J. Braddell (Singapore: Oxford University Press, 1991 [1921]); Cecil C. Smith, "Military Contribution," in *Proceedings of the Legislative Council of the Straits Settlements for the Year 1891* (Singapore: Straits Settlements Government Printing Office, 1892), C3–C8.

95. Harumi Goto-Shibata, "Empire on the Cheap: The Control of Opium Smoking in the Straits Settlements, 1925–1939," *Modern Asian Studies* 40, no. 1 (2006): 59–80.

96. Mitchell Dean, *Governmentality: Power and Rule in Modern Society* (London: Sage, 1999).

97. Prakash, *Another Reason*, 123–58. See also James S. Duncan, *In the Shadows of the Tropics: Climate, Race and Biopower in Nineteenth Century Ceylon* (Aldershot: Ashgate, 2007); Peter Redfield, "Foucault in the Tropics: Displacing the Panopticon," in *Anthropologies of Modernity*, ed. Jonathan Xavier Inda (Malden, MA: Blackwell, 2005).

98. Ann Laura Stoler, *Race and the Education of Desire: Foucault's History of Sexuality and the Colonial Order of Things* (Durham: Duke University Press, 1995).

99. Foucault, *Society Must Be Defended*, 254.

100. "Colony Cavalcade: Another Chinatown Tour—the Brighter Side from the Back-Yard—Lanes in Human Antheaps," *Straits Times*, May 24, 1936.

101. "Another Big Step Forward in Slum Clearance Scheme," *Straits Times*, July 2, 1937; "From Hovels to Modern Housing in Singapore," *Straits Times*, July 3, 1937.

102. See also David Cannadine, *Ornamentalism: How the British Saw Their Empire* (Oxford: Oxford University Press, 2007).

Chapter 3   Colonial Anxiety Counted

*   The authors thank Trevor Barnes, Robert Peckham, and David Pomfret for comments on a first draft. The research for this chapter was supported by the Social Sciences and Humanities Research Council of Canada.

1. The browsing that unearthed the censuses was guided by Partho Datta, to whom we owe thanks. See also the "incredulous" comment by Kingsley Davis in *The Population of India and Pakistan* (New York: Russel and Russel, 1951), 4.

2. On the urban impact of and colonial responses to the so-called Third Plague Pandemic, see Myron Echenberg, *Plague Ports: The Global Urban Impact of Bubonic Plague, 1894–1901* (New York: New York University Press, 2007).

3. C. A. Bayly, *Empire and Information: Intelligence Gathering and Social Communication in India, 1780–1870* (Cambridge: Cambridge University Press, 2000).

4. However, on the unforeseen consequences of these technologies, see D. K. Lahiri-Choudhury, *Telegraphic Imperialism: Crisis and Panic in the Indian Empire, c.1830–1920* (Basingstoke: Palgrave Macmillan, 2010).

5. Arjun Appadurai, "Number in the Colonial Imagination," in *Orientalism and the Postcolonial Predicament: Perspectives in South Asia*, ed. C.A. Breckenridge and P. van der Veer (Philadelphia: University of Pennsylvania Press, 1993), 316.

6. Bernard Cohn, "Introduction," in *Colonialism and Its Forms of Knowledge: The British in India*, ed. Bernard Cohn (Princeton, NJ: Princeton University Press, 1996), 8.

7. Margo Anderson, *The American Census: A Social History* (New Haven: Yale University Press, 1988), 85. Also see Matthew Hannah, *Governmentality and the Mastery of Territory in Nineteenth-Century America* (New York: Cambridge University Press, 2000), 114–49.

8. Roger Owen, "The Population Census of 1917 and its Relationship to Egypt's Three 19th Century Statistical Regimes," *Journal of Historical Sociology* 9, no. 4 (1996): 457–72.

9. T. S. Weir, *Census of the City and Island of Bombay Taken on the 17th of February, 1881* (Bombay: Times of India Steam Press, 1883).

10. H. Maguire, *Report on the Census of Calcutta Taken on the 26th of February 1891* (Calcutta: Bengal Secretariat Press, 1891).

11. Calculated from Census of India, 1901. Vol. 7 [J. R. Blackwood] *Census of Calcutta. Town and Suburbs. Part II. Report (Administrative)* (Calcutta: Bengal Secretariat Press, 1902), 27.

12. N. Gerald Barrier, "Introduction," in *The Census in British India. New Perspectives*, ed. N. Gerald Barrier (New Delhi: Monohar, 1981), ix.

13. Tabular data were reported in Census of India, 1901, Vol. 11A [S. M. Edwardes] *Bombay (Town and Island) Part VI. Tables* (Bombay: Times of India Press, 1901). For the city of Calcutta see Census of India, 1901, Vol. 7 [J. R. Blackwood] *Calcutta Town and Suburbs. Part III. Tabular Statistics* (Calcutta: Bengal Secretariat Press, 1902). For the suburbs, see Census of India, 1901, Vol. 6A, *The Lower Provinces of Bengal and Their Feudatories. Part II. The Imperial Tables* (Calcutta: Bengal Secretariat Press, 1902); Census of India, 1901, Vol. 6B, *The Lower Provinces of Bengal and Their Feudatories. Part II. Provincial Tables* (Calcutta: Bengal Secretariat Press, 1902).

14. Nancy Krieger, "A Century of Census Tracts: Health and the Body Politic (1906–2006)," *Journal of Urban Health* 83 (2006): 335–41.

15. The distinction was primarily based on quality and permanence. Dandapani Natarajan, *Indian Census through a Hundred Years*, Census of India Centenary Monograph 2 (New Delhi: Office of the Registrar General, 1972), 184–204, 471–503.

16. Census of India, 1901, Vol. 7, *Census of Calcutta. Part II*, 25, 27.

17. Ian Hacking, *The Taming of Chance* (Cambridge: Cambridge University Press, 1990), 3.

18. Benedict Anderson, *Imagined Communities. Reflections on the Origins and Spread of Nationalism* (London: Verso, 1991), 166.

19. Dipesh Chakrabarty, "Modernity and Ethnicity in India," in *Multicultural States. Rethinking Difference and Identity*, ed. David Bennett (London: Routledge, 1998), 97.

20. Nicholas Dirks, *Castes of Mind: Colonialism and the Making of Modern India* (Princeton: Princeton University Press, 2001), 9.

21. In Britain, households were counted during the Napoleonic wars and the census developed progressively into a centralized state project, For an account of the history of the census in Victorian Britain, see Kathrin Levitan, *A Cultural History of the British Census: Envisioning the Multitude in the Nineteenth Century* (Basingstoke: Palgrave Macmillan, 2011).

22. Nicholas Thomas, *Colonialism's Culture: Anthropology, Travel and Government* (Cambridge: Polity, 1994), 4.

23. Bruce Curtis, *The Politics of Population* (Toronto: University of Toronto Press, 2001).

24. Gyan Prakash, *Another Reason. Science and the Imagination of Modern India* (Princeton, NJ: Princeton University Press, 1999), 126; Talal Asad, "Ethnographic Research, Statistics and Modern Power," *Social Research* 61 (1994): 56.

25. David Ludden, "Orientalist Empiricism," in *Orientalism and the Postcolonial Predicament: Perspectives on South Asia*, ed. Carol A. Breckenridge and Peter van der Veer (Philadelphia: University of Pennsylvania Press, 1993), 267.

26. Stephen Legg, "Foucault's Population Geographies. Classification, Biopolitics and Governmental Spaces," *Space and Place* 11 (2005): 145.

27. Bernard Cohn, "The Census, Social Structure and Objectification in South Asia," in *An Anthropologist among Historians, and Other Essays*, ed. Bernard Cohn (Delhi:

Oxford University Press, 1987), 248; Barrier, "Introduction," xi; Chakrabarty, "Modernity and Ethnicity in India," 99.

28. Prakash, *Another Reason*, 135.

29. J. A. Baines, "Administration of the Imperial Census of India, 1891," *Journal of the Society of Arts* 40, no. 2064 (June 10, 1892): 718; Barrier, "Introduction," viii; Legg, "Foucault's Population Geographies," 145.

30. Stuart Elden, "Plague, Panopticon, Police," *Surveillance and Society* 1 (2003): 249. See Michel Foucault, *Discipline and Punish: The Birth of the Prison* (New York: Vintage, 1979).

31. Foucault, *Discipline and Punish*, 195–97. Foucault speaks of how orders define an "enclosed, segmented space, observed at every point . . . in which the slightest movements are supervised" (197). That might have been the goal, but was never the reality.

32. Cf. Prasannan Parthasarathi, "The State of Indian Social History," *Journal of Social History* 37 (2003): 47–54.

33. Prakash, *Another Reason*.

34. Barbara and Thomas Metcalfe, *A Concise History of India* (Cambridge: Cambridge University Press, 2004), 138–39.

35. Padmanabh Samarendra, "Classifying Caste. Census Surveys in India in the Late Nineteenth and Early Twentieth Centuries," *South Asia: Journal of South Asian Studies* 26, no. 2 (2003): 141–64.

36. Priscilla Wald, *Constituting Americans: Cultural Anxiety and Narrative Form* (Durham, NC: Duke University Press, 1995).

37. Rajnarayan Chandavarkar, "Plague Panic and Epidemic Politics in India, 1896–1914," in *Imperial Power and Popular Politics: Class, Resistance and the State in India, c. 1850–1950*, ed. Rajnarayan Chandavarkar (Cambridge: Cambridge University Press, 1998), 264.

38. U. Kalpagam, "The Colonial State and Statistical Knowledge," *History of the Human Sciences* 13 (2000): 49.

39. R. H. Hooker, "Modes of Census-Taking in the British Dominions," *Journal of the Royal Statistical Society* 57, no. 2 (1894): 313; Baines, "Administration," 722–23.

40. Ibid.

41. Dirks, *Castes of Mind*, 201. On caste, see Cohn, "The Census," 238–41; Chakrabarty, "Modernity and Ethnicity," 98; Rashmi Pant, "The Cognitive Status of Caste in Colonial Ethnography. A Review of Some Literature of the North-West Provinces and Oudh," *Indian Economic and Social History Review* 24, no. 3 (1987): 145–62; Samarendra, "Classifying Caste."

42. Baines, "Administration"; J. A. Baines, "On Census-taking and its Limitations," *Journal of the Royal Statistical Society* 63, no. 1 (1900): 41–71; Hooker, "Modes of Census-Taking."

43. Barrier, "Introduction," viii; Susan Bayly, "Caste and 'Race' in the Colonial Ethnography of India," in *The Concept of Race in South Asia*, ed. Peter Robb (Delhi: Oxford University Press, 1995), 165–218. The Institute of Actuaries of Great Britain and Ireland also pressed for a better census, although they were chiefly interested

in selling life insurance to "government servants or non-officials of the same social standing." Lord Curzon and others, to Lord George Hamilton, October 25, 1900. Finance and Commerce, No. 352, Proceedings of the Home Department (hereafter PHDC), Census, P/5885, 276, India Office Records, British Library (hereafter IOBL).

44. Forster to Secretary of State for India, December 1899, in "Proposals of the British Association Regarding Ethnography, Etc., in Connection with the Census of 1901," Pro. No. 6, PHDC, Census, 153–54, P/5885, IOBL.

45. E. H. H. Collen, A. C. Trever, and T. Raleigh, to Lord George F. Hamilton, November 1, 1900, IOBL, No. 368 of 1900, Finance and Commerce, Census, 268. Reprinted in Natarajan, *Indian Census*, 545–50.

46. Cohn, "Introduction," 8.

47. On the ethnography of caste, see Census of India, 1901, Vol.1 [H. H. Risley], *India. Ethnographic Appendices. Being the data upon which the caste chapter of the Report is based* (Calcutta: Office of the Superintendent of Government Printing, 1903).

48. Dirks, *Castes of Mind*, 48, 220.

49. Quoted in Richard Saumarez Smith, "Rule-by-records and Rule-by-reports. Complementary Aspects of the British Imperial Rule of Law," *Contributions to Indian Sociology*, n.s., 19 (1985): 153–76.

50. Ibid.

51. Hewitt, to Chief Secretary to the Government of Bombay, July 12, 1900, PHDC, Census P/5885, IOBL.

52. The history of Bombay appeared as Census of India, 1901, Vol. 10 [S. M. Edwardes], *Part IV The Rise of Bombay. A Retrospect* (Bombay: Times of India Press, 1902). The interpretation of data appeared as Census of India, 1901, Vol. 11 [S. M. Edwardes], *Bombay. (Town and Island). Part V. Report* (Bombay: Times of India Press, 1901). On administrative procedures, see Census of India, 1901, Vol. 9, *Bombay (Town and Island). Part V. Report* (Bombay: Times of India Press, 1901).

53. Census of India, 1901, Vol. 7 [A. K. Ray], *Calcutta Town and Suburbs. Part I. A Short History of Calcutta* (Calcutta: Bengal Secretariat Press, 1902); Census of India, 1901, Vol. 7 [J. R. Blackwood], *Calcutta Town and Suburbs. Part IV. Report (Statistical)* (Calcutta: Bengal Secretariat Press, 1902). On the suburbs, see Census of India, 1901, Vol. 6 [E. A. Gait], *The Lower Provinces of Bengal and Their Feudatories. Part I. Report* (Calcutta: Bengal Secretariat Press, 1902).

54. Ibid.

55. Rebsch to Provincial Superintendent of the Census, Bombay Presidency, No. 1834, August 27, 1900. PHDC, Census, 291–292, P/5885, IOBL.

56. Atkins to Secretary of the Government of India, No. 4905, September 17, 1900, PHDC, Census, 287, P/5885, IOBL.

57. H. S. Risley, "Note by the Census Commissioner for India Regarding the Census of Calcutta, February 1, 1901, PHDC, Census, 1901, 53 P/6121, IOBL.

58. Methods in Calcutta were adapted from India-wide guidelines and those for Bengal. Census of India, 1901, Vol. 1, *Administrative Volume with Appendices* (Calcutta: Office of the Superintendent of Government Printing, 1901); E. A. Gait,

Report on the Census of Bengal, 1901. Administrative Volume (Calcutta: Bengal Secretariat Press, 1902); Census of India, 1901, Vol. 7, *Census of Calcutta. Part II.*

59. Ibid.

60. Hooker, "Modes of Census-Taking," 345; Baines, "On Census-Taking"; R. E. Enthoven, to the Secretary of the Government of Bombay, No. 536, August 31, 1900, PHDC, Census, P/5885, 289–91, IOBL; W. L. Harvey to the Secretary of the Government of Bombay, No. 13253, August 23, 1900, PHDC, Census P/5885, 288–89, IOBL.

61. Harvey to Secretary to the Government of Bombay, No. 13253, August 23, 1900, PHDC, Census, 288–289, P/5885, IOBL.

62. Extract from the Proceedings of the Government of India, in the Home Department (Census), – under date Simla, the 3rd. August 1900." PHDC, Census, P/5885, IOBL.

63. Atkins, to Secretary of the Government of India, September 17, 1900, No. 4905, PHDC, Census, 287, P/5885, IOBL.

64. On workers and housing conditions in Calcutta, see Subho Basu, "Strikes and 'Communal' Riots in Calcutta in the 1890. Industrial Workers, Bhadralok Nationalist Leadership and the Colonial State," *Modern Asian Studies* 32 (1998): 949; Christine Furedy, "Whose Responsibility? Dilemmas of Calcutta's Bustee Policy in the Nineteenth Century," *South Asia* 5 (1982): 24–46. On Bombay, see A. R. Burnett-Hurst, *Labour and Housing in Bombay* (London: King and Sons, 1925); Rajnarajan N. Chandavarkar, *Origins of Industrial Capitalism in India. Business Strategies and Working Classes in Bombay, 1900–1940* (Cambridge: Cambridge University Press, 1994); Frank F. Conlon, "Industrialization and the Housing Problem in Bombay 1850–1940," in *Changing South Asia. Economy and Society Vol. 4*, ed. Kenneth Ballhatchet and David Taylor (London: Centre for South Asian Studies, School of Oriental and African Studies, 1984), 153–68; Prashant Kidambi, *The Making of an Indian Metropolis. Colonial Governance and Public Culture in Bombay, 1890–1920* (Abingdon: Ashgate, 2007), 71–113; Shaski Bhushan Upadhyaya, "Cotton Mill Workers in Bombay, 1875–1918. Conditions of Work and Life," *Economic and Political Weekly* 25 (1990): 87–99.

65. Ira Klein, "Urban Development and Death. Bombay City, 1870–1914," *Modern Asian Studies* 20 (1986): 729; Census of India, 1901, Vol. 7, *Calcutta Town and Suburbs. Part IV. Report (Statistical)*, 17. Figures have been rounded.

66. Census of India, 1901, Vol. 7, *Calcutta Town and Suburbs. Part IV. Report (Statistical)*, 4, 10–11.

67. Census of India, 1901, Vol. 11, *Bombay (Town and Island). Part V. Report*, 12. The head of the Improvement Trust later reported trends in residential densities. J. P. Orr, *Density of Population in Bombay. Lecture Delivered to the Bombay Cooperative Housing Association* (Bombay, 1914). Klein reports a higher figure for 1881 in "Urban Development and Death," 733.

68. Census of India, 1901, Vol. 7, *Calcutta Town and Suburbs. Part IV. Report (Statistical)*, 2.

69. Census of India, 1901, Vol. 11, *Bombay (Town and Island). Part V. Report*, 68.
70. Kidambi, *Making of an Indian Metropolis*, 38.
71. Prashant Kidambi, "'The Ultimate Masters of the City': Police, Public Order and the Poor in Colonial Bombay, c.1893–1914," *Crime, History and Societies* 8 (2004): 27–47.
72. Paul Bairoch, *Cities and Economic Development. From the Dawn of History to the Present* (Chicago: University of Chicago Press, 1988), 402, 450.
73. Klein, "Urban Development and Death," 729.
74. Chandavarkar, "Plague Panic"; Klein, "Urban Development and Death"; Echenberg, *Plague Ports*; Mridula Ramanna, *Western Medicine and Public Health in Colonial Bombay* (London: Sangam, 2002), 159.
75. Reported in Klein, "Plague Policy, and Popular Unrest in British India," *Modern Asian Studies* 22, no. 4 (1988): 726.
76. Ibid., 729.
77. Chandavarkar, "Plague Panic," 234.
78. For a discussion about the motives behind segregation, see Philip Curtin, "Medical Knowledge and Urban Planning in Tropical Africa," *American Historical Review* 90 (1985): 594–613; John W. Cell, "Anglo-Indian Medical Theory and the Origins of Segregation in West Africa," *American Historical Review* 91 (1986): 307–35; Robert Home, *Of Planting and Planning. The Making of British Colonial Cities* (London: E&FN Spon, 1997), 122–27; Chandavarkar, *Origins of Industrial Capitalism*, 41–42; Mark Harrison, *Public Health in British India. Anglo-Indian Preventive Medicine 1859–1914* (Cambridge: Cambridge University Press, 1994), 229.
79. E. P. Richards, *Report, by Request of the Trust, On the Condition, Improvement and Town Planning of the City of Calcutta and Contiguous Areas* (Hertfordshire: Jennings, 1914), 31.
80. Ibid.
81. A. J. Christopher, "Urban Segregation Levels in the British Overseas Empire and Its Successors, in the Twentieth Century," *Transactions, Institute of British Geographers*, n.s., 17 (1992): 101. For similar assessments, see Rajat Ray, *Urban Roots of Indian Nationalism: Pressure Groups and Conflict of Interests in Calcutta City Politics, 1875–1939* (New Delhi: Vikas, 1979), 1–9.
82. Ibid.
83. Carl Nightingale, *Segregation: A Global History of Divided Cities* (Chicago: University of Chicago Press, 2012).
84. Cell, "Anglo-Indian Medical Theory," 321.
85. Echenberg, *Plague Ports*, 55.
86. Rusi Daruwala, *The Bombay Chamber Story: 150 Years* (Bombay: Bombay Chamber of Commerce and Industry, 1986), 55.
87. Census of India, 1901, Vol. 11, *Bombay (Town and Island), Part V, Report*, 44.
88. Chandavarkar, "Plague Panic."
89. Mary Sutphen, "Not What, but Where: Bubonic Plague and the Reception of Germ Theories in Hong Kong and Calcutta, 1894–1897," *Journal of the History of*

Medicine 52 (1997): 107. Simpson was influential in promoting racial segregation, notably in Africa. Home, *Of Planting and Planning*, 43–44.

90. I. J. Catanach, "Plague and the Tensions of Empire: India, 1896–1918," in *Imperial Medicine and Indigenous Societies*, ed. David Arnold (Manchester: Manchester University Press, 1988), 149–71; Chandavarkar, "Plague Panic"; Mary Sutphen, "Not What, but Where"; Klein, "Plague Policy and Popular Unrest." For contemporary reports and accounts, see Herbert M. Crake, *The Calcutta Plague 1896–1907 with Some Observations on the Epidemiology of Plague* (Calcutta: Criterion, 1908); T. Frederick Pearse, *Report of Plague in Calcutta for the Year Ending 30th June 1904* (Calcutta: Bengal Secretariat Press, 1905); P. C. H. Snow, *Report on the Outbreak of Bubonic Plague in Bombay, 1896–97* (Bombay), 2 vols.

91. Prakash, *Another Reason*, 134–35, 139–41.

92. For descriptions, see David Arnold, *Colonizing the Body: State Medicine and Epidemic Disease in Nineteenth-century India* (Berkeley: University of California Press, 1993); M. E. Couchman, *Account of Plague Administration in the Bombay Presidency from September 1896 till May 1897* (Bombay: Government Central Press, 1897); Echenberg, *Plague Ports*, 57–59; William F. Gatacre, *Report on the Bubonic Plague in Bombay, 1896–97* (Bombay: Times of India, 1897); Kidambi, *Making of an Indian Metropolis*, 56–67; Snow, *Report on the Outbreak*.

93. Chandavarker, "Plague Panic," 237.

94. Echenberg, *Plague Ports*, 64–65; Kidambi, "Ultimate Masters," 31.

95. Arnold, *Colonising the Body*, 211. See also Basu, "Strikes and 'Communal' Riots."

96. Census of India, 1901, Vol. 10, Part 4, *Rise of Bombay*, 334.

97. Harrison, *Public Health in British India*, 229.

98. Conlon, "Industrialization and the Housing Problem," 161; Echenberg, *Plague Ports*, 75; Sandip Hazareesingh, *The Colonial City and the Challenge to Modernity. Urban Hegemonies and Civic Confrontations in Bombay City 1900–1925* (Delhi: Orient Longman, 2007), 27; Home, *Of Planting and Planning*, 171; Prashant Kidambi, "Housing the Poor in a Colonial City: The Bombay Improvement Trust, 1898–1918," *Studies in History* 17, no. 1 (2001), 58, 60; Kidambi, *Making of an Indian Metropolis*, 71.

99. Chandavarkar, *Origins of Industrial Capitalism*, 43–44.

100. S. Rebsch, August 27, 1900, in Census of India, 1901, Vol. 1, *Administrative Volume*, 200–201; Kidambi, "Housing the Poor," 60.

101. Hewitt, to Chief Secretary of the Government of Bombay, July 12, 1900, 137–8, PHDC, Census P/5885, IOBL.

102. Kidambi, *Making of an Indian Metropolis*, 6.

103. Extract from the Proceedings of the Government of India, in the Home Department (Census), – under date Simla, the 3rd. August 1900." PHDC, Census, P/5885, IOBL.

104. Ibid.

105. Edward Higgs, *Making Sense of the Census: The Manuscript Returns for England Wales, 1801–1901* (London: HMSO, 1989), 15.

106. Orr, "Density of Population"; Richard, *Calcutta Improvement Trust Report*, maps 1, 7, 9; H. V. Lanchester, *Town Planning in Madras* (London: Constable and Co., 1918); Pearse, *Report on Plague in Calcutta*; Bombay Improvement Trust, *Administrative Report for the Year Ending 31st March* (Bombay, 1901), annual; S. M. Edwardes, *The Gazetteer of Bombay City and Island* (Bombay: Times Press, 1909), 3 vols.

Chapter 4   "Beyond Risk of Contagion"

*   Research for this chapter, which relates to a larger project on the history of young people in colonial contexts, was generously supported by an RGC/CERG grant (HKU7455/05H).

1.   See, for example, Elizabeth Buettner, *Empire Families: Britons and Late Imperial India* (Oxford: Oxford University Press, 2004); Laura Briggs, *Reproducing Empire: Race, Sex, Science and US Imperialism in Puerto Rico* (Berkeley: University of California Press, 2002); Julia Clancy-Smith and Frances Gouda, ed., *Domesticating the Empire: Race, Gender and Family Life in French and Dutch Colonialism* (Charlottesville: University Press of Virginia, 1998); Durba Ghosh, *Sex and the Family in Colonial India: The Making of Empire* (Cambridge: Cambridge University Press, 2006); Mary A. Procida, *Married to the Empire: Gender Politics and Imperialism in India, 1883–1947* (Manchester: Manchester University Press, 2000); Ann Laura Stoler, *Carnal Knowledge and Imperial Power: Race and the Intimate in Colonial Rule* (Berkeley: University of California Press, 2002); Ann Laura Stoler, *Race and the Education of Desire: Foucault's History of Sexuality and the Colonial Order of Things* (Durham, NC: Duke University Press, 1995).

2.   Carolyn Steedman, *Strange Dislocations: Childhood and the Idea of Human Interiority, 1780–1930* (Cambridge: Harvard University Press, 1994), 130–49.

3.   On the hill station in Asia, see J. E. Spencer and W. L. Thomas, "The Hill Stations and Summer Resorts of the Orient," *Geographical Review* 38 (1948): 637–51. On their decline and as "nurseries of the ruling race," see Dane Kennedy, *The Magic Mountains: Hill Stations and the British Raj* (Delhi: Oxford University Press, 1996), 118, 204. On the generally observed decline in mortality, see Philip Curtin, *Death by Migration: Europe's Encounter with the Tropical World in the Nineteenth Century* (New York: Cambridge University Press, 1989).

4.   Biswamoy Pati and Mark Harrison, *The Social History of Health and Medicine in Colonial India* (New York: Routledge, 2009); David Arnold, *Colonizing the Body: State, Medicine and Epidemic Disease in Nineteenth-Century India* (Berkeley: University of California Press, 1993), 7–10; Daniel R. Headrick, *The Tools of Empire: Technology and European Imperialism in the Nineteenth Century* (New York and Oxford: Oxford University Press, 1981).

5.   Warwick Anderson, *Colonial Pathologies: American Tropical Medicine, Race, and Hygiene in the Philippines* (Durham, NC: Duke University Press, 2006).

6.   Mark Harrison, *Public Health in British India: Anglo-Indian Preventative Medicine, 1859–1914* (Cambridge: Cambridge University Press, 1994).

7. For Atkinson, the meeting represented the culmination of a professional career that had begun in 1887 as superintendent of Hong Kong's Government Civil Hospital, and had progressed in 1895 following his promotion to the new post of principal civil medical officer. The Far Eastern Association for Tropical Medicine was founded in Manila in 1904. Originally known as the Philippine Island Medical Association, its name was changed in 1909 to the "Far Eastern Association for Tropical Medicine." The association was founded to foster scientific collaboration, to coordinate the dissemination of common practice in medical science, and to instruct public opinion in the prevention of disease in the Far East. The first congress was held in Manila in 1910.

8. On the visual nature of the new medicine in Hong Kong, see "The Plague at Hongkong," *Lancet*, August 11, 1894, 325; "Discovery of the Plague Bacillus. Interview with Professor Kitasato," *China Mail*, June 20, 1894. On the acceptance of germ theory in Hong Kong, see Mary Sutphen, "Not What but Where: Bubonic Plague and the Reception of Germ Theories in Hong Kong and Calcutta, 1894–1897," *Journal of the History of Medicine* 52, no. 1 (1997): 81–113. See also, Nancy Leys Stepan, *Picturing Tropical Nature* (Chicago: University of Chicago Press, 2001).

9. See, for example, Leonore Manderson, *Sickness and the State: Health and Illness in Colonial Malaya, 1870–1940* (Cambridge: Cambridge University Press, 1996), 8–10; Harrison, *Public Health*, 3.

10. Chamberlain established a malaria commission in West Africa to examine the application of the new knowledge. Patrick Manson, chief medical advisor to the colonial office from 1897, successfully encouraged Joseph Chamberlain to establish a School of Tropical Medicine in London in 1899. Philip H. Manson-Bahr and A. Alcock, *The Life and Work of Sir Patrick Manson* (London: Cassell and Company Limited, 1927), 217.

11. In 1901, the findings of the Colonial Office malaria commission in West Africa prompted the colonial secretary, Chamberlain, to promote the application of segregationist ideas in colonial urban planning. Governors were advised that, *new* buildings should be located away from native quarters and where possible on high ground. Stephen Frenkel and John Western, "Pretext or Prophylaxis? Racial Segregation and Malarial Mosquitos in a British Tropical Colony: Sierra Leone," *Annals of the Association of American Geographers* 78, no. 2 (June 1988): 216; On these changes as identified by Americans in the Philippines, see Warwick Anderson, "'Where Every Prospect Pleases and Only Man is Vile': Laboratory Medicine as Colonial Discourse," *Critical Enquiry* 18 (Spring 1992): 507–8; Maynard W. Swanson, "The Sanitation Syndrome: Bubonic Plague and Urban Native Policy in the Cape Colony, 1900–1909," *Journal of African History* 18, no. 3 (1977): 387–410; Philip D. Curtin, "Medical Knowledge and Urban Planning in Tropical Africa," *American Historical Review* 90, no. 3 (June 1985): 594–613; John W. Cell, "Anglo-Indian Medical Theory and the Origins of Segregation in West Africa," *American Historical Review* 91, no. 2 (April 1986): 307–35.

12. S. Marks and W. Anderson, "Typhus and Social Control: South Africa, 1917–1950," in *Disease, Medicine and Empire*, ed. R. MacLeod and M. Lewis (London: Routledge, 1988), 257–83.

13. May to Lucas, June 19, 1904, Great Britain, Colonial Office, Original Correspondence: Hong Kong, 1841–1951, Series 129 CO129/323, 137, Public Record Office, Kew, London (hereafter PRO).

14. Ambe Njoh, *Planning Power: Town Planning and Social Control in Colonial Africa* (New York: Routledge, 2007), 206.

15. Chamberlain to Blake, September 12, 1902, PRO CO129/311, 48.

16. May to Lyttelton, May 21, 1904, CO129/322, 779, PRO; Roger Bristow, *Land Use Planning in Hong Kong: History, Policies and Procedures* (Hong Kong: Oxford University Press, 1984), 39–40; Ka-che Yip, "Colonialism, Disease and Public Health: Malaria in the History of Hong Kong," in *Disease, Colonialism and the State: Malaria in Modern East Asian History*, ed. Ka-che Yip (Hong Kong: Hong Kong University Press, 2009), 20.

17. Blake to Lucas, April 17, 1904, PRO CO129/327, 37.

18. Sutphen, "Not What but Where," 81–113.

19. May to Lucas, June 19, 1904, PRO CO129/323, 135.

20. John M. Carroll, *Edge of Empires: Chinese Elites and British Colonials in Hong Kong* (Harvard: Harvard University Press, 2005), 93.

21. "Legislative Council, No. 7," *Papers Laid Before the Legislative Council of Hongkong*, April 26, 1904.

22. "Report of the Meeting of the Legislative Council," *Papers Laid Before the Legislative Council of Hongkong*, April 19, 1904, 18–19.

23. An Ordinance for the Reservation of a Residential Area in the Hill District," *The Hongkong Government Gazette*, April 29, 1904, 752; "Report of the Meeting of the Legislative Council," *Papers Laid Before the Legislative Council of Hongkong*, April 19, 1904, 20. Ho Kai's father had been the first ordained Chinese pastor in the London Missionary Society's (LMS) Hong Kong mission and he was himself a member of the LMS church, a member of the Sanitary Board 1886–96 and Legislative Council from 1890–1914.

24. David Sibley, *Geographies of Exclusion: Society and Difference in the West* (London: Routledge, 1995), 39.

25. David M. Pomfret, "'Raising Eurasia': Age, Gender and Race in Hong Kong and Indochina," *Comparative Studies in Society and History* 51, no. 2 (April 2009), 324–25.

26. Kennedy, *Magic Mountains*, 204.

27. Report on Ordinance 14 of 1919, September 10, 1919, PRO CO129/455, 344.

28. "Cheung Chau (Residence) Ordinance," *Papers Laid Before the Legislative Council of Hongkong*, August 28, 1919, 63–64.

29. Ibid., 64.

30. Ibid., 64–65.

31. Ibid., 64.

32. Laurence Monnais-Rousselot, "'Modern Medicine' in French Colonial Vietnam: From the Importation of a Model to its Nativisation," in *The Development of Modern Medicine in Non-Western Countries*, ed. Hormoz Ebrahimnejad (London: Routledge, 2008), 130–32.

33. Yersin, as serving vice-president, hosted the third biennial congress of the Far Eastern Association of Tropical Medicine in Saigon. *Comptes rendus des travaux du troisième congrés biennial de la Far Eastern Association of Tropical Medicine* (Saigon: Imprimerie Nouvelle Albert Portail, 1914).

34. A Pasteur Institute was established in Saigon under the supervision of Albert Calmette in 1890, only four years after the Pasteur Institue had opened in Paris. The Faculty of Medicine at the University of Hanoi, the Pasteur institutes and several zoological laboratories cooperated closely in the first half of the twentieth century. P-Noël Bernard, ed., *Les Instituts Pasteur d'Indochine* (Saigon: Imprimerie Nouvelle Albert Portail, 1922).

35. Ibid., 24.

36. Monnais-Rousselot, "Modern Medicine," 127, 138; Laurence Monnais-Rousselot, "La médicalisation de la mère et de son enfant: l'exemple du Vietnam sous domination française, 1860–1939," *Canadian Bulletin for the History of Medicine/ Bulletin Canadien d'Histoire de la Medecine* 19 (2002): 47–94.

37. Michael G. Vann, "Building Colonial Whiteness on the Red River: Race, Power and Urbanism in Paul Doumer's Hanoi, 1897–1902," *Historical Reflections/Réflexions Historiques* 33 (Summer 2007): 277–304.

38. Beylié, Pennequin, and Bizar led missions exploring the plateau. "Rapport de l'inspecteur général des travaux publics sur le sanatorium du Lang Bian (Dalat), 1915," September 24, 1915, 4092, Fonds de la Résidence Supérieure d'Annam (hereafter RSA), HC, National Archives of Vietnam IV, Dalat, Vietnam (hereafter VNNA4).

39. Pasquier, "Note postale," January 29, 1920, 1020/RSA/HC, VNNA4.

40. "Rapport de l'inspecteur général des travaux publics, Saigon," September 24, 1915, 37, 4092/RSA/HC, VNNA4.

41. Ibid.

42. For a discussion of Hébrard's work in Indochina see Gwendolyn Wright, *The Politics of Design in French Colonial Urbanism* (Chicago: University of Chicago Press, 1991), 232.

43. "Decisions prises par le Gouverneur Général de l'Indochine," August 16, 1924, 4109/RSA/HC, VNNA4.

44. "L'Urbanisme—Dalat," *L'Eveil Economique*, October 21, 1923, 7.

45. Ibid.

46. Perot to Rivet, May 30, 1916, VIA8/263(4), National Archives of Vietnam II, Ho Chi Minh City, Vietnam (hereafter VNNA2).

47. Merlin to Pasquier, January 16, 1924, 1447/RSA/HC, VNNA4; Deletie to Pasquier, January 26, 1924, 1447/RSA/HC, VNNA4.

48. Pierre Pasquier, hurrying to meet the governor's requirements, demanded that the boarding school, planned for 30 pupils, be implemented "urgently," "without too

much of delay," and "in the briefest possible time." Deletie to Pasquier, February 12, 1924, 1447/RSA/HC, VNNA4; Pasquier to Merlin, May 16, 1924, 1447/RSA/HC, VNNA4.

49. The "Commissaire Délégué" of Dalat, Léon Garnier, complained repeatedly to the High Resident of Annam about the deficiencies of workers and the lack of building materials. Garnier to Pasquier, January 12, 1924, 4101/RSA/HC, VNNA4.

50. Engineer-in-Chief, Annam, to Pasquier, July 22, 1925, 4120/RSA/HC, VNNA4.

51. "Réunions de la Commission Municipale, 1926," Municipal Commission, Dalat, November 25, 1926, 4118/RSA/HC, VNNA4; "Décisions, A.S. de l'exécution des travaux à Dalat," March 13, 1925, 4109/RSA/HC, VNNA4.

52. Charles Grall, *Hygiène coloniale appliquée. Hygiène de l'Indochine* (Librairie J.-B. Baillère et Fils: Paris, 1908), 9–53.

53. Etienne Tardif, *La Naissance de Dalat: Annam (1899-1900) Capitale de l'Indochine* (Vienne: Ternet-Martin, 1949), 38–39.

54. Bernard, *Les Instituts Pasteur*, 126.

55. "Rapport sur l'organisation médicale de Dalat 1923–24," 1924, 1333/RSA/HC, VNNA4.

56. "Procès verbal de la commission de contrôle du Langbian Palace," August 6, 1924, 4109/RSA/HC, VNNA4.

57. Ibid.

58. Vassal had also conducted studies on children's blood in 1905. Dr. Joseph-Emile Borel, "Résultats d'une enquête malériologique à Dalat (Cochinchine)," *Extrait du Bulletin de la Société de Patholoqie Exotique* 20, no. 5 (11 May 1927): 429, 431–32.

59. Ibid.

60. Direction General de l'instruction Publique, *Le Petit Lycée de Dalat* (Hanoi: Imprimerie d'Extrème-Orient, 1930), 10.

61. Ibid., 7.

62. Ibid., 20.

63. Ibid., 21.

64. Laurent Joseph Gaide, *Les Stations climatiques en Indochine* (Hanoi: Imprimerie d'Extrème-Orient, 1930), 28–29.

65. Terrisse to Commissaire Délégué, December 15, 1926, VNNA4 4113/RSA/HC. In the face of resistance from commercial interests, the deputy commissioner, Terrisse, demanded that the Municipal Hygiene Commission to agree in 1925 that all "Asiatics" hailing from outside Dalat should undergo medical inspection on arrival, "in order protect public health." After the hotelier, Desanti, and Commissaire Adjoint Elie Cunhac strongly opposed this on the grounds that it would harm tourism the measure was to be applied only to those suspected of having frequented "dangerous milieux." "Procès verbal, Commission municipale d'hygiène," January 16, 1925, 4113/RSA/HC, VNNA4.

66. "Décision du 16 août 1924 de M le Gouverneur Général concernant divers travaux à Dalat," August 16, 1924, 4109/RSA/HC, VNNA4.

67. Dr Guérin, director of the Pasteur Institute, proposed that Borel join Dalat's Comité de Salubrité. Terrisse to Commissaire Délégué, December 15, 1926, 4113/RSA/HC, VNNA 4.

68. Completed in 1926, this project added momentum to that of relocating the *village annamite*. "Procès verbal des réunions des 13 & 14 novembre 1926," Comité de salubrité de Dalat, 4116/RSA/HC, VNNA4.

69. Terrisse to Commissaire Délégué, December 15, 1926, Bureau municipal d'hygiene de Dalat 1925, 4113/RSA/HC, VNNA4.

70. "Ordre du jour, délibérations, session ordinaire," Municipal Commission, Dalat, September 17, 1928, 4122/RSA/HC, VNAA4.

71. Robert Reed, "From Highland Hamlet to Regional Capital: Reflections on the Colonial Origins, Urban Transformation and Environmental Impact of Dalat," in Terry Rambo et al., *The Challenges of Highland Development in Vietnam* (Honolulu: East-West Center, 1995), 51.

72. "Procès verbal des deliberations," Municipal Commission, Dalat, June 27, 1934, 4124/RSA/HC, VNNA4; "Ordre du jour, deliberations," Municipal Commission, Dalat, February 23, 1935, 4122/RSA/HC, VNNA4.

73. Pasquier to Billotte, December 1, 1930, 2762/RSA/HC, VNNA4.

74. Ibid. In 1935, the Resident Mayor of Dalat, Lucien Auger, boasted that the *lycée* would reopen with 300 pupils. "Procès verbaux de la Commission municipale et commission sanitaire de Dalat," Municipal Commission, Dalat, August 17, 1935, 4124/RSA/HC, VNNA4.

75. "Procès verbal des déliberations," Municipal Commission, Dalat, December 5, 1936, 4130/RSA/HC, VNNA4.

76. On July 1, 1936, the total population of Dalat was 7,191 people, of which 6,273 were Vietnamese. "Procès verbal des déliberations," Municipal Commission, Dalat, March 20, 1937," 38–9, 4133/RSA/HC, VNNA4.

77. Gaide, *Les Stations climatiques*, 47; at a ceremony held in honor of Yersin, the resident mayor reiterated that "the *lycée* is fundamentally linked to the development of the Hill Station." "Procès verbal des déliberations," Municipal Commission, Dalat, May 25 1935, 4126/RSA/HC, VNNA4.

78. "Procès verbal des déliberations," Municipal Commission, Dalat, September 14, 1928, 2, 4122/RSA/HC, VNNA4. The Municipal Commission proudly reported that the opening of the school: "confirms at what a high level the view is entertained" that Dalat was the pre-eminent hill station in the peninsula. "Ordre du jour, delibérations," Municipal Commission, Dalat, September 14, 1928, 4122/RSA/HC, VNNA4.

79. Eric T. Jennings, "Urban Planning, Architecture and Zoning at Dalat, Indochina, 1900–1944," *Historical Reflections/Reflexions Historiques* 33, no. 2 (2007): 343. See also Eric Jennings' forthcoming book on Dalat. Eric T. Jennings, *Imperial Heights: Dalat and the Making and Undoing of French Indochina* (Berkeley: University of California Press, forthcoming).

80. "Procès verbal," Hygiene Committee, Dalat, 2–3 June 1925, 9. 4112/RSA/HC, VNNA4.

81. Jennings, "Urban Planning," 341.

82. *Allocution prononcée par Monsieur Jules Brévié, Gouverneur Général de l'Indochine, Commandeur de la Légion d'honneur à la distribution des prix du Lycée Yersin à Dalat le 12 juillet 1938* (Saigon: Imprimerie A. Portail, 1938), 9.

83. These included cults of celebrity that cohered around acrobats, boxers, and other sportsmen and women; *Les Fêtes de Dalat en l'honneur de M. Yersin à l'occasion du baptême du lycée* (Hanoi: Imprimerie d'Extrême-Orient, June 28, 1935), 3.

84. *Allocution prononcée par Monsieur Jules Brévié*, 9.

85. Andrew Cunningham, "Transforming Plague," in *The Laboratory Revolution in Medicine*, ed. Andrew Cunningham and Perry Williams (Cambridge: Cambridge University Press, 1992), 240.

86. Eric T. Jennings, "Dalat, Capital of Indochina: Remolding Frameworks and Spaces in the Late Colonial Era," *Journal of Vietnamese Studies* 4, no. 2 (2009): 12.

87. Type A1 bungalow style houses, for example, had a very large *salle commune* occupied by four beds for children and "a bedroom of modest size for the parents," while type A2 had "a bedroom for the children (3 beds), a little bedroom for the parents." *Dalat Cite Jardin Amiral Decoux* (Hanoi, n.d., c.1942); see also Jean Decoux, *A la barre de l'Indochine: Histoire de mon gouvernement général, 1940–1945* (Paris: Plon, 1959), 461–62.

Chapter 5   Planning Social Hygiene

1. Michel Foucault, *The History of Sexuality*, Vol. 1, *An Introduction*, trans. Robert Hurley (London: Allen Lane, 1979).

2. Thomas Metcalf, *Imperial Connections: India in the Indian Ocean Arena, 1860–1920* (Berkeley: University of California Press, 2007).

3. David Arnold, *Colonizing the Body: State Medicine and Epidemic Disease in Nineteenth-century India* (Berkeley: University of California Press, 1993), 1.

4. Edward Blunt, *Social Service in India: An Introduction to Some Social and Economic Problems of the Indian People* (London: Her Majesty's Stationery Office, 1938), 192.

5. Mark Harrison, *Climates and Constitutions: Health, Race, Environment and British Imperialism in India 1600–1850* (New Delhi: Oxford University Press, 1999).

6. James S. Duncan, *In the Shadows of the Tropics: Struggles over Bio-power in Nineteenth Century Ceylon* (Aldershot: Ashgate, 2007).

7. Arnold, 33.

8. Ibid., 194.

9. Duncan, 103.

10. Mariam Dossal, *Imperial Design and Indian Realities: The Planning of Bombay City, 1845–1875* (Bombay: Oxford University Press, 1991).

11. Blunt, *Social Service in India*, 360.

12. Philip Howell, *Geographies of Regulation: Policing Prostitution in Nineteenth-Century Britain and the Empire* (Cambridge: Cambridge University Press, 2009); Kenneth Ballhatchet, *Race, Sex and Class under the Raj: Imperial Attitudes and Policies and Their Critics, 1793–1905* (London: Weidenfeld and Nicolson, 1980); Philippa Levine, *Prostitution, Race and Politics: Policing Venereal Disease in the British Empire* (London: Routledge, 2003).

13. Stephen Legg, "Stimulation, Segregation and Scandal: Geographies of Prostitution Regulation in British India, between Registration (1888) and Suppression (1923)," *Modern Asian Studies* (2012 advance online publication).

14. Stephen Legg, "Governing Prostitution in Colonial Delhi: From Cantonment Regulations to International Hygiene (1864–1939)," *Social History* 34, no. 4 (2009): 447–67.

15. David Armstrong, "Public Health Spaces and the Fabrication of Identity," *Sociology* 27, no. 3 (1993): 393–410.

16. Michel Foucault, *Security, Territory, Population: lectures at the Collège de France 1977–78*, trans. Graham Burchell (Basingstoke; New York: Palgrave Macmillan, 2007), chapter 1.

17. Michel Foucault, *Discipline and Punish: The Birth of the Prison* (Harmondsworth: Penguin, 1977), 195.

18. Brenda S. A. Yeoh, *Contesting Space: Power Relations and the Urban Built Environment in Colonial Singapore* (New York and Oxford: Oxford University Press, 1996), 82.

19. Ibid., 146.

20. Michel Foucault, *The Birth of Biopolitics: Lectures at the Collège de France, 1978–79*, trans. Graham Burchell (Basingstoke: Palgrave Macmillan, 2008).

21. Alison Bashford and Claire Hooker, "Introduction: Contagion, Modernity, and Postmodernity," in *Contagion: Historical and Cultural Studies*, ed. Alison Bashford and Claire Hooker (London and New York: Routledge, 2001), 1.

22. Stephen Legg, *Spaces of Colonialism: Delhi's Urban Governmentalities* (Oxford: Blackwell, 2007), 21.

23. Alison Bashford, *Imperial Hygiene: A Critical History of Colonialism, Nationalism and Public Health* (Basingstoke: Palgrave Macmillan, 2004).

24. Ibid., 1.

25. Deana Heath, "Sanitizing Modernity: Imperial Hygiene, Obscenity, and Moral Regulation in Colonial India," in *Enchantments of Modernity: Empire, Nation, Globalization*, ed. Saurabh Dube (London and New York: Routledge, 2009), 117.

26. David Arnold, "British India and the 'Beriberi Problem,' 1798–1942," *Medical History* 54, no. 3 (2010): 295–314. I am indebted to Joanna Barnard for this point, the result of her doctoral research on beriberi in colonial Burma.

27. Mark Swislocki, "Nutritional Governmentality: Food and the Politics of Health in Late Imperial and Republican China," *Radical History Review* 2011, no. 110 (2011): 9–35.

28. Warwick Anderson, *Colonial Pathologies: American Tropical Medicine, Race, and Hygiene in the Philippines* (Durham, NC: Duke University Press, 2006).

29. Warwick Anderson, "Immunization and Hygiene in the Colonial Philippines," *Journal of the History of Medicine and Allied Sciences* 62, no. 1 (2007): 1–20.

30. Laura Briggs, *Reproducing Empire: Race, Sex, Science and US Imperialism in Puerto Rico* (Berkeley, CA: University of California Press, 2002).

31. Sarah Hodges, *Contraception, Colonialism and Commerce: Birth Control in South India, 1920–40* (Aldershot: Ashgate, 2008).

32. Ibid., 7.

33. Ann Laura Stoler, *Carnal Knowledge and Imperial Power: Race and the Intimate in Colonial Rule* (Berkeley; Los Angeles; London: University of California Press, 2002).

34. Hodges, *Contraception, Colonialism and Commerce*, 8.

35. Sunil Amrith, *Decolonizing International Health: India and Southeast Asia, 1930–65* (Basingstoke: Palgrave Macmillan, 2006).

36. Madho Pershad, *The History of the Delhi Municipality 1863–1921* (Allahabad: Pioneer Press, 1921).

37. Ibid., 8.

38. Reginald Craufuird Sterndale, *Municipal Work in India; or, Hints on Sanitation, General Conservancy and Improvements in Municipalities, Towns and Villages* (Calcutta: Thacker, Spink and Co., 1881).

39. Ibid., 3.

40. Ibid., 19.

41. Ibid., 24.

42. Ibid., 25.

43. Rajnarayan Chandavarkar, *Imperial Power and Popular Politics: Class, Resistance and the State in India, c. 1850–1950* (Cambridge: Cambridge University Press, 1998), 235.

44. Pershad, 146.

45. Chief Commissioner's files, (Education)/1924/6B, Delhi State Archives, New Delhi (hereafter DA/CC).

46. Education, Health and Lands/1936-H/23-10, National Archives of India, New Delhi (hereafter NAI).

47. See Legg, *Spaces of Colonialism*, 159.

48. *Report on the Administration of the Delhi Municipality for the Years 1929–30*, vol. 2, *Annual Report of the Medical Officer for Health for 1929* (Delhi: Delhi Municipal Press, 1930), 63.

49. *Report on the Administration of the Delhi Municipality for the Years 1937–38*, vol. 2, *Annual Report of the Medical Officer for Health for 1937* (Delhi: Delhi Municipal Press, 1938), 66.

50. Legg, *Spaces of Colonialism*, chapter 4; Stephen Legg, "Ambivalent Improvements: Biography, Biopolitics, and Colonial Delhi," *Environment and Planning A* 39 (2008): 37–56.

51. Legg, "Governing Prostitution in Colonial Delhi."

52. Stephen Legg, "An Intimate and Imperial Feminism: Meliscent Shephard and the Regulation of Prostitution in Colonial India," *Environment and Planning D: Society and Space* 28, no. 1 (2010): 68–94.

53. Bashford and Hooker, "Introduction: Contagion, Modernity, and Postmodernity," 4.

54. Foucault, *The History of Sexuality*, Vol. 1, *An Introduction*.

55. Bashford, *Imperial Hygiene*, 164.

56. Havelock Ellis, *Studies in the Psychology of Sex*, Vols. 1–6 (Philadelphia: FA Davis Company, 1910 [1925]); Havelock Ellis, *The Task of Social Hygiene* (London: Constable & Company Ltd, 1927 [1912]).

57. Bashford, *Imperial Hygiene*, 167.

58. David J. Pivar, *Purity and Hygiene: Women, Prostitution, and the 'America Plan,' 1900–30* (Westport, CT: Greenwood Press, 2002); Greta Jones, *Social Hygiene in Twentieth Century Britain* (Wolfeboro, NH: Croom Helm, 1986).

59. Alan Hunt, *Governing Morals: A Social History of Moral Regulation* (Cambridge: Cambridge University Press, 1999), 183.

60. *Fifth Annual Report of the National Council for Combating Venereal Diseases, 1919–20* (London: National Council for Combating Venereal Disease, 1920), 9.

61. Imperial and International Questions Committee minutes, September 25, 1923, SA/BSH/B1/3: box 17, Wellcome Trust Library, London (hereafter WTL).

62. *Sixth Annual Report of the National Council for Combating Venereal Diseases, 1920–21* (London, National Council for Combating Venereal Disease, 1920), 9–10.

63. *Twelfth Annual Report of the British Social Hygiene Council, 1926–27* (London: British Social Hygiene Council, 1927), 24.

64. India Sub-Committee minutes, January 27, 1925 and March 20, 1925, SA/BSH/G2, WTL.

65. Sybil Neville-Rolfe, "Preface," in *Imperial Social Hygiene Congress*, ed. NCCVD (London National Council for Combating Venereal Diseases, 1924).

66. L. S. Amery, "Imperial Questions," in *Imperial Social Hygiene Congress*, ed. NCCVD (London: National Council for Combating Venereal Diseases, 1924), 210.

67. Ibid., 210–11.

68. Rachel Crowdy, "The League of Nations: International Positions with Regard to Prostitution and the Suppression of the Traffic in Women and Children," in *Imperial Social Hygiene Congress* (London: National Council for Combating Venereal Disease, 1924).

69. Basil Blackett, "Foreword: Imperial Citizenship," in *Empire Social Hygiene Year-Book* (London: George Allen & Unwin Ltd., 1934).

70. Hebe Spaull, "Social Hygiene and the League of Nations," *The Shield*, third series, 4, no. 1 (1923): 15–18.

71. Paul Weindling, ed., *International Health Organisations and Movements, 1918–39* (Cambridge: Cambridge University Press, 1995).

72. Stephen Legg, "Of Scales, Networks and Assemblages: The League of Nations Apparatus and the Scalar Sovereignty of the Government of India," *Transactions of the Institute of British Geographers*, n.s., 34, no. 2 (2009): 234–53.
73. For a detailed case study, see Ashwini Tambe, *Codes of Misconduct: Regulating Prostitution in Late Colonial Bombay* (Minneapolis: University of Minnesota Press 2009).

Chapter 6 Matshed Laboratory

1. See, for example, the accounts of Yersin's improvised laboratory in Noël Bernard, *Yersin: pionnier – savant – explorateur, 1863–1943* (Paris: La Colombe, 1955), 91; Henri H. Mollaret and Jacqueline Brossollet, *Alexandre Yersin ou le vainqueur de la peste* (Paris: Fayard, 1985), 137; Pierre Le Roux, *Alexandre Yersin, un passe-muraille (1863–1943). Vainqueur de la peste et de la diphtérie, explorateur des hauts plateaux d'Indochine* (Paris: Connaissance et Savoirs, 2007), 48.
2. On the tension between the adventurous explorer and the scientific traveler, see Felix Driver, *Geography Militant: Cultures of Exploration and Empire* (Oxford: Blackwell, 2001).
3. Peter Galison, "Buildings and the Subject of Science," in *The Architecture of Science*, ed. Peter Galison and Emily Thompson (Cambridge, MA: MIT Press, 1999), 1.
4. Ruth Rogaski, *Hygienic Modernity: Meanings of Health and Disease in Treaty-Port China* (Berkeley: University of California Press, 2004).
5. Paul Weindling, "Scientific Elites and Laboratory Organisation in Fin de Siècle Paris and Berlin: The Pasteur Institute and Robert Koch's Institute for Infectious Diseases Compared," in *The Laboratory Revolution in Medicine*, ed. Andrew Cunningham and Perry Williams (Cambridge: Cambridge University Press, 1992), 170–88.
6. Andrew Cunningham, "Transforming Plague: The Laboratory and the Identity of Infectious Disease," in ibid, 209–44.
7. Driver, *Geography Militant*, 10.
8. Mark Harrison, *Public Health in British India: Anglo-Indian Preventive Medicine, 1859–1914* (Cambridge: Cambridge University Press, 1994), 150–51.
9. Warwick Anderson, *Colonial Pathologies: American Tropical Medicine, Race, and Hygiene in the Philippines* (Durham, NC: Duke University Press, 2006). However, on the resurgent interest in the history of the laboratory and its relations to the field, see Robert E. Kohler, *Landscapes and Labscapes: Exploring the Lab-Field Border in Biology* (Chicago: University of Chicago Press, 2002); see also the special issue of *Isis* 99, no. 4 (December 2008) devoted to the theme.
10. Frank A. J. L. James, ed. *The Development of the Laboratory: Essays on the Place of Experiment in Industrial Civilization* (Basingstoke: Macmillan, 1989), 2. As Peter Galison observes, there is "no single transtemporal, transcultural entity that is the 'laboratory'"; see Galison, "Buildings and the Subject of Science," 1.
11. A relationship described by Roy MacLeod as the "moving metropolis"; see "On Visiting the 'Moving Metropolis': Reflections on the Architecture of Imperial

Science," in *Scientific Colonialism: A Cross-Cultural Comparison*, ed. Nathan Reingold and Marc Rothenberg (Washington, DC: Smithsonian Institution Press, 1987), 217–49.

12. Diarmid A. Finnegan, "The Spatial Turn: Geographical Approaches in the History of Science," *Journal of the History of Biology* 41, no. 2 (2008): 382.

13. Ibid., 369.

14. David N. Livingstone, *Putting Science in its Place: Geographies of Scientific Knowledge* (Chicago: University of Chicago Press, 2003), 4.

15. Londa Schiebinger, *Plants and Empire: Colonial Bioprospecting in the Atlantic World* (Cambridge, MA: Harvard University Press, 2004), 82–89; see Finnegan, who cites Schiebinger, "The Spatial Turn," 382; on the standardizaton and replication of experiments and experimental instruments, see Livingstone, *Putting Science in its Place*.

16. Finnegan, "The Spatial Turn." On the shifting border between field and lab, see Kohler, *Landscapes and Labscapes*.

17. Carol Benedict, *Bubonic Plague in Nineteenth-Century China* (Stanford: Stanford University Press, 1996), 49. See the summary of William J. Simpson's report, "Plague in Hong Kong," *British Medical Journal* 1, no. 2204 (March 28, 1903): 755–57.

18. "Government Proclamation No. 3," *Hongkong Government Gazette*, May 10, 1894; see also "Government Notification No. 175," *Hongkong Government Gazette*, May 11, 1894, 375–76. The minutes of the meeting were printed in the newspaper along with the proclamation; "A Meeting of the Sanitary Board," *Hongkong Daily Press*, May 11, 1894, 2. On the various theories of the disease's origins, see Robinson to Lord Ripon, June 20, 1894, *China. British Parliamentary Papers: Correspondence, Annual Reports, Conventions, and Other Papers Relating to the Affairs of Hong Kong, 1882–1899*, vol. 26 (Shannon: Irish University Press, 1971), 411–16. Dr James Lowson in his report, "The Epidemic of Bubonic Plague in Hongkong, 1894," suggested that the disease had been brought to the colony by the Chinese fleeing the epidemic in Canton; *Hongkong Sessional Papers for 1895*, 179.

19. On the founding of the Institute of Infectious Diseases, Koch, and Kitasato's training in Germany, see James R. Bartholomew, *The Formation of Science in Japan* (New Haven, CT: Yale University Press, 1989), 72–77, 100–01, passim.

20. S. Kitasato, "The Bacillus of Bubonic Plague," *Lancet* 2, no. 3704 (August 25, 1894): 428–30. See also the interview with Kitasato published in the *China Mail* on June 20, 1894, which was sent as an enclosure in Robinson to Lord Ripon, June 22, 1894, Great Britain, Colonial Office, General Correspondence: Hong Kong, 1841–1951, Series 129, CO129/163, 490–93, Public Record Office, Kew, London (hereafter PRO).

21. "The Plague at Hong Kong," *Lancet* 1, no. 3695 (June 23, 1894): 1581–82. A fuller account was provided on August 11, 1894: see "The Plague at Hong-Kong," *Lancet* 2, no. 3702: 325.

22. Jean Cantlie Stewart, *The Quality of Mercy: The Lives of Sir James and Lady Cantlie* (London: George Allen & Unwin, 1983), 68.

23. James Cantlie, "A Lecture on the Spread of Plague Delivered before the Epidemiological Society on Dec. 18th, 1896," *Lancet* 1, no. 3828 (January 9, 1897): 90.

24. John Thomson, *Through China with a Camera* (London and New York: Harper and Brothers, 1899), 29.

25. Osbert Chadwick, "Report on the Sanitary Condition of Hong Kong," *British Parliamentary Papers*, 99.

26. Cantlie, "A Lecture on the Spread of Plague," 90.

27. Cantlie described Hong Kong as "an El Dorado to the leprous Chinaman"; *Leprosy in Hong Kong* (Hong Kong: Kelley & Walsh, 1890), 1.

28. Robinson to Lord Ripon, June 20, 1894, *British Parliamentary Papers*, 415. See also the Letter from Robinson to Chamberlain dated July 10, 1895, which was prefixed to the Blue Book for 1894, *British Parliamentary Papers*, 429–37.

29. Ibid., 413.

30. Ibid., 412. Lowson notes that the Kennedy Town police barracks were converted into a hospital on May 14, the glassworks hospital opened on May 21, and the slaughterhouse hospital opened on June 8; see "The Epidemic of Bubonic Plague," 203–6.

31. Edward H. Paterson, *A Hospital for Hong Kong: The Centenary History of the Alice Ho Miu Ling Nethersole Hospital* (Hong Kong: Alice Ho Miu Ling Nethersole Hospital, 1987), 35–39.

32. Elizabeth Sinn, *Power and Charity: A Chinese Merchant Elite in Colonial Hong Kong* (Hong Kong: Hong Kong University Press, 2003 [1989]), 159–61.

33. "The Plague," *British Medical Journal* 1, no. 1884 (February 6, 1897): 358.

34. There is surely a connection here to the complex, mutual implications of humanitarian and military interventions explored in *Contemporary States of Emergency: The Politics of Military and Humanitarian Interventions*, ed. Didier Fassin and Mariella Pandolfi (New York: Zone Books, 2010).

35. Alexandre Yersin, "La peste bubonique à Hong-Kong," *Annales de l'Institut Pasteur* 8 (1894): 662. Descriptions of 'native' habitation recur in Yersin's travel writing; see, for example, his account of indigenous dwellings "élevées sur pilotis" ("raised on stilts") in Alexandre Yersin, "Sept mois chez les Moïs," reproduced in Le Roux, *Alexandre Yersin*, 95–123.

36. "The Plague," *British Medical Journal*, 357.

37. See Charles Nicholl, *Somebody Else: Arthur Rimbaud in Africa 1880–91* (London: Vintage, 1998), 151–58.

38. Patrice Debré, *Louis Pasteur*, trans. Elborg Forster (Baltimore, MD: Johns Hopkins University Press, 1998), 487.

39. Laurence Monnais-Rousselot, *Médecine et colonisation. L'aventure Indochinoise, 1860–1939* (Paris: CNRS Editions, 1999), 403.

40. "The Bacteriology of Plague," *British Medical Journal* 1, no. 1882 (January 23, 1897): 238. Lowson was critical of Cantlie's medical views on the plague; see, for example, his response to Cantlie in "Some Remarks on Plague," *Lancet* 1, no. 3833 (February 13, 1897): 439–42.

41. "The Plague at Hongkong," *Straits Times*, July 16, 1894, 3.

42. Edward Eigen expatiates on the 'economy' of laboratory space in his perceptive essay "The Place of Distribution: Episodes in the Architecture of Experiment," in *Architecture and the Sciences: Exchanging Metaphors*, ed. Antoine Picon and Alessandra Ponte (New York: Princeton Architectural Press, 2003), 52–79.

43. Sections of Yersin's unedited journal, "Mon voyage à Hongkong au sujet de la peste" are reproduced in Bernard, *Yersin*, 83–92.

44. Debré, *Louis Pasteur*, 191.

45. When Yersin moved in, the institute was still full of workmen putting finishing touches to the building; see Mollaret and Brossollet, *Alexandre Yersin*, 73–74. On the architectural and functional features of the new institute, see "L'Institut Pasteur," *Annales de l'Institut Pasteur* 3 (1889): 1–14.

46. Bernard, *Yersin*, 91.

47. Alexandre Yersin, "Voyage de NhaTrang à Stung Streng," *Bulletin de la Société de Géographie Commerciale de Paris* 15 (1892–93): 82. On the illustration of Yersin in front of a native hut, see Raoul Jolly, "Le docteur Yersin chez les Moïs," *Journal des Voyages et des Aventures de Terre et de Mer* 36 and 37, no. 26 (1895): 933–58.

48. "Dr Yersin Interviewed," *Singapore Free Press and Mercantile Advertiser* (February 23, 1897), 2.

49. Mollaret and Brossollet, *Alexandre Yersin*, 134–35. In contrast to this image of the solitary researcher, Cantlie noted that he "worked with Dr. Yersin in his laboratory at Hong Kong for six weeks"; see "The Bacteriology of Plague," 238.

50. James William Norton-Kyshe, *The History of the Laws and Courts of Hong Kong from the Earliest Period to 1898*, with a new foreword by Sir Ivo Rigby (Hong Kong: Vetch and Lee, 1971), 70.

51. J. A. Turner, *Kwang Tung: Or, Five Years in South China*, with an introduction by H. J. Lethbridge (London: S.W. Partridge, 1894), 132.

52. "Hong Kong," *British Medical Journal* 1, no. 2091 (January 26, 1901): 246.

53. On colonial perceptions of "loitering" and "criminal" Chinese labourers, see Christopher Munn, *Anglo-Chinese People and British Role in Hong Kong, 1841–1880* (Hong Kong: Hong Kong University Press, 2009 [2001]), 81; see also "The Eviction of Squatters at Kennedy Town," September 17, 1886, *Hongkong Sessional Papers for 1887*, 175–79.

54. Christopher Cowell, *Form Follows Fever: Malaria and the Making of Hong Kong, 1841–1848* (unpublished M.Phil. dissertation, University of Hong Kong, 2009), 280–81, 289, 292.

55. Lowson, "The Epidemic of Bubonic Plague," 181.

56. For a description of the characteristics and construction methods of the "misérables paillottes," see Charles Garnier and Auguste Ammann, *L'habitation humaine* (Paris: Librairie Hachette, 1892), 846–48.

57. Philippe Papin, *Des 'villages dans la ville' aux 'villages urbains'. L'espace et les formes du pouvoir à Hà-Nôi de 1805 à 1940* (unpublished Ph.D. dissertation, Université de Paris 7, 1997). On the perceived threat of indigenous dwellings for colonial authorities in Hanoi, see generally Michael G. Vann, *White City on the Red River:*

Race, Culture, and Power in Colonial Hanoi, 1872–1954 (unpublished Ph.D. dissertation, University of California, Santa Cruz, 1999), 19–83; Philippe Papin, *Histoire de Hanoi* (Paris: Fayard, 2001), 248–9.

58. See J. Gonzalès, "Histoire de la naissance et du développement de l'École de Médecine de Hanoï," *Histoire des Sciences Médicales* 301 (1996): 61–70.

59. Michael G. Vann, "'All the World's a Stage', Especially in the Colonies: *L'Exposition de Hanoï*, 1902–3," in *Empire and Culture: The French Experience, 1830–1940*, ed. Martin Evans (Basingstoke and New York: Palgrave Macmillan, 2004), 181–83.

60. See Alain Ruscio, "Du village à l'exposition: les Français à la rencontre des Indochinois," in *Zoos humains: au temps des exhibitions humaines*, ed. Nicolas Bancel, Pascal Blanchard and Sandrine Lemaire (Paris: La Découverte, 2004), 267–74. On the Hanoi Exhibition of 1902–03, see Vann, "'All the World's a Stage', Especially in the Colonies."

61. Ibid. The culmination of such exotic representations was the *Exposition Coloniale Internationale* of 1931. There, the showcasing of Indochinese animals in *paillotes* further reinforced the association of indigenous culture with animality; see Penny Edwards, *Cambodge: The Cultivation of a Nation, 1860–1945* (Honolulu: University of Hawaii Press, 2007), 160–62; Patricia A. Morton, *Hybrid Modernities: Architecture and Representation at the 1931 Colonial Exposition, Paris* (Cambridge, MA: MIT Press, 2000), 35. See also Ruscio, "Du village à l'exposition."

62. Gwendolyn Wright, *The Politics of Design in French Colonial Urbanism* (Chicago: University of Chicago Press, 1991), 230.

63. Eric Thomas Jennings, "Conservative Confluences, 'Nativist' Synergy: Reinscribing Vichy's National Revolution in Indochina, 1940–1945," *French Historical Studies* 27, no. 3 (2004): 601–35.

64. On the "filthy" condition of Chinese dwellings and the link with plague, see Lowson, "The Epidemic of Bubonic Plague," 182.

65. Ibid., 205; see also Colonial Surgeon's Report of 1893 (July 11, 1894), "Government Notification – No. 455," *Hongkong Government Gazette*, December 1, 1894, 976, in which he noted that "Coloured Troops" are housed in "mat huts," as opposed to the "White Troops," who are put up in "old barracks and Chinese houses converted into barracks."

66. Robinson to Lord Ripon, June 20, 1894, *British Parliamentary Papers*, 413. Similar matsheds were used to house the families and victims of plague in India; see "The Plague: Chronicle of the Epidemic," *British Medical Journal* 1, no. 1892 (April 3, 1897): 873.

67. James Cantlie, "A Lecture on the Plague," *Lancet* 1, no. 3827 (January 2, 1897): 6.

68. "Hong Kong Plague Items," *Daily Advertiser* (June 15, 1894), 3.

69. Cantlie, "A Lecture on the Plague," 7.

70. Quoted in Shiona Airlie, *Thistle and Bamboo: The Life and Times of Sir James Stewart Lockhart* (Oxford: Oxford University Press, 1989), 58.

71. Gerald H. Choa, *The Life and Times of Sir Kai Ho Kai* (Hong Kong: Chinese University Press, 2000 [1981]), 3.

72. Cowell, *Form Follows Fever*, 281; G. B. Endacott, *A Biographical Sketch-Book of Early Hong Kong*, with a new introduction by John M. Carroll (Hong Kong: Hong Kong University Press, 2005 [1962]), 61.

73. Vann, *White City on the Red River*, 29, 51.

74. Eigen, "The Place of Distribution," 70.

75. Ibid., 69–71.

76. Karin Knorr-Cetina, "The Couch, the Cathedral, and the Laboratory: On the Relationship between Experiment and Laboratory in Science," in *Science as Practice and Culture*, ed. Andrew Pickering (Chicago: University of Chicago Press, 1992), 118.

77. Ibid.

78. Arjun Appadurai, "Disjuncture and Difference in the Global Cultural Economy," in *Modernity at Large: Cultural Dimensions of Globalization* (Minneapolis: University of Minnesota Press, 1996), 27–47.

79. See, in this context, Anthony King's account of the Anglo-Indian 'bungalow' and its integration into suburban English architecture; *The Bungalow: The Production of a Global Culture*, 2nd ed. (Oxford: Oxford University Press, 1984); *Spaces of Global Cultures: Architecture, Urbanism, Identity* (London and New York: Routledge, 2004), 171–82.

80. Wright, *The Politics of Design*; Thomas R. Metcalf, *An Imperial Vision: Indian Architecture and Britain's Raj* (Berkeley and London: University of California Press). For an account of the conflict between the British and the local Chinese in relation to the construction of a matshed police headquarters in Tai Po Hui in the recently acquired New Territories (1899), see Peter Wesley-Smith, *Unequal Treaty, 1898–1997: China, Great Britain, and Hong Kong's New Territories*, rev. ed. (Hong Kong and Oxford: Oxford University Press, 1998 [1983]), 79–83.

81. Quoted in Eigen, "The Place of Distribution," 53.

82. Chadwick, "Report on the Sanitary Condition of Hong Kong," 125. For the make-shift "cabins," see the plans of a house in Kaiming Lane, 101.

83. Yersin's original letter with translation in E. Lagrange, "Concerning the Discovery of the Plague Bacillus," *Journal of Tropical Medicine and Hygiene* 29, no. 17 (1926): 302.

84. Claude Bernard, *An Introduction to the Study of Experimental Medicine*, trans. H. C. Greene (New York: Dover Publications, 1957 [1927]), 146.

85. Laura Otis, *Membranes: Metaphors of Invasion in Nineteenth-Century Literature, Science, and Politics* (Baltimore, MD: Johns Hopkins University Press, 1999), 1–7.

86. Ibid, 8.

87. Ashley Miles, "Reports by Louis Pasteur and Claude Bernard on the Organization of Scientific Teaching and Research," *Notes and Records of the Royal Society of London* 37, no. 1 (1982): 112.

88. René Vallery-Radot, *The Life of Pasteur*, trans. Mrs R. L. Devonshire (New York: Doubleday, Page & Company, 1928), 151.

89. Ibid., 152.

90. Bruno Latour, *The Pasteurization of France*, trans. Alan Sheridan and John Law (Cambridge, MA: Harvard University Press, 1988), 43–49; *Science in Action: How to Follow Scientists and Engineers Through Society* (Cambridge, MA: Harvard University Press, 1987), 162.

91. George Weisz, "Reform and Conflict in French Medical Education, 1870–1914," in *The Organization of Science and Technology in France 1808–1914*, ed. Robert Fox and George Weisz (Cambridge and New York: Cambridge University Press, 1980), 71.

92. Stanley J. Reiser, *Medicine and the Reign of Technology* (Cambridge: Cambridge University Press, 1978), 140.

93. Vallery-Radot, *The Life of Pasteur*, 152.

94. Ibid.

95. Despite the drive for reform, the extent to which real changes were effected remains debatable; see Abraham Flexner, *Medical Education in Europe: A Report to the Carnegie Foundation for the Advancement of Teaching*, introduction by Henry S. Pritchett (New York: Carnegie Foundation for the Advancement of Teaching, 1912), 220–26.

96. See Raoul Girardet, *L'idée coloniale en France de 1871 à 1962* (Paris: Hachette, 1972).

97. Jean-Pierre Dedet, "The Overseas Pasteur Institutes, with Special Reference to their Role in the Diffusion of Microbiological Knowledge: 1887–1975," *Research in Microbiology* 159, no. 1 (2008): 31–35; Annick Guénel, "The Creation of the First Overseas Pasteur Institute, or the Beginning of Albert Calmette's Pastorian Career," *Medical History* 43 (1999): 1–25.

98. "Inauguration de l'Institut Pasteur," *Annales de l'Institut Pasteur* 2 (1888): 29–30. However, Pasteur qualified this notion of borderless, "international" science by stating: "Si la science n'a pas de patrie, l'homme de science doit en avoir une, et c'est à elle qu'il doit reporter l'influence que ses travaux peuvent avoir dans le monde" ("Science has no country, but the man of science must have one, and it is to his country that he should bring all the influence that his works might have in the world").

99. Heather Bell, *Frontiers of Medicine in the Anglo-Egyptian Sudan, 1899–1940* (Oxford: Oxford University Press, 1999), 55.

100. Camille Limoges, "The Development of the Musée d'Histoire Naturelle of Paris, c.1800–1914," in *The Organization of Science and Technology in France*, 237.

101. Anne Marie Moulin, "Bacteriological Research and Medical Practice in and out of the Pastorian School," in *French Medical Culture in the Nineteenth Century*, ed. Ann La Berge and Mordechai Feingold (Amsterdam and Atlanta: Rodopi, 1994), 342. On the multi-function of the Pasteur institutes as dispensaries, research centers, and educational institutions, see the vision enunciated by Pasteur in "Inauguration de l'Institut Pasteur," 29.

102. Anne Marcovich, "French Colonial Medicine and Colonial Rule: Algeria and Indochina," in *Disease, Medicine and Empire*, ed. Roy MacLeod and Milton Lewis (New York and London: Routledge, 1988), 110.

103. Latour, *The Pasteurization of France*, 19–20.

104. Moulin, "Bacteriological Research and Medical Practice," 342.

105. Driver, *Geography Militant*, 8.

106. Latour, *The Pasteurization of France*, 45, 63, 79; Bruno Latour, "Give Me a Laboratory and I will Raise the World," in *Science Observed, Perspectives on the Study of Science*, ed. Michael Mulkay and Karin Knorr-Cetina (London: Sage, 1983), 154.

107. On Yersin's agronomic activities, see Mollaret and Brossollet, *Alexandre Yersin*, 183–86, 205–24.

108. Latour, *The Pasteurization of France*, 94–100.

109. Yersin, "La peste bubonique à Hong-Kong," 662.

110. Yersin, "Sept mois chez les Moïs," 96.

111. Ibid.

112. "The Plague," *British Medical Journal*, 357.

113. Frédéric Thomas, "L'invention des 'Hauts Plateaux' en Indochine: conquête coloniale et production de savoirs," *Ethnologie Française* 34, no. 4 (2004): 641.

114. Ibid., 645. For a general account of colonialism and tropical geography in France, see Paul Claval, "Colonial Experience and the Development of Tropical Geography in France," *Singapore Journal of Tropical Geography* 26, no. 3 (2005): 289–303.

115. Nicola Cooper, *France in Indochina: Colonial Encounters* (Oxford: Berg, 2001), 145–71.

116. As contemporaries pointed out, this assault on boundaries was a fundamental feature of microbes themselves. Although the role of microbes in breaking down living things was viewed as destructive, the ability of microbes to decompose matter was also recognized as a necessary precondition for life. See L. Capitan, "Le rôle des microbes dans la société," *Bulletin de la Société d'Anthropologie de Paris* 4, no. 4 (1893): 765.

117. Albert Calmette, "Les missions scientifiques de l'Institut Pasteur et l'expansion coloniale de la France," *Revue Scientifique* 3, no. 2 (1912): 129. See also his essay "Le rôle des sciences médicales dans la colonisation," *Revue Scientifique* 8, no. 4 (1905): 417–21.

118. Yersin, "La peste bubonique à Hong-Kong," 662.

119. J. Andrew Mendelsohn, "The Microscopist of Modern Life," *Osiris* 18 (2003): 151.

120. Ibid., 154.

121. "Dr Yersin Interviewed," *Singapore Free Press and Mercantile Advertiser*.

122. Cunningham, "Transforming Plague."

123. Quoted in William F. Bynum, *Science and the Practice of Medicine in the Nineteenth Century* (Cambridge: Cambridge University Press, 1994), 100.

124. Cunningham and Williams, "Introduction," in *The Laboratory Revolution in Medicine*, 1–13.

125. Thomas Lamarre, "Bacterial Cultures and Linguistic Colonies: Mori Rintarō's Experiments with History, Science, and Language," *Positions* 6, no. 3 (1998): 620.

126. Monnais-Rousselot, *Médecine et colonisation*, 404.

127. Thomson, *Through China with a Camera*, 7.

128. Driver, *Geography Militant*, 2.

129. Ibid.

130. Mary Robinson, *Vie de Emile Duclaux* (Laval: Barnéoud, 1906), 161; English translation in Moulin, "Bacteriological Research and Medical Practice," 328. On July
30, 1894, Émile Duclaux had read extracts from Yersin's letters to the Academy of
Sciences in Paris announcing Yersin's discovery; see, "Sur la peste de Hong Kong,"
Comptes rendus de l'Académie des sciences 119 (1894): 356.

131. Blake to Chamberlain, June 12, 1901, CO129/305, 350–51, PRO; see the discussion
in Arthur Starling et al., eds., *Plague, SARS and the Story of Medicine in Hong Kong*
(Hong Kong: Hong Kong Museum of Medical Sciences Society and Hong Kong
University Press, 2006), 148–51.

132. Patrick Manson, "The Science and Practice of Western Medicine in China," *The
China Review, or Notes & Queries on the Far East* 16, no. 2 (September 1887): 67.

133. Blake to Chamberlain, September 2, 1901, CO129/306, 298, PRO.

134. William Hunter, "Report of the Government Bacteriologist, for the Year 1902,"
Hongkong Sessional Papers for 1902, 211.

135. William Hunter, "Report of the Government Bacteriologist, for the Year 1903,"
Hongkong Sessional Papers for 1903, 261.

136. Vann, *White City on the Red River*, 51.

137. Eigen, "The Place of Distribution," 53.

Chapter 7   "Contagion of the Depot"

1.   Adam McKeown, "Global Migration, 1846–1940," *Journal of World History* 15, no.
2 (2004): 155–89.

2.   Sunil S. Amrith, *Migration and Diaspora in Modern Asia* (Cambridge: Cambridge
University Press, 2011).

3.   Alison Bashford, *Imperial Hygiene: A Critical History of Colonialism, Nationalism
and Public Health* (Basingstoke: Palgrave Macmillan, 2004); Warwick Anderson,
The Cultivation of Whiteness: Science, Health and Racial Destiny in Australia
(Durham, NC: Duke University Press, 2006); Adam McKeown, *Melancholy Order:
Asian Migration and the Globalization of Borders* (New York: Columbia University
Press, 2008); Marilyn Lake and Henry Reynolds, *Drawing the Global Colour
Line: White Men's Countries and the International Challenge of Racial Equality*
(Cambridge: Cambridge University Press, 2008).

4.   Sunil S. Amrith, "Indians Overseas? Governing Tamil Migration to Malaya, 1870–
1941," *Past and Present*, 208 (August 2010): 231–61.

5.   Eric Tagliacozzo, *Secret Trades, Porous Borders: Smuggling and States along a
Southeast Asian Frontier, 1865–1915* (New Haven, CT: Yale University Press, 2005).

6.   Amitav Ghosh, *Sea of Poppies* (London: John Murray, 2008), 258–59.

7.   Markus Rediker, *The Slave Ship: A Human History* (New York: Viking, 2008), 265.

8. Hugh Tinker, *A New System of Slavery: The Export of Indian Labour Overseas 1830–1920* (Oxford: Oxford University Press, 1974), 111, 137.

9. Giorgio Agamben, *Homo Sacer: Sovereign Power and Bare Life*, trans. Daniel Heller-Roazen (Stanford: Stanford University Press, 1998).

10. Wynne to Under Secretary to Government, December 13, 1880, Proceedings 17–23, April 1881, Emigration Branch, Home, Revenue and Agriculture Department, National Archives of India, New Delhi (hereafter NAI).

11. Tinker, *New System of Slavery*, 157–58.

12. Official Resident Councillor, Prince of Wales Island to Fort Saint George, December 12, 1848, Madras Public Proceedings (hereafter MPP), vol. 832, Tamil Nadu State Archives, Chennai (hereafter TNSA).

13. Governor of Prince of Wales Island to Montgomery, 15 May 1849, MPP, vol. 836, TNSA.

14. Straits Settlements, Ordinance XIX of 1886, in C. G. Garrard, ed., *The Acts and Ordinances of the Legislative Council of the Straits Settlements*, 2 vols. (London: 1898), 970–72.

15. For broader perspectives, see Alison Bashford and Carolyn Strange, eds., *Isolation: Places and Practices of Exclusion* (London: Routledge, 2003); and Alison Bashford and Claire Hooker, eds., *Contagion: Historical and Cultural Studies* (London: Routledge, 2001).

16. Tinker, *New System of Slavery*, v.

17. "A Bill for Regulating the Immigration of Native Labourers from British India," Proceedings 1–11, June, 1872, Emigration Branch, Department of Revenue Agriculture & Commerce (hereafter RAC), NAI.

18. For a fuller discussion of these points, see Amrith, "Indians Overseas?"

19. Lieutenant-Governor of Penang to Colonial Secretary, Straits Settlements, March 26, 1875, Proceedings 10–21, November 1875, Emigration Branch, RAC, NAI.

20. Ibid.

21. Fischer to Protector of Emigrants, Madras, Letter No. 282, Karikal, April 1, 1873, Proceedings 38–48, February 1874, Emigration Branch, RAC, NAI. My emphasis.

22. Charles Taylor, "What is Human Agency?" in *Philosophical Papers*, Vol. 1, *Human Agency and Language* (Cambridge: Cambridge University Press, 1985).

23. Amrith, "Indians Overseas?"

24. Hume to Colonial Secretary, Singapore, June 9, 1874, Proceedings June 10–13, 1874, Emigration Branch, RAC, NAI.

25. Ibid.

26. Coghill to Magistrate of Police, Province Wellesley, November 16, 1873, Proceedings 10–13, June 1874, Emigration Branch, RAC, NAI.

27. A. E. Anson, Memorandum, Number 4223, December 4, 1873, Proceedings 10–13, June 1874, Emigration Branch, RAC, NAI.

28. W. E. Maxwell and others, Memorandum, December 15, 1873, Proceedings 10–13, June 1874, Emigration Branch, RAC, NAI.

29. Amarjit Kaur, "Indian Labour, Labour Standards, and Workers' Health in Burma and Malaya, 1900–1940," *Modern Asian Studies* 40, no. 2 (2006): 425–75 (469).

30. Kaur, "Indian Labour," 466.

31. Michel Foucault, *Society Must Be Defended: Lectures at the College de France, 1976*, trans. David Macey (London: Penguin, 2003).

32. For an expanded perspective, see Sunil S. Amrith, "Eugenics in Postcolonial Southeast Asia," in *The Oxford Handbook of the History of Eugenics*, ed. Alison Bashford and Philippa Levine (Oxford: Oxford University Press, 2010), chapter 17.

33. Didier Fassin, "Humanitarianism as a Politics of Life," *Public Culture* 19, no. 3 (2007): 500–501.

34. Straits Settlements, *Report on Indian Immigration for the Year 1881* (Singapore, 1882).

35. See Madhavi Kale, *Fragments of Empire: Capital, Slavery and Indian Indentured Labour* (Philadelphia: University of Pennsylvania Press, 1998); John D. Kelly, *A Politics of Virtue: Hinduism, Sexuality and Countercolonial Discourse in Fiji* (Chicago: University of Chicago Press, 1991); and Marina Carter and Khal Torabully, *Coolitude: An Anthology of the Indian Labour Diaspora* (London: Anthem Press, 2002).

36. Johnson, to The Collector, Tanjore, May 7, 1908, Proceedings, 2–5 (A), July 1908, Emigration Branch, Department of Commerce and Industry (hereafter DCI), NAI.

37. J. D. Samy, "The Indian Coolies in the Federated Malay States: The Perils of Ignorance," reproduced in Proceedings 2–3 (B), July 1914, Emigration Branch, DCI, NAI.

38. Karl Marx, *Capital: A Critique of Political Economy*, trans. Ben Fowkes (Harmondsworth: Penguin, 1976), 130, 134.

39. On the "value" of slave bodies, see Rediker, *Slave Ship*, 273, and Megan Vaughan, "Slavery, Smallpox and Revolution: 1792 in Ile de France (Mauritius)," *Social History of Medicine* 13, no. 3 (2000): 411–28.

40. Agamben, *Homo Sacer*.

41. Kelly, *A Politics of Virtue*; Amrith, "Indians Overseas?"

42. The phrase from James Clifford, "Traveling Culture," in *Routes: Travel and Translation in the Late Twentieth Century* (Cambridge, MA: Harvard University Press, 1997), 17–46.

43. James Low, *The British Settlement of Penang* (Singapore: Singapore Free Press, 1836); for further discussion, see Sunil S. Amrith, "Tamil Diasporas Across the Bay of Bengal," *American Historical Review* 114, no. 3 (June 2009): 547–72.

44. Brenda S. A. Yeoh, *Contesting Space: Power Relations and the Urban Built Environment in Colonial Singapore* (Oxford: Oxford University Press, 1996).

45. C. Snouck Hurgronje, *Mekka in the Latter Part of the 19ᵗʰ Century: Daily Life, Customs and Learning; the Moslims of the East Indian Archipelago*, trans. J.H. Monahan (Leyden: E. J. Brill, 1931); W. Blythe, *The Impact of Chinese Secret Societies in Malaya* (Oxford: Oxford University Press, 1969).

Chapter 8   Carter and Contagion in India

1. On the "webs" of empire, see the introduction to this volume and the works by Tony Ballantyne, *Between Colonialism and Diaspora: Sikh Cultural Formations in an Imperial World* (Durham, NC: Duke University Press, 2001), 30–31; *Orientalism and Race: Aryanism in the British Empire* (Basingstoke: Palgrave Macmillan, 2002), 3–4, 14–15.

2. See, for example, Jo Robertson's discussion on the pressures brought to bear on the Leprosy Investigation Commission to India in 1890–91; "In Search of *M. Leprae*: Medicine, Public Debate, Politics and the Leprosy Commission to India," in *Economies of Representation, 1790–2000: Colonialism and Commerce*, ed. Leigh Dale and Helen Gilbert (Aldershot: Ashgate, 2007), 41–58.

3. See Douglas M. Haynes, *Imperial Medicine: Patrick Manson and the Conquest of Tropical Disease* (Pennsylvania: University of Pennsylvania Press, 2001).

4. On colonialism, compassion and the development of "Imperial Humanitarianism," see Michael Barnett, *Empire of Humanity: A History of Humanitarianism* (Ithaca, NY: Cornell University Press, 2011), 60–75.

5. E. A. Parkes, "Address in Medicine," *British Medical Journal* 2, no. 658 (August 9, 1897): 141–46.

6. Ibid., 144.

7. Ibid.

8. Ibid.

9. Ibid.

10. G. Drews, "The Roots of Medical Microbiology and the Influence of Ferdinand Cohn on the Microbiology of the 19th century," *FEMS Microbiology Reviews* 24 (2000): 225–49. See also D. Jokl, "Robert Koch's Debt to Ferdinand Cohn," *Documenta Ophthalmologica* 99, no. 3 (1999): 285–92. Parkes died in 1876.

11. Editorial, "Killed in Action [Otto Obermeier]," *International Journal of Medical Microbiology* 295 (2005): 513–18.

12. Carter's visit is fully described in Henry Vandyke Carter, *Report on Leprosy and Leper-Asylums in Norway, with references to India* (London: India Office, 1874).

13. D. C. Danielssen and C. W. Boeck, *Om Spedalsked* (Grondhal, Christiania, 1847), published in French the following year, *Traité de la Spédalskhed ou Eléphantiasis des Grecs* (Paris, Bailliere, 1848). Virchow thought highly of the book; see L. M. Irgens, "The Discovery of Mycobacterium Leprae," *American Journal of Dermatopathology* 6, no. 4 (1984): 337–43. See also T. M. Vogelsgang, "Leprosy in Norway," *Medical History* 9 (1965): 29–35.

14. M. Maiden, "Putting Leprosy on the Map," *Nature Genetics* 41 (2009): 1264–66.

15. On the revulsion and fear provoked by leprosy and the responses to the disease in Britain and its empire, see Rod Edmond, *Leprosy and Empire: A Medical and Cultural History* (Cambridge: Cambridge University Press, 2006).

16. Carter, *Report on Leprosy and Leper-Asylums in Norway*. For information on the Bergen Leprosy Museum, see http://www.bergen-guide.com/54.htm

17. Henry Vandyke Carter, *Reports on Leprosy*, second series (London: Her Majesty's Stationery Office, 1876).

18. Carter, *Report on Leprosy and Leper-Asylums in Norway*, 27. Hansen and Carter remained in touch for the rest of Carter's working life, and possibly afterwards.

19. Henry Vandyke Carter, "Reflections," March 18, 1854, Carter Papers, Wellcome Western Manuscripts, MS.5819, Wellcome Trust Library, London (hereafter WTL).

20. S. H. Brown, "British Army Surgeons Commissioned 1840–1909," *Medical History* 37 (1993): 416.

21. Ruth Richardson, *The Making of Mr Gray's Anatomy: Bodies, Books, Fortune, Fame* (Oxford: Oxford University Press, 2008).

22. Henry Vandyke Carter, Journal, April 15, 1858, Carter Papers, Wellcome Western Manuscripts, MS.5818, WTL.

23. See, for example, Robert Liveing, *Elephantiasis Graecorum, or True Leprosy* (London: Longmans, Green and Co, 1873), 86.

24. Henry Vandyke Carter, *Symptoms & Morbid Anatomy of Leprosy* (Bombay: Bombay Medical & Physical Society, 1862).

25. Henry Vandyke Carter, *On Mycetoma, or the Fungus Disease of India* (London: Churchill, 1874).

26. Carter, *Report on Leprosy and Leper-Asylums in Norway*, 24.

27. Henry Vandyke Carter, *Modern Indian Leprosy: Being the Report of a Tour in Kattiawar, 1876 with Addenda on Norwegian, Cretan and Syrian Leprosy* (Bombay, 1876); *Reports on Leprosy (Second Series) Comprising Notices of the Disease as it Now Exists in North Italy, the Greek Archipelago, Palestine and Part of the Bombay Presidency* (Great Britain, India Office, 1876).

28. Carter, *Report on Leprosy and Leper-Asylums in Norway*, 27.

29. Ibid., 30. The disease is indeed now extinct in Norway.

30. Ibid., 9.

31. Editorial, *Lancet* 2, no. 3022 (July 30, 1881): 184–85.

32. Henry Vandyke Carter, *Leprosy and Elephantiasis* (London: Her Majesty's Stationery Office, 1874), Appendix I.

33. The death rate for the fever seems to have been very high in Bombay. Many immigrants became ill on the roads into the city, and hunger and privation among them were exacerbated on their arrival by the insanitary and malaria-infested area chosen by the imperial authorities for a "camp of refuge," and by a concurrent epidemic of typhus.

34. Henry Vandyke Carter, "Spirilla in Tropical Fevers," *Lancet* 1, no. 2806 (June 9, 1877): 859. *Indian Medical Gazette* (November 1, 1877): 275.

35. S. Pandya, "Regularly Brought-up Medical Men," *Indian Economic and Social History Review* 41, no. 3 (2004): 308.

36. Henry Vandyke Carter, "Notes on the Spirillum Fever of Bombay, 1877," *British Medical Journal* 1, no. 910 (June 8, 1878): 839.

37. Henry Vandyke Carter, "Contributions to the Experimental Pathology of Spirillum Fever: Its Communicability by Inoculation to the Monkey," *British Medical Journal* (March 28, 1880): 327.

38. Henry Vandyke Carter, "Contribution to the History of the Epidemic Fever prevailing in the Country districts of the Bombay Presidency during the Famineperiod of 1876–8," *Transactions of the Epidemiological Society of London* (1881): 580–96.

39. Henry Vandyke Carter, *Spirillum Fever* (London: Churchill, 1882). The Stewart Pathology Prize award was reported in the *British Medical Journal* (August 12, 1882): 276.

40. "Sir William Guyer Hunter K.C.M.G." *British Medical Journal* (February 16, 1884): 329. See also D'Arcy Power and P. Wallis, "Sir W.G. Hunter," in *Oxford Dictionary of National Biography* (Oxford: Oxford University Press, 2004) [article 34065 accessed online, November 27, 2009].

41. Carter exhibited the bacilli of leprosy and tuberculosis, the spirillum of relapsing fever, and the "seeds of mycetoma" at a meeting of the Bombay Medical and Physical Society in June 1883. A colored zincograph of a drawing by Carter of the two first organisms, showing their comparative size and similarity of appearance, was attached to his *Memorandum on the Prevention of Leprosy by Segregation* (Bombay: Bombay Government, 1884).

42. Carter displayed Koch's comma-bacillus at a meeting of the Bombay Medical and Physical Society in May 1884. See *British Medical Journal* (August 30, 1884): 435.

43. W. S. Osler, "An Address on the Haematozoa of Malaria," *British Medical Journal* (March 12, 1887): 556–62. The *British Medical Journal* (January 15, 1887), 121–2, had also published a report of Osler's presentation of his findings in Philadelphia the previous November.

44. Henry Vandyke Carter, "The Blood Organisms in Ague," in *Scientific Memoirs by Medical Officers of the Army of India* (Calcutta, 1888).

45. Carter drew Indian government attention to the decline in the number of cases of leprosy in Norway by publishing Hansen's latest figures. See, for example: Carter, *Memorandum on the Prevention of Leprosy*; and Henry Vandyke Carter, *Observations on the Prevention of Leprosy by Segregation* (Bombay: Bombay Government, 1887).

46. "A Victim of Leprosy," *British Medical Journal* (January 26, 1889): 2.

47. Robert Louis Stevenson, *Father Damien: An Open Letter to the Rev. Dr. Hyde of Honolulu* (London: Chatto & Windus, 1890).

48. H. P. Wright, *Leprosy, an Imperial Danger* (London: Churchill, 1889).

49. Robertson, "In Search of *M. Leprae*," 41.

50. L. M. Irgens, "The Discovery of Mycobacterium Leprae," *American Journal of Dermatopathology* 6, no. 4 (1984): 337–43.

51. Jane Buckingham, *Leprosy in Colonial South India: Medicine and Confinement* (Basingstoke: Palgrave Macmillan, 2002).

52. "Indian Leprosy," *Times* [London] (April 10, 1876), 4.

Chapter 9   Epidemics of Famine and Obesity

1.   "The Fat of the Lands," *Economist*, February 23, 2002, 81–82.
2.   Ali H. Mokdad et al., "The Spread of the Obesity Epidemic in the United States, 1991–1998," *Journal of the American Medical Association* 282, no. 16 (1999): 1519–22.
3.   Annabel Ferriman, "The man who will try to persuade us to give up some of life's good things," *Times* [London], (August 7, 1981), 12.
4.   Longde Wang et al., "Preventing Chronic Diseases in China," *Lancet* 366, no. 9499 (November 19, 2005); see also Dongfeng Gu et al., "Prevalence of the Metabolic Syndrome and Overweight Among Adults In China," *Lancet* 365, no. 9468 (April 16, 2005): 1398–1405.
5.   G. S. Ma, et al., "The Prevalence of Body Overweight and Obesity and Its Changes Among Chinese People during 1992 to 2002," [in Chinese] *Zhonghua Yu Fang Yi Xue Za Zhi* [Chinese journal of preventive medicine] 39 (2005): 311–15.
6.   Xiaoping Weng and Benjamin Caballero, *Obesity and Its Related Diseases in China: The Impact of the Nutrition Transition in Urban and Rural Adults* (Youngstown, NY: Cambria Press, 2007), 1.
7.   W. P. Jia, K. S. Xiang, L. Chen, J. X. Lu, and Y. M. Wu, "Epidemiological Study on Obesity and Its Comorbidities in Urban Chinese Older than 20 Years of Age in Shanghai, China," *Obesity Reviews* 3 (2002): 157–65.
8.   For example, Joseph S. Alter, ed., *Asian Medicine and Globalization* (Philadelphia, PA: University of Pennsylvania Press, 2005).
9.   James L. Watson, "Food as a Lens: The Past, Present, and Future of Family Life in China," in *Feeding China's Little Emperors: Food, Children, and Social Change*, ed. Jun Jing (Stanford: Stanford University Press, 2000), 208.
10. Heinrich, *Afterlife of Images*.
11. Lillian M. Li, *Fighting Famine in North China: State, Market, and Environmental Decline, 1690s–1990s* (Stanford: Stanford University Press, 2007), 264; Robert Marks, *Tigers, Rice, Silk, and Silt: Environment and Economy in Late Imperial South China* (Cambridge: Cambridge University Press, 1998), 148.
12. William Hamilton Jefferys and James L. Maxwell, *The Diseases of China: Including Formosa and Korea* (London: Bale & Danielsson, 1911), 48.
13. "Preliminary Report of Committee on Infant and Invalid Diet," *China Medical Journal* 26 (1912): 133–44.
14. For a discussion of sweetened milk as therapy for hospital patients and of the craze for condensed milk as "modern" see Frank Dikötter, *Exotic Commodities: Modern Objects and Everyday Life in China* (New York: Columbia University Press, 2007), 220, 224.
15. Hannah Velten, *Milk: A Global History* (London: Reaktion, 2010).
16. S. Weir Mitchell, *Fat and Blood* (New York: Lippincott, 1900), 119.
17. U.S. Congress Senate Committee on Finance, *Testimony taken by the subcommittee on the tariff of the Senate Committee on the Tariff* (Washington, DC: Government Printing Office, 1885), 835.

18. N. Kretchmer, "Lactose and Lactase," *Scientific American* 227, no. 4 (1972): 71–78.

19. Jefferys and Maxwell, *Diseases of China*, 259.

20. Ibid.

21. Mary Stone, "Hospital Dietary in China," *China Medical Journal* 26 (1912): 299.

22. Amartya Sen has more recently argued that famine occurs not from a lack of food, but from inequalities built into mechanisms for distributing food. Amartya Sen, *Poverty and Famines: An Essay on Entitlement and Deprivation* (Oxford: Clarendon Press, 1981); B.E. Read, "Some Factors Controlling the Food Supply in China," *China Medical Journal* 25 (1921): 1–7.

23. Hartley Embrey and Tsou Ch'ing Wang, "Analysis of Some Chinese Foods," *China Medical Journal* 35 (1921): 247–57.

24. W. H. Adolph and P. C. Kiang, "The Nutritive Value of Soy Bean Products," *China Medical Journal* 34 (1920): 268–75; William H. Adolph, "Diet Studies in Shantung," *China Medical Journal* 37 (1923): 1013–19.

25. Thus the journal regularly reprints summaries of Western medical essays such as one taken from the *Berliner Klinische Wochenschrift* of March 1914, advocating "cream and bed rest." *China Medical Journal* 29 (1915): 419–20.

26. Jean I. Dow, "Maternity Famine Relief," *China Medical Journal* 36 (1922): 59–67.

27. Letter to the editor by Sargent, "The Trade in Chinese Children," *China Medical Journal* 34 (1920): 695.

28. Thus, in an editorial, the concern is about diseases ranging from appendicitis to gallstones to cancer. "Relation of Oriental Diet to Disease," *China Medical Journal* 38 (1924): 834–36.

29. J.-P. Beaude, "Obésité," in J.-P. Beaude, ed., *Dictionnaire de médecine usuelle à l'usage des gens du monde*, vol. 2 (Paris: Didier, 1849), 529–30.

30. Rousselot de Surgy, *Mélanges intéressans et curieux*, vol. 4 (Paris: Lacombe, 1766), 190.

31. Frederic W. Farrar, "Aptitudes of Races," *Transactions of the Ethnological Society of London* 5 (1867): 124.

32. Arthur de Gobineau, *Essai sur l'inégalité des races humaines*, vol. 1 (Paris: Librairie de Firmin Didot Frères, 1853), 352.

33. Thomas King Chambers, "On the Pathology of Obesity," *Boston Medical and Surgical Journal* 43 (1851): 9–16.

34. J. Richardson Parke, *Human Sexuality: A Medico Literary Treatise* (Philadelphia: Spinoza Professional Publishing Company, 1912), 74.

35. Jefferys and Maxwell, *Diseases of China*, 320.

36. Thomas B. Futcher, "Diabetes Mellitus and Ixsipidus," in *Modern Medicine: Its Theory And Practice*, ed. William Osler, vol. 1 (Philadelphia and New York: Lea & Febiger 1914), 674–75.

37. Osler, *Modern Medicine*, 751.

38. Quoted in Vivienne Lo and Penelope Barrett, "Cooking up Fine Remedies: On the Culinary Aesthetic in a Sixteenth-century *Materia Medica*," *Medical History* 49 (2005): 417.

39. Watson, "Food as a Lens," 208.

40. Wang Dungen "Reforming the Human Body" ("Renti Gailiang"), *Shenbao Ziyoutan* (August 29, 1911), 3.

41. Mao Zedong, "A Study of Physical Education" (April 1917), in *Mao's Road to Power: Revolutionary Writings 1912–1949*, ed. Stuart R. Schram, vol. 1 (Armonk, NY: M.E. Sharpe, 1992): 113–27.

42. Watson, "Food as a Lens," 208.

43. Shu Hui and Wei Seng, "On Obesity" ("Lun Feipang Zhi Bing"), *Funu Shibao* [*Women's Newspaper*] (April 10, 1913), 26–28.

44. Wilhelm Ebstein, *Die Fettleibigkeit (Corpulenz) und ihre Behandlung nach physiologischen Grundstätzen*, 6th ed. (Wiesbaden: J.F. Bergmann, 1884), 10.

45. Dai Zuo, "Jianshou Ja" [Keep the body slim], *Jiating zazhi* [Family magazine] 3 (1922): 1–4 (1).

46. W.S. Hedley, *Therapeutic Electricity and Practical Muscle Testing* (Philadelphia: P. Blakiston's Son and Co., 1900), 209–10.

47. Zhou Zhenyu, "Funü Feipang De Yuanyin He Haichu" [The cause and danger of female obesity], *Xin Nüxing* [The new woman] (Shanghai) 1 (1926): 42–45.

48. "What Causes Obesity?" *Journal of the American Medical Association* 83, no. 13 (September 27, 1924): 1003.

49. Qi Hui, "Canzhuoshang De Beiju" [Tragedy at the dinner table], *Liangyou* 167 (June 1941), unpaginated.

50. Ibid.

51. Ibid.

Chapter 10   'Rails, Roads, and Mosquito Foes'

1. Daniel Headrick, *The Tools of Empire. Technology and European Imperialism in the Nineteenth Century* (Oxford: Oxford University Press, 1981); William B. Cohen, "Malaria and French Imperialism," *Journal of African History* 24 (1983): 23–36; David Arnold, ed., *Imperial Medicine and Indigenous Societies* (Manchester: Manchester University Press, 1988), 10–11; Mark Harrison, "'Hot Beds of Disease': Malaria and Civilization in Nineteenth Century India," *Parassitologia* 40 (1998): 11–18.

2. Alice Conklin, *A Mission to Civilize: The Republican Idea of Empire in France and West Africa, 1895–1930* (Stanford: Stanford University Press, 1997).

3. Laurence Monnais, *Médecine et colonisation. L'aventure indochinoise, 1860–1939* (Paris : CNRS Editions, 1999), 35–37.

4. Jules Boissière, "Dans la forêt," in *Indochine. Un rêve d'Asie*, ed. A. Quella-Villégier (Paris : Omnibus, 1995 [1896]), 12–13.

5. Dr De Fornel, "Etat sanitaire du Tonkin pendant l'année 1889," *Archives de Médecine Navale* 57 (1892): 244–62.

6. Edouard Jeanselme, "Les principaux facteurs de la morbidité et de la mortalité indochinoise," Congrès colonial français, Paris, May 29–June 5, 1904.

7. Monnais, *Médecine et colonisation*, 53.

8. Constant Mathis and Maurice Léger, "Le paludisme au Tonkin. Index épidémiologique aux différentes saisons," *Annales d'Hygiène et de Médecine Coloniales* (hereafter *AHMC*) 14 (1911): 294–316 and 523–48.

9. In fact, Alphonse Laveran identified the *Falciparum* (or *Praecox*) *plasmodium* responsible for a serious form of malaria. Three other hematozoans were discovered during the colonial period: *Plasmodium vivax, Plasmodium malariae,* and *Plasmodium ovale*.

10. "Sur les mesures à prendre pour développer dans les colonies françaises l'usage préventif de la quinine contre le paludisme," *Bulletin de la Société de Pathologie Exotique* (hereafter *BSPE*) 2 (1909): 225–34.

11. Dr. Vassal, "Géographie médicale de Nha Trang," *AHMC* 9 (1906): 481–511.

12. Noël Bernard, "Rapport médical sur l'application du programme d'organisation ouvrière aux chantiers de la ligne de Yen Bay à Lao Kay, Tonkin, 1er octobre 1904 – 1er octobre 1905," *AHMC*, 10 (1907): 432.

13. René Montel, "Un essai de quinine préventive à Hatien (Cochinchine)," *BSPE* 3 (1910): 626–28.

14. Dr Boyé, "Relations entre la consommation de quinine et la fréquence de la fièvre bilieuse hémoglobinurique au Tonkin," *AHMC* 17 (1914): 71.

15. File 65324, Fonds du Gouvernement général de l'Indochine (hereafter Gougal), Centre des Archives d'Outre-Mer, Aix-en-Provence (hereafter CAOM).

16. Dossier 2787, Fonds des Amiraux (hereafter Amiraux), CAOM.

17. On the history of pharmaceuticals in colonial Vietnam, see Laurence Monnais, *Médicaments coloniaux. Circulation, distribution et consommation de médicaments au Viêt nam, 1905–40* (Paris: Les Indes Savantes, forthcoming).

18. The independence of the Indochinese health budget would never allow it to be large enough to support the sanitary system that was envisioned. In 1913, this budget was worth 1.7 million piastres (Indochinese currency); in 1931, three million, which was equivalent to a maximum of 3.8 percent of the general colonial budget. On average, half of this budget went towards the construction and maintenance of the sanitary infrastructure, 25 percent to environmental sanitation. The portion of the budget dedicated to materials, including the supply of the SQS, represented a maximum of 0.3 percent of the total budget.

19. Pierre Hermant, "Note sur l'organisation de la vente de la quinine d'Etat dans la province de Nghe An," *Bulletin de la Société Médico-chirurgicale de l'Indochine* (*BSMI*) 3 (1912): 231–33.

20. Drs Guillon and Kéruzoré, "Quelques précisions sur la quinine et ses sels et leur emploi en thérapeutique coloniale," *Archives de Médecine et de Pharmacie Coloniales* (hereafter *AMPC*) 24 (1926): 516.

21. Dr Allain, "Paludisme et quinine d'Etaten Annam pendant l'année 1912: Rapports des provinces collationnés," *BSPE* 6 (1913): 730–44.

22. Dr Havet, "Rapport médical concernant la province de Tay Ninh," *Bulletin de la Société des Etudes Indochinoises* (1916–17): 190–91.

23. Allain, "Paludisme et quinine d'Etat," 646.

24. Dossier 379, Fonds de la Direction locale de la santé du Tonkin (hereafter DLS), National Archives of Vietnam I, Hanoi (hereafter VNNA1).

25. Hermant, "Note sur l'organisation de la vente de la quinine d'Etat," 117.

26. Nha Que, "La quinine d'Etat," L'Echo Annamite, July 8, 1922.

27. Dossier 34, Fonds de l'Inspection Générale de l'Hygiène et de la Santé publique (hereafter IGHSP), VNNA1.

28. Dossier 4, Fonds IGHSP, VNNA1.

29. It is unclear as to why Annam was penalized in this way, though perhaps it was because as a predominantly rural pays it was considered less valuable to the colonial government in terms of economic exploitation and development.

30. Carton 189, dossier 2787, Amiraux, CAOM.

31. Marie-Etienne Farinaud, Constantin Toumanoff, and Hoang Thuy Ba, "Le paludisme à Tuyên Quang. Enquête malariologique," BSMI 10 (1932): 66–128.

32. Joseph-Emile Borel, "Anophèles et paludisme dans la région de Chaudoc (Cochinchine). Résultats d'une enquête faite du 16 au 21 janvier 1926," BSPE 19 (1926): 806; Dorolle, Pierre, "Le paludisme à Ha Giang (Tonkin)," BSPE 20 (1927): 921.

33. Dossier 380, 383, 384, 385, DLS, VNNA1.

34. Dr Lecomte, "L'assistance médicale en Cochinchine pendant l'année 1924," AMPC, 26 (1926): 137.

35. Dossier 3829, Fonds de la Résidence Supérieure du Tonkin Nouveau Fonds (hereafter RSTNF), CAOM; dossier 2931, Gougal Service Economique (hereafter SE), CAOM; dossier 4 IGHSP, VNNA1.

36. Allain, "Paludisme et quinine d'Etat," 643; Dr Audibert, "Les maladies endémo-épidémiques observés en Indochine pendant l'année 1921 (extraits du rapport annuel)," AMPC 21 (1923): 64.

37. Dossier 581, DLS, VNNA1.

38. Pierre Hermant, "A propos d'une note récente sur la Quinine d'Etat," BSMI 3 (1912): 344.

39. Henry G.S. Morin and Louis Bordes, "Développement de la lutte anti-malarienne en Indochine," Archives des Instituts Pasteur d'Indochine 12 (1931): 81.

40. "Contre le paludisme," L'Echo Annamite, September 23, 1927.

41. "Pour la santé publique en Cochinchine. Distribution de la Quinine d'Etat," L'Echo Annamite, January 3, 1929.

42. Splenomegaly is the enlargement of the spleen palpable under the left side of the ribs, a sympton indicating that malaria has set in.

43. Maurice Blanchard, "Les insuccès de la quinine préventive dus à l'insolubilité des comprimés," BSPE 15 (1922): 293–95.

44. Boyé, "Relations"; Louis Normet, "Le traitement du paludisme," AMPC 19 (1921): 202–7; Jean Legendre, "A propos de l'efficacité de la quinine préventive," BSPE 18 (1925): 272. Hemoglobinuric fever is in fact a serious complication related to problems of non-adherence to anti-malarial treatment.

45. Marcel Autret, "La fraude sur la quinine en Indochine," *Revue Médicale Française d'Extrême-Orient* 17 (1939): 925–28.
46. Monnais, *Médecine et colonisation*, 389.
47. Joseph-Emile Borel, "Contribution à l'étude de la mortalité infantile en Cochinchine," *BSPE* 20 (1927): 52–55; "Enquête malariologique à la station d'essai de Giaray (Cochinchine)," *BSPE* 21 (1928): 312–14.
48. Dossier 47474, Gougal, CAOM; Fonds de la Résidence Supérieure de l'Annam (hereafter RSA) HC 3373, National Archives of Vietnam II, Ho Chi Minh City (hereafter VNNA2).
49. Annick Guénel, "Malaria, Colonial Economics, and Migrations in Vietnam," Fourth Conference of the European Association of Southeast Asian Studies, Paris, September 1–4, 2004, 3.
50. Louis Bordes, *Le paludisme en Indochine* (Hanoi: Imprimerie d'Extrême-Orient, 1931), 14.
51. Randall Packard, *The Making of a Tropical Disease: A Short History of Malaria* (Baltimore, MD: Johns Hopkins University Press, 2007), 7–8, 102, 113.
52. Laurent Gaide, "Le paludisme en Annam et au Tonkin," *AHMC* 12 (1909): 288–89.
53. 22b, Fonds de la Commission Guernut, CAOM.
54. Joseph-Emile Borel, "Paludisme en Cochinchine. Résultats de mesures prophylactiques à la plantation de Suzannah (11 au 13 août 1926)," *BSPE* 19 (1926): 811–15.
55. Numerous experiments were undertaken by the Pasteur institutes in order to acclimatize cinchona trees in Indochina but they never succeeded.
56. Quinine has a schizonticid action (i.e., a destructive action on asexual forms of plasmodium). So does Quinacrine (Rhône-Poulenc), the brand name of Atebrin synthesized in 1930. In contrast, Plasmochine (Bayer), the brand name of Praequine synthesized in 1925, and Rhodoquine (Rhône-Poulenc), both have a gametocid action, i.e., a destructive action on sexual forms of plasmodium. Therefore they have to be taken in conjunction with quinine.
57. Dossier 3710, RST NF, CAOM; dossier 3783, RSTNF, CAOM.
58. Pierre Hermant, "La lutte contre le paludisme dans les Etats malais fédérés," *La Presse Médicale*, October 18, 1930; Annick Guénel, "Malaria Control, Land Occupation, and Scientific Developments in Vietnam in the 20th Century," 51st Annual Meeting of the Association for Asian Studies (AAS), Boston (United States), March 11–14, 1999; Ku Ya Wen, "Anti-Malaria Policy and Its Consequences in Colonial Taiwan," in *Disease, Colonialism, and the State. Malaria in Modern East Asian History*, ed. Ka-Che Yip (Hong Kong: Hong Kong University Press, 2009), 39–42.
59. Annick Guénel, "The 1937 Bandung Conference on Rural Hygiene: Towards a New Vision of Health Care?" in *Global Movements, Local Concerns: Medicine and Health in Southeast Asia*, ed. Laurence Monnais and Harold J. Cook (Singapore: NUS Press, forthcoming), 62–80.
60. Société des Nations, Organisation d'Hygiène, *Enquête sur les besoins en quinine des pays impaludés et sur l'extension du paludisme dans le monde* (Geneva: SDN, 1932).

Colonial sources do not agree on the total amount of quinine distributed that year; depending on the source it varies between 3,092 and 3,874 kilos—compared to 294 in 1917 and 1,638 in 1921.

61.   At least no more than it was in British India: Arnold, *Imperial Medicine and Indigenous Societies*, 202; Harrison, "'Hot Beds of Disease,'" 11.

62.   Conklin, *A Mission to Civilize*, 6.

Afterword

1.   *The Declaration of Alma-Ata* in *Concepts and Practice of Humanitarian Medicine*, ed. S. William A. Gunn and Michele Masellis (New York: Springer, 2008): 21–23.

2.   Margaret Chan, "Return to Alma-Ata," *Lancet* 372, no. 9642 (September 13, 2008): 865.

3.   Ibid., 865.

4.   Sunil Amrith, *Decolonizing International Health: India and Southeast Asia, 1930–65* (Basingstoke: Palgrave Macmillan, 2006).

5.   Cyrus Edson, "The Microbe as Social Leveller," *North American Review* 161, no. 467 (October 1895): 421–26, 425.

6.   See, for example, Warwick Anderson, "Immunities of Empire: Race, Disease, and the New Tropical Medicine, 1900–1920," *Bulletin of the History of Medicine* 70, no. 1 (1996): 94–118.

7.   See also, in this context, the essays in D. Ann Herring and Alan C. Swedlund, eds., *Plagues and Epidemics: Infected Spaces Past and Present* (Oxford and New York: Berg, 2010).

8.   The conference was co-sponsored by the National Institute of Allergy and Infectious Disease, Rockefeller University, and the Fogarty International Center. It was the brainchild largely of Joshua Lederberg and Stephen Morse.

9.   That geography is evident, for example, in many of the essays in two collections that emerged from the conference: Committee on Emerging Microbial Threats to Health, *Emerging Infections: Microbial Threats to Health in the United States* (Washington, DC: National Academies Press, 1992) and Stephen Morse, ed., *Emerging Viruses* (New York: Oxford University Press, 1993) as well as in such works as Laurie Garrett's *The Coming Plague: Newly Emerging Diseases in a World Out of Balance* (1994), which was inspired at least in part by the conference.

10.   Richard Preston, *The Hot Zone* (New York: Doubleday, 1994), 18.

11.   See my *Contagious: Cultures, Carriers, and the Outbreak Narrative* (Durham, NC: Duke University Press, 2008).

12.   G. Cowley, "How Progress Makes Us Sick," *Newsweek*, May 5, 2003, 35.

13.   Melinda Liu, "The Flimsy Wall of China," *Newsweek*, October 31, 2005, 28; Anita Manning, "Asia: The 'Perfect Incubator,'" *USA Today*, February 28, 2005, 6; Michael Specter, "Nature's Bioterrorist: Is There Any Way to Prevent a Deadly Avian-Flu Pandemic?" *The New Yorker*, February 28, 2005, 50–61.

14. Madeline Drexler, *Secret Agents: The Menace of Emerging Infections* (New York: Penguin Books, 2002), 3, 8, 9, and 11 respectively.

15. Joshua Lederberg, "Infectious Disease—A Threat to Global Health and Security," *Journal of the American Medical Association* 276, no. 5 (August 7, 1996): 417–19, 418, 417.

16. Preston, *The Hot Zone*, 85.

17. Richard M. Krause, "The Origin of Plagues: Old and New," *Science* 257 (August 21, 1992): 1073.

18. Laurie Garrett, *The Coming Plague: Newly Emerging Diseases in a World Out of Balance* (New York: Penguin Books, 1995 [1994]), 618.

19. Ibid., 6.

20. Paul Farmer, *Pathologies of Power: Health, Human Rights, and the New War on the Poor* (Berkeley: University of California Press, 2004), 140.

21. The Declaration of Alma-Ata is motivated partly by that assumption, and it has the support, as Paul Farmer suggests, of economists, such as Amartya Sen.

Bibliography

Agamben, Giorgio. *Homo Sacer: Sovereign Power and Bare Life.* Translated by Daniel Heller-Roazen. Stanford: Stanford University Press, 1998.

Airlie, Shiona. *Thistle and Bamboo: The Life and Times of Sir James Stewart Lockhart.* Oxford: Oxford University Press, 1989.

Amrith, Sunil S. *Decolonizing International Health: India and Southeast Asia, 1930–65.* Basingstoke: Palgrave Macmillan, 2006.

———. "Tamil Diasporas Across the Bay of Bengal." *American Historical Review* 114, no. 3 (June 2009): 547–72.

———. "Indians Overseas? Governing Tamil Migration to Malaya, 1870–1941." *Past and Present* 208 (August 2010): 231–61.

———. *Migration and Diaspora in Modern Asia.* Cambridge: Cambridge University Press, 2011.

Anderson, Benedict. *Imagined Communities. Reflections on the Origins and Spread of Nationalism.* London: Verso, 1991.

Anderson, Margo. *The American Census: A Social History.* New Haven, CT: Yale University Press, 1988.

Anderson, Warwick. "'Where Every Prospect Pleases and Only Man is Vile': Laboratory Medicine as Colonial Discourse." *Critical Enquiry* 18 (Spring 1992): 507–8.

———. "Immunities of Empire: Race, Disease, and the New Tropical Medicine, 1900–1920." *Bulletin of the History of Medicine* 70, no. 1 (1996): 94–118.

———. "Excremental Colonialism: Public Health and the Poetics of Pollution." In *Contagion: Historical and Cultural Studies,* ed. Alison Bashford and Claire Hooker, 76–105. London and New York: Routledge, 2001.

———. *Colonial Pathologies: American Tropical Medicine, Race, and Hygiene in the Philippines.* Durham, NC: Duke University Press, 2006.

———. *The Cultivation of Whiteness: Science, Health and Racial Destiny in Australia.* Durham, NC: Duke University Press, 2006.

———. "Immunization and Hygiene in the Colonial Philippines." *Journal of the History of Medicine and Allied Sciences* 62, no. 1 (2007): 1–20.

Appadurai, Arjun. "Number in the Colonial Imagination." In *Orientalism and the Postcolonial Predicament: Perspectives in South Asia,* ed. C.A. Breckenridge and P. van der Veer, 314–40. Philadelphia: University of Pennsylvania Press, 1993.

————. *Modernity at Large: Cultural Dimensions of Globalization*. Minneapolis: University of Minnesota Press, 1996.

Armstrong, David. "Public Health Spaces and the Fabrication of Identity." *Sociology* 27, no. 3 (1993): 393–410.

Arnold, David, ed. *Imperial Medicine and Indigenous Societies*. Manchester: Manchester University Press, 1988.

————. *The Problem of Nature: Environment, Culture and European Expansion*. Oxford: Blackwell, 1996.

————. *Colonizing the Body. State Medicine and Epidemic Disease in Nineteenth-century India*. Berkeley: University of California Press, 1993.

————. "British India and the 'Beriberi Problem', 1798–1942." *Medical History* 54, no. 3 (2010): 295–314.

Asad, Talal. "Ethnographic Representation, Statistics and Modern Power." *Social Research* 61 (1994): 55–88.

Au, Sokhieng. *Mixed Medicines: Health and Culture in French Colonial Cambodia*. Chicago: University of Chicago Press, 2011.

Autret, Marcel. "La fraude sur la quinine en Indochine." *Revue médicale française d'Extrême-Orient* 17 (1939): 925–28.

Bairoch, Paul. *Cities and Economic Development. From the Dawn of History to the Present*. Chicago: University of Chicago Press, 1988.

Baker, R.A., and R.A. Bayliss. "William John Ritchie Simpson (1855–1931): Public Health and Tropical Medicine." *Medical History* 31 (1987): 450–65.

Ballantyne, Tony. *Between Colonialism and Diaspora: Sikh Cultural Formations in an Imperial World*. Durham, NC: Duke University Press, 2001.

————. *Orientalism and Race: Aryanism in the British Empire*. Basingstoke: Palgrave Macmillan, 2002.

Ballhatchet, Kenneth. *Race, Sex and Class under the Raj: Imperial Attitudes and Policies and their Critics, 1793–1905*. London: Weidenfeld and Nicolson, 1980.

Ballhatchet, Kenneth, and David Taylor, eds. *Changing South Asia. Economy and Society*, Vol. 4. London: Centre for South Asian Studies, School of Oriental and African Studies, 1984.

Barnet, Michael. *Empire of Humanity: A History of Humanitarianism*. Ithaca, NY: Cornell University Press, 2011.

Barrier, N. Gerald, ed. *The Census in British India. New Perspectives*. New Delhi: Monohar, 1981.

Bartholomew, James R. *The Formation of Science in Japan*. New Haven, CT: Yale University Press, 1989.

Bashford, Alison. *Imperial Hygiene: A Critical History of Colonialism, Nationalism and Public Health*. Basingstoke: Palgrave Macmillan, 2004.

Bashford, Alison, and Claire Hooker. "Introduction: Contagion, Modernity, and Postmodernity." In *Contagion: Historical and Cultural Studies*, ed. Alison Bashford and Claire Hooker, 1–12. London and New York: Routledge, 2001

————. eds. *Contagion: Historical and Cultural Studies*. London: Routledge, 2001.

Bashford, Alison, and Philippa Levine, eds. *The Oxford Handbook of the History of Eugenics*. Oxford: Oxford University Press, 2010.

Bashford, Alison, and Carolyn Strange, eds. *Isolation: Places and Practices of Exclusion*. London: Routledge, 2003.

Basu, Subho. "Strikes and 'Communal' Riots in Calcutta in the 1890s. Industrial Workers, Bhadralok Nationalist Leadership and the Colonial State." *Modern Asian Studies* 32 (1998): 949–83.

Bayly, Christopher A. *Empire and Information: Intelligence Gathering and Social Communication in India, 1780–1870*. Cambridge: Cambridge University Press, 2000.

Bayly, Susan. "Caste and 'Race' in the Colonial Ethnography of India." In *The Concept of Race in South Asia*, ed. Peter Robb, 165–218. Delhi: Oxford University Press, 1995.

Bell, Heather. *Frontiers of Medicine in the Anglo-Egyptian Sudan, 1899–1940*. Oxford: Oxford University Press, 1999.

Benedict, Carol. *Bubonic Plague in Nineteenth-Century China*. Stanford: Stanford University Press, 1996.

Bennett, David, ed. *Multicultural States. Rethinking Difference and Identity*. London: Routledge, 1998.

Bernard, Noël. *Yersin: pionner–savant–explorateur, 1863–1943*. Paris: La Colombe, 1955.

Bhabha, Homi K. *The Location of Culture*. London: Routledge, 2004 [1994].

Bibel, David J., and T. H. Chen. "Diagnosis of Plague: An Analysis of the Yersin-Kitasato Controversy." *Bacteriological Review* 40 (1976): 633–51.

Blythe, W. *The Impact of Chinese Secret Societies in Malaya*. Oxford: Oxford University Press, 1969.

Breckenridge, Carol A., and Peter van der Veer, eds. *Orientalism and the Postcolonial Predicament: Perspectives on South Asia*. Philadelphia: University of Pennsylvania Press, 1993.

Briggs, Laura. *Reproducing Empire: Race, Sex, Science and US Imperialism in Puerto Rico*. Berkeley: University of California Press, 2002.

Bristow, Michael R. "Early Town Planning in British South East Asia, 1910–1939." *Planning Perspectives* 15, no. 2 (2000): 139–60.

Bristow, Roger. *Land Use Planning in Hong Kong: History, Policies and Procedures*. Hong Kong: Oxford University Press, 1984.

Bruegmann, Robert. "Architecture of the Hospital: 1770–1870." Unpublished Ph.D. dissertation, University of Pennsylvania, 1976.

Buckingham, Jane. *Leprosy in Colonial South India: Medicine and Confinement*. Basingstoke: Palgrave Macmillan, 2002.

Buettner, Elizabeth. *Empire Families: Britons and Late Imperial India*. Oxford: Oxford University Press, 2004.

Bynum, William F. *Science and the Practice of Medicine in the Nineteenth Century*. Cambridge: Cambridge University Press, 1994.

Cannadine, David. *Ornamentalism: How the British Saw Their Empire*. Oxford: Oxford University Press, 2007.

Carroll, John M. *Edge of Empires: Chinese Elites and British Colonials in Hong Kong.* Cambridge, MA: Harvard University Press, 2005.

Carter, Marina, and Khal Torabully. *Coolitude: An Anthology of the Indian Labour Diaspora.* London: Anthem Press, 2002.

Çelik, Zeynep. *Empire, Architecture and the City: French-Ottoman Encounters, 1830–1914.* Seattle: University of Washington Press, 2008.

Cell, John W. "Anglo-Indian Medical Theory and the Origins of Segregation in West Africa." *American Historical Review* 91 (1986): 307–35.

Chakrabarty, Dipesh. *Provincializing Europe: Postcolonial Thought and Historical Difference.* Princeton, NJ: Princeton University Press, 2000.

Chandavarkar, Rajnarayan. "Plague Panic and Epidemic Politics in India, 1896–1914." In *Imperial Power and Popular Politics: Class, Resistance and the State in India, c. 1850–1950,* ed. Rajnarayan Chandavarkar, 234–65. Cambridge: Cambridge University Press, 1998.

Chandavarkar, Rajnarajan, ed. *Origins of Industrial Capitalism in India. Business Strategies and Working Classes in Bombay, 1900–1940.* Cambridge: Cambridge University Press, 1994.

———. *Imperial Power and Popular Politics: Class, Resistance and the State in India, c. 1850–1950.* Cambridge: Cambridge University Press, 1998.

Chang, Jiat-Hwee. *No Boundaries: The Lien Villas Collective.* Singapore: Pesaro, 2010.

———. "Tropicalising Technologies of Environment and Government: The Singapore General Hospital and the Circulation of the Pavilion Plan Hospital in the British Empire, 1860–1930." In *Re-Shaping Cities: How Global Mobility Transforms Architecture and Urban Form,* ed. Michael Guggenheim and Ola Söderström, 123–42. London: Routledge, 2009.

Chang, Jiat-Hwee, and Anthony D. King. "Towards a Genealogy of 'Tropical Architecture': Historical Fragments of Power-Knowledge, Built Environment, and Climate in the British Colonial Territories." *Singapore Journal of Tropical Geography* 32, no. 3 (2011): 283–300.

Chattopadhyay, Swati. *Representing Calcutta: Modernity, Nationalism, and the Colonial Uncanny.* London: Routledge, 2005.

Choa, G. H. *The Life and Times of Sir Kai Ho Kai.* Hong Kong: Chinese University Press, 1981.

Christopher, A. J. "Urban Segregation Levels in the British Overseas Empire and Its Successors, in the Twentieth Century." *Transactions, Institute of British Geographers,* n.s., 17 (1992): 95–107.

Clancy-Smith, Julia, and Frances Gouda, ed. *Domesticating the Empire: Race, Gender and Family Life in French and Dutch Colonialism.* Charlottesville: University Press of Virginia, 1998.

Claval, Paul. "Colonial Experience and the Development of Tropical Geography in France." *Singapore Journal of Tropical Geography* 26, no. 3 (2005): 289–303.

Clifford, James. *Routes: Travel and Translation in the Late Twentieth Century.* Cambridge, MA: Harvard University Press, 1997.

Cohen, Ed. *A Body Worth Defending: Immunity, Biopolitics and the Apotheosis of the Modern Body*. Durham, NC: Duke University Press, 2009.

Cohen, William B. "Malaria and French Imperialism." *Journal of African History* 24 (1983): 23–36.

Cohn, Bernard S., ed. *An Anthropologist Among the Historians, and Other Essays*. Delhi: Oxford University Press, 1987.

———. "The Census, Social Structure and Objectification in South Asia." In *An Anthropologist among Historians, and Other Essays*, ed. Bernard Cohn, 224–54. Delhi: Oxford University Press, 1987.

———. ed. *Colonialism and Its Forms of Knowledge. The British in India*. Princeton, NJ: Princeton University Press, 1996.

Collier, Stephen J., and Aihwa Ong. "Global Assemblages, Anthropological Problems." In *Global Assemblages: Technology, Politics, and Ethics as Anthropological Problems*, ed. Aihwa Ong and Stephen J. Collier, 3–21. Malden, MA: Blackwell Publishing, 2005.

———. eds. *Global Assemblages: Technology, Politics, and Ethics as Anthropological Problems*. Malden, MA: Blackwell Publishing, 2005.

Committee on Emerging Microbial Threats to Health. *Emerging Infections: Microbial Threats to Health in the United States*. Washington, DC: National Academies Press, 1992.

Conklin, Alice. *A Mission to Civilize: The Republican Idea of Empire in France and West Africa, 1895–1930*. Stanford: Stanford University Press, 1997.

Cooper, Frederick. *Colonialism in Question: Theory, Knowledge, History*. Berkeley: University of California Press, 2005.

Cooper, Frederick, and Ann Laura Stoler, eds. *Tensions of Empire: Colonial Cultures in the Bourgeois World*. Berkeley: University of California Press, 1997.

Cooper, Nicola. *France in Indochina: Colonial Encounters*. Oxford: Berg, 2001.

Cowell, Christopher. *Form Follows Fever: Malaria and the Making of Hong Kong, 1841–1848*. Unpublished M.Phil. dissertation, University of Hong Kong, 2009.

Cunningham, Andrew. "Transforming Plague: The Laboratory and the Identity of Infectious Disease." In *The Laboratory Revolution in Medicine*, ed. Andrew Cunningham and Perry Williams, 209–44. Cambridge: Cambridge University Press, 1992.

Cunningham, Andrew, and Perry Williams, eds. *The Laboratory Revolution in Medicine*. Cambridge: Cambridge University Press, 1992.

Curtin, Philip. "Medical Knowledge and Urban Planning in Tropical Africa." *American Historical Review* 90 (1985): 594–613.

———. *Death by Migration: Europe's Encounter with the Tropical World in the Nineteenth Century*. Cambridge: Cambridge University Press, 1989.

Curtis, Bruce. *The Politics of Population*. Toronto: University of Toronto Press, 2001.

Dale, Leigh, and Helen Gilbert, eds. *Economies of Representation, 1790–2000: Colonialism and Commerce*. Aldershot: Ashgate, 2007.

Daruwala, Rusi. *The Bombay Chamber Story: 150 Years*. Bombay: Bombay Chamber of Commerce and Industry, 1986.

De Bevoise, Ken. *Agents of Apocalypse: Epidemic Disease in the Colonial Philippines*. Princeton, NJ: Princeton University Press, 1995.

Dean, Mitchell. *Governmentality: Power and Rule in Modern Society*. London: Sage, 1999.

Debré, Patrice. *Louis Pasteur*. Translated by Elborg Forster. Baltimore, MD: Johns Hopkins University Press, 1998.

Dedet, Jean-Pierre. "The Overseas Pasteur Institutes, with Special Reference to their Role in the Diffusion of Microbiological Knowledge: 1887–1975." *Research in Microbiology* 159, no. 1 (2008): 31–35.

della Dora, Veronica. "Making Mobile Knowledges: The Educational Cruises of the *Revue Générale des Sciences Pures et Appliquées*, 1897–1914." *Isis* 101 (2010): 467–500.

Digby, Anne, Waltraud Ernst, and Projit B. Mukharji, eds. *Crossing Colonial Historiographies: Histories of Colonial and Indigenous Medicine in Transnational Perspective*. Newcastle: Cambridge Scholars, 2010.

Dikötter, Frank. *Exotic Commodities: Modern Objects and Everyday Life in China*. New York: Columbia University Press, 2007.

Dirks, Nicholas. *Castes of Mind. Colonialism and the Making of Modern India*. Princeton, NJ: Princeton University Press, 2001.

Dossal, Miriam. *Imperial Design and Indian Realities: The Planning of Bombay City, 1845–1875*. Bombay: Oxford University Press, 1991.

Drews, G. "The Roots of Medical Microbiology and the Influence of Ferdinand Cohn on the Microbiology of the 19th century." *FEMS Microbiology Reviews* 24 (2000): 225–49.

Drexler, Madeline. *Secret Agents: The Menace of Emerging Infections*. New York: Penguin Books, 2002.

Driver, Felix. "Moral Geographies: Social Science and the Urban Environment in Mid-Nineteenth Century England." *Transactions of the Institute of British Geographers* 13, no. 3 (1988): 275–87.

———. *Geography Militant: Cultures of Exploration and Empire*. Oxford: Blackwell, 2001.

Dube, Saurabh, ed. *Enchantments of Modernity: Empire, Nation, Globalization*. New Delhi: Routledge, 2009.

Duncan, James S. *In the Shadows of the Tropics: Climate, Race and Biopower in Nineteenth Century Ceylon*. Aldershot: Ashgate, 2007.

Ebrahimnejad, Hormoz, ed. *The Development of Modern Medicine in Non-Western Countries*. London: Routledge, 2008.

Echenberg, Myron. *Plague Ports. The Global Urban Impact of Bubonic Plague, 1894–1901*. New York: New York University Press, 2007.

Edmond, Rod. *Leprosy and Empire: A Medical and Cultural History*. Cambridge: Cambridge University Press, 2006.

Edwards, Penny. *Cambodge: The Cultivation of a Nation, 1860–1945*. Honolulu: University of Hawaii Press, 2007.

Eigen, Edward. "The Place of Distribution: Episodes in the Architecture of Experiment." In *Architecture and the Sciences: Exchanging Metaphors*, ed. Antoine Picon and Alessandra Ponte, 52–79. New York: Princeton Architectural Press, 2003.

Elden, Stuart. "Plague, Panopticon, Police." *Surveillance and Society* 1 (2003): 240–53.

Endacott, G. B. *A Biographical Sketch-Book of Early Hong Kong*. With a new introduction by John M. Carroll. Hong Kong: Hong Kong University Press, 2005 [1962].

Ernst, Waltraud, and Projit B. Mukharji, eds. *Crossing Colonial Historiographies: Histories of Colonial and Indigenous Medicine in Transnational Perspective*. Cambridge: Cambridge University Press, 2010.

Evans, Emery. "The Foundation of Hong Kong: A Chapter of Accidents." In *Hong Kong: The Interaction of Traditions and Life in the Towns*, ed. Marjorie Toplie, 1–41. Hong Kong: Hong Kong Branch of the Royal Asiatic Society, 1975.

Evans, Martin, ed. *Empire and Culture: The French Experience, 1830–1940*. Basingstoke and New York: Palgrave Macmillan, 2004.

Evans, Robin. *Translations from Drawing to Building and Other Essays*. London: Architectural Associations, 1997.

Fan, Fa-ti. *British Naturalists in Qing China: Science, Empire, and Cultural Encounter*. Cambridge, MA: Harvard University Press, 2004.

Farmer, Paul. *Pathologies of Power: Health, Human Rights, and the New War on the Poor*. Berkeley: University of California Press, 2004.

Farrar, Frederic W. "Aptitudes of Races." *Transactions of the Ethnological Society of London* 5 (1867): 115–26.

Fassin, Didier. "Humanitarianism as a Politics of Life." *Public Culture* 19, no. 3 (2007): 500–501.

Fassin, Didier, and Mariella Pandolfi, eds. *Contemporary States of Emergency: The Politics of Military and Humanitarian Interventions*. New York: Zone Books, 2010.

Finnegan, Diarmid A. "The Spatial Turn: Geographical Approaches in the History of Science." *Journal of the History of Biology* 41, no. 2 (2008): 369–88.

Foucault, Michel. *Discipline and Punish: The Birth of the Prison*. Translated by Alan Sheridan. Harmondsworth: Penguin, 1977.

———. *The History of Sexuality*, Vol. 1, *An Introduction*. Translated by Robert Hurley. New York: Vintage, 1990 [1978].

———. *Society Must Be Defended: Lectures at the College de France, 1976*. Translated by David Macey. London: Penguin, 2003.

———. *Security, Territory, Population: Lectures at the Collège de France 1977–78*. Translated by Graham Burchell. Basingstoke and New York: Palgrave Macmillan, 2007.

———. *The Birth of Biopolitics: Lectures at the Collège de France, 1978–79*. Basingstoke: Palgrave Macmillan, 2008.

Foucault, Michel, et al. *The Foucault Effect: Studies in Governmentality*. Chicago: University of Chicago Press, 1991.

Fox, Robert, and George Weisz, eds. *The Organization of Science and Technology in France 1808–1914*. Cambridge and New York: Cambridge University Press, 1980.

Frenkel, Stephen, and John Western. "Pretext or Prophylaxis? Racial Segregation and Malarial Mosquitos in a British Tropical Colony: Sierra Leone." *Annals of the Association of American Geographers* 78, no. 2 (June 1988): 211–28.

Furedy, Christine. "Whose Responsibility? Dilemmas of Calcutta's Bustee Policy in the Nineteenth Century." *South Asia* 5 (1982): 24–46.

Galison, Peter. "Buildings and the Subject of Science." In *The Architecture of Science*, ed. Peter Galison and Emily Thompson, 1–25. Cambridge, MA: MIT Press, 1999.

Galison, Peter, and Emily Thompson, eds. *The Architecture of Science*. Cambridge, MA: MIT Press, 1999.

Gandy, Matthew. "Planning, Anti-Planning and the Infrastructure Crisis Facing Metropolitan Lagos." *Urban Studies* 43 (2006): 371–96.

Garrett, Laurie. *The Coming Plague: Newly Emerging Diseases in a World Out of Balance*. New York: Farrar, Straus and Giroux, 1994.

Ghosh, Amitav. *Sea of Poppies*. London: John Murray, 2008.

Ghosh, Durba. *Sex and the Family in Colonial India: The Making of Empire*. Cambridge: Cambridge University Press, 2006.

Girardet, Raoul. *L'idée coloniale en France de 1871 à 1962*. Paris: Hachette, 1972.

Glover, William. *Making Lahore Modern: Constructing and Imagining a Colonial City*. Minneapolis: University of Minnesota Press, 2008.

Gonzalès, J. "Histoire de la naissance et du développement de l'École de Médecine de Hanoï." *Histoire des Sciences Médicales* 30 (1996): 61–70.

Goto-Shibata, Harumi. "Empire on the Cheap: The Control of Opium Smoking in the Straits Settlements, 1925–1939." *Modern Asian Studies* 40, no. 1 (2006): 59–80.

Griffiths, D. A., and S. P. Lau, "The Hong Kong Botanical Gardens: A Historical Overview." *Journal of the Royal Asiatic Society Hong Kong Branch* 26 (1986): 55–77.

Gu, Dongfeng, Kristi Reynolds, Xigui Wu, Jing Chen, Xiufang Duan, Robert F. Reynolds, Paul K Whelton, and Jiang He. "Prevalence of the Metabolic Syndrome and Overweight among Adults in China." *The Lancet* 365 (April 2005): 1398–1405.

Guénel, Annick. "The 1937 Bandung Conference on Rural Hygiene: Towards a New Vision of Health Care?" In *Global Movements, Local Concerns: Medicine and Health in Southeast Asia*, ed. Laurence Monnais and Harold J. Cook. Singapore: NUS Press, forthcoming.

———. "The Creation of the First Overseas Pasteur Institute, or the Beginning of Albert Calmette's Pastorian Career." *Medical History* 43 (1999): 1–25.

Guggenheim, Michael, and Ola Söderström, eds. *Re-Shaping Cities: How Global Mobility Transforms Architecture and Urban Form*. London: Routledge, 2009.

Gunn, S. William A., and Michele Masellis, eds. *The Declaration of Alma-Ata in Concepts and Practice of Humanitarian Medicine*. New York: Springer, 2008.

Haas, Peter, and Emanuel Adler. "Do Regimes Matter? Epistemic Communities and Mediterranean Pollution Control." *International Organization* 43, no. 3 (1992): 377–403.

Hacking, Ian. *The Taming of Chance*. Cambridge: Cambridge University Press, 1990.

Hamlin, Christopher. *Public Health and Social Justice in the Age of Chadwick: Britain, 1800–1854*. Cambridge: Cambridge University Press, 1998.

Hannah, Matthew. *Governmentality and the Mastery of Territory in Nineteenth-Century America*. New York: Cambridge University Press, 2000.

Hardt, Michael, and Antonio Negri. *Empire*. Cambridge, MA: Harvard University Press, 2000.

Harris, Richard. "Development and Hybridity Made Concrete in the Colonies." *Environment and Planning A* 40 (2008): 15–36.

Harrison, Mark. *Public Health in British India. Anglo-Indian Preventive Medicine 1859–1914*. Cambridge: Cambridge University Press, 1994.

———. "'Hot Beds of Disease': Malaria and Civilization in Nineteenth-Century India." *Parassitologia* 40 (1998): 11–18.

———. *Climates and Constitutions: Health, Race, Environment and British Imperialism in India 1600–1850*. New Delhi: Oxford University Press, 1999.

Haupt, Heinz-Gerhard, and Jürgen Kocka, eds. *Comparative and Transnational History: Central European Approaches and New Perspectives*. Oxford: Berghahn, 2009.

Haynes, Douglas M. "The Social Production of Metropolitan Expertise in Tropical Diseases: The Imperial State, Colonial Service and Tropical Diseases Research Fund." *Science, Technology & Society* 4, no. 2 (1999): 205–38.

———. *Imperial Medicine: Patrick Manson and the Conquest of Tropical Disease*. Philadelphia: University of Pennsylvania Press, 2001.

Hazareesingh, Sandip. *The Colonial City and the Challenge to Modernity. Urban Hegemonies and Civic Confrontations in Bombay City 1900–1925*. Delhi: Orient Longman, 2007.

Headrick, Daniel R. *The Tools of Empire. Technology and European Imperialism in the Nineteenth Century*. Oxford: Oxford University Press, 1981.

———. *The Tentacles of Progress: Technology Transfer in the Age of Imperialism, 1850–1940*. New York: Oxford University Press, 1988.

Heath, Deana. "Sanitizing Modernity: Imperial Hygiene, Obscenity, and Moral Regulation in Colonial India." In *Enchantments of Modernity: Empire, Nation, Globalization*, ed. Saurabh Dube, 113–29. London amd New York: Routledge, 2009.

Heinrich, Larissa N. *The Afterlife of Images: Translating the Pathological Body between China and the West*. Durham, NC: Duke University Press, 2008.

Hernández, Felipe. "Introduction: Transcultural Architectures in Latin America." In *Transculturation: Cities, Spaces and Architectures in Latin America*, ed. Felipe Hernández, Mark Millington, and Iain Borden, ix–xxv. New York: Rodopi, 2005.

Hernández, Felipe, Mark Millington, and Iain Borden, eds. *Transculturation: Cities, Spaces and Architectures in Latin America*. New York: Rodopi, 2005.

Herring, D. Ann, and Alan C. Swedlund, eds. *Plagues and Epidemics: Infected Spaces Past and Present*. Oxford and New York: Berg, 2010.

Heteren, G. M. van, M. J. D. Poulissen, A. de Knecht-van Eekelen, and A. M. Luyendijk-Elshout, eds. *Dutch Medicine in the Malay Archipelago, 1816–1942*. Amsterdam: Rodopi, 1989.

Higgs, Edward. *Making Sense of the Census: The Manuscript Returns for England Wales, 1801–1901*. London: HMSO, 1989.

Hodges, Sarah. *Contraception, Colonialism and Commerce: Birth Control in South India, 1920–40*. Aldershot: Ashgate, 2008.

Home, Robert K. *Of Planting and Planning: The Making of British Colonial Cities*. London: E&FN Spon, 1997.

Hosagrahar, Jyoti. *Indigenous Modernities: Negotiating Architecture and Urbanism*. London and New York: Routledge, 2005.

Howard-Jones, Norman. "Was Shibasaburo Kitasato the Co-discoverer of the Plague Bacillus?" *Perspectives in Biology and Medicine* 16 (1973): 292–305.

Howell, Philip. *Geographies of Regulation: Policing Prostitution in Nineteenth-Century Britain and the Empire*. Cambridge: Cambridge University Press, 2009.

Hunt, Alan. *Governing Morals: A Social History of Moral Regulation*. Cambridge: Cambridge University Press, 1999.

Inda, Jonathan Xavier, ed. *Anthropologies of Modernity*. Malden, MA: Blackwell, 2005.

Irgens, L. M. "The Discovery of Mycobacterium Leprae." *American Journal of Dermatopathology* 6, no. 4 (1984): 337–343.

James, A.J.L., ed. *The Development of the Laboratory: Essays on the Place of Experiment in Industrial Civilization*. Basingstoke: Macmillan, 1989.

Jefferys, William Hamilton, and James L. Maxwell. *The Diseases of China: Including Formosa and Korea*. London: Bale & Danielsson.

Jennings, Eric T. "Conservative Confluences, 'Nativist' Synergy: Reinscribing Vichy's National Revolution in Indochina, 1940–1945." *French Historical Studies* 27, no. 3 (2004): 601–35.

―――. "Urban Planning, Architecture and Zoning at Dalat, Indochina, 1900–1944." *Historical Reflections/Reflexions Historiques* 33, no. 2 (2007): 343, 346.

―――. "Dalat, Capital of Indochina: Remolding Frameworks and Spaces in the Late Colonial Era." *Journal of Vietnamese Studies* 4, no. 2 (2009): 12.

―――. *Imperial Heights: Dalat and the Making and Undoing of French Indochina*. Berkeley: University of California Press, 2011.

Jia, W. P., K. S. Xiang, L. Chen, J. X. Lu, and Y. M. Wu. "Epidemiological Study on Obesity and its Comorbidities in Urban Chinese Older than 20 Years of Age in Shanghai, China." *Obesity Reviews* 3 (2002): 157–65.

Jing, Jun, ed., *Feeding China's Little Emperors: Food, Children, and Social Change*. Stanford: Stanford University Press, 2000.

Johnson, Ryan, and Amna Khalid, eds. *Public Health in the British Empire: Intermediaries, Subordinates and Public Health Practice, 1850–1960*. London: Routledge, 2011.

Jokl, D. "Robert Koch's Debt to Ferdinand Cohn." *Documenta Ophthalmologica* 99, no. 3 (1999): 285–92.

Jones, Greta. *Social Hygiene in Twentieth Century Britain*. Wolfeboro, NH: Croom Helm, 1986.

Joyce, Patrick. *The Rule of Freedom: Liberalism and the Modern City*. London and New York: Verso, 2003.

Kale, Madhavi. *Fragments of Empire: Capital, Slavery and Indian Indentured Labour*. Philadelphia: University of Pennsylvania Press, 1998.

Kalpagam, U. "The Colonial State and Statistical Knowledge." *History of the Human Sciences* 13 (2000): 37–55.

Kaur, Amarjit. "Indian Labour, Labour Standards, and Workers' Health in Burma and Malaya, 1900–1940." *Modern Asian Studies* 40, no. 2 (2006): 425–75.

Kelly, John D. *A Politics of Virtue: Hinduism, Sexuality and Countercolonial Discourse in Fiji.* Chicago: University of Chicago Press, 1991.

Kennedy, Dane. *The Magic Mountains: Hill Stations and the British Raj.* Delhi: Oxford University Press, 1996.

Kidambi, Prashant. "Housing the Poor in a Colonial City: The Bombay Improvement Trust, 1898–1918." *Studies in History* 17, no. 1 (2001): 57–79.

———. "'The Ultimate Masters of the City.' Police, Public Order and the Poor in Colonial Bombay, c.1893–1914." *Crime, History and Societies* 8 (2004): 27–47.

———. *The Making of an Indian Metropolis. Colonial Governance and Public Culture in Bombay, 1890–1920.* Abingdon: Ashgate, 2007.

King, Anthony D. "Hospital Planning: Revised Thoughts on the Origin of the Pavilion Principle in England." *Medical History* 10, no. 6 (1966): 360–73.

———. *Colonial Urban Development: Culture, Social Power, and Environment.* London: Routledge & Kegan Paul, 1976.

———. *The Bungalow: The Production of a Global Culture.* 2nd ed. Oxford: Oxford University Press, 1984.

———. "Colonial Cities: Global Pivots of Change". In *Colonial Cities: Essays on Urbanism in a Colonial Context*, ed. R. J. Ross and G. J. Telkamp, 7–32. Dordrecht: Martinus Nijhoff, 1985.

———. *Spaces of Global Cultures: Architecture, Urbanism, Identity.* London and New York: Routledge, 2004.

Klein, Ira. "Urban Development and Death. Bombay City, 1870–1914." *Modern Asian Studies* 20, no. 4 (1986): 725–54.

———. "Plague Policy, and Popular Unrest in British India." *Modern Asian Studies* 22, no. 4 (1988): 723–55.

Knorr-Cetina, Karin. "The Couch, the Cathedral, and the Laboratory: On the Relationship between Experiment and Laboratory in Science." In *Science as Practice and Culture*, ed. Andrew Pickering, 113–38. Chicago: Chicago University Press, 1992.

Kohler, Robert E. *Landscapes and Labscapes: Exploring the Lab-Field Border in Biology.* Chicago: University of Chicago Press, 2002.

Krause, Richard M. "The Origin of Plagues: Old and New." *Science* 257 (August 21, 1992): 1073–77.

Kretchmer, N. "Lactose and Lactase." *Scientific American* 227, no. 4 (1972): 71–78.

Krieger, Nancy. "A Century of Census Tracts: Health and the Body Politic (1906–2006)." *Journal of Urban Health* 83 (2006): 335–41.

Kusno, Abidin. *Behind the Postcolonial: Architecture, Urban Space, and Political Cultures in Indonesia.* New York: Routledge, 2000.

La Berge, Ann, and Mordechai Feingold, eds. *French Medical Culture in the Nineteenth Century.* Amsterdam and Atlanta: Rodopi, 1994.

Lahiri Choudhury, Deep Kanta. *Telegraphic Imperialism: Crisis and Panic in the Indian Empire, c.1830–1920*. Basingstoke: Palgrave Macmillan, 2010.

Lake, Marilyn, and Henry Reynolds. *Drawing the Global Colour Line: White Men's Countries and the International Challenge of Racial Equality*. Cambridge: Cambridge University Press, 2008.

Lamarre, Thomas. "Bacterial Cultures and Linguistic Colonies: Mori Rintarō's Experiments with History, Science, and Language." *Positions* 6, no. 3 (1998): 597–635.

Latour, Bruno. "Give Me a Laboratory and I will Raise the World." In *Science Observed, Perspectives on the Study of Science*, ed. Michael Mulkay and Karin Knorr-Cetina, 141–70. London: Sage, 1983.

———. *The Pasteurization of France*. Translated by Alan Sheridan and John Law. Cambridge, MA: Harvard University Press, 1984.

———. *Science in Action: How to Follow Scientists and Engineers through Society*. Cambridge, MA: Harvard University Press, 1987.

———. *We Have Never Been Modern*. Translated by Catherine Porter. Cambridge, MA: Harvard University Press, 1993.

Le Roux, Pierre. *Alexandre Yersin, un passe-muraille (1863–1943). Vainqueur de la peste et de la diphtérie, explorateur des hauts plateaux d'Indochine*. Paris: Connaissance et Savoirs, 2007.

Lederberg, Joshua. "Infectious Disease—A Threat to Global Health and Security." *Journal of the American Medical Association* 276, no. 5 (August 7, 1996): 417–19.

Leeming, Frank. *Street Studies in Hong Kong: Localities in a Chinese City*. Hong Kong and New York: Oxford University Press, 1977.

Legg, Stephen. "Foucault's Population Geographies. Classification, Biopolitics and Governmental Spaces." *Space and Place* 11 (2005): 137–56.

———. *Spaces of Colonialism: Delhi's Urban Governmentalities*. Oxford: Blackwell, 2007.

———. "Of Scales, Networks and Assemblages: The League of Nations Apparatus and the Scalar Sovereignty of the Government of India." *Transactions of the Institute of British Geographers*, n.s., 34, no. 2 (2009): 234–53.

———. "Ambivalent Improvements: Biography, Biopolitics, and Colonial Delhi." *Environment and Planning A* 39 (2008): 37–56.

———. "Governing Prostitution in Colonial Delhi: From Cantonment Regulations to International Hygiene (1864–1939)." *Social History* 34, no. 4 (2009): 447–67.

———. "An Intimate and Imperial Feminism: Meliscent Shephard and the Regulation of Prostitution in Colonial India." *Environment and Planning D: Society and Space* 28, no. 1 (2010): 68–94.

———. "Stimulation, Segregation and Scandal: Geographies of Prostitution Regulation in British India, between Registration (1888) and Suppression (1923)." *Modern Asian Studies* (2012 advance online publication).

Lester, Alan. *Imperial Networks: Creating Identities in Nineteenth-Century South Africa and Britain*. London and New York: Routledge, 2001.

Leung, Angela Ki Che, and Charlotte Furth, eds. *Health and Hygiene in Chinese East Asia: Policies and Publics in the Long Twentieth Century.* Durham, NC: Duke University Press, 2010.

Levin, Miriam R., Sophie Forgan, Martina Hessler, Robert H. Kargon, and Morris Low. *Urban Modernity: Cultural Innovation in the Second Industrial Revolution.* Cambridge, MA: MIT Press, 2010.

Levine, Philippa. *Prostitution, Race and Politics: Policing Venereal Disease in the British Empire.* London: Routledge, 2003.

Levitan, Kathrin. *A Cultural History of the British Census: Envisioning the Multitude in the Nineteenth Century.* Basingstoke: Palgrave Macmillan, 2011.

Li, Lillian M. *Fighting Famine in North China: State, Market, and Environmental Decline, 1690s–1990s.* Stanford: Stanford University Press, 2007.

Liao, Ping-hui, and David Der-wei Wang. *Taiwan under Japanese Colonial Rule, 1895–1945: History, Culture, Memory.* New York: Columbia University Press, 2006.

Limoges, Camille. "The Development of the Musée d'Histoire Naturelle of Paris, c.1800–1914." In *The Organization of Science and Technology in France*, ed. Robert Fox and George Weisz, 211–40. Cambridge and New York: Cambridge University Press, 1980.

Livingstone, David N. *Putting Science in its Place: Geographies of Scientific Knowledge.* Chicago: Chicago University Press, 2003.

Lo, Vivienne, and Penelope Barrett. "Cooking up Fine Remedies: On the Culinary Aesthetic in a Sixteenth-century *Materia Medica*." *Medical History* 49 (2005): 395–422.

Logan, William S. *Hanoi: Biography of a City.* Seattle: University of Washington Press, 2000.

Lowe, Kate, and Eugene McLaughlin. "Sir John Pope Hennessy and the 'Native Race Craze': Colonial Government in Hong Kong, 1877–1882." *Journal of Imperial and Commonwealth History* 20, no. 2 (May 1992): 223–47.

Löwy, Ilana. 'Making Plagues Visible: Yellow Fever, Hookworm, and Chagas' Disease, 1900–1950." In *Plagues and Epidemics: Infected Spaces Past and Present*, ed. D. Ann Herring and Alan C. Swedlund, 269–85. Oxford and New York: Berg, 2010.

Lu, Duanfang. "Travelling Urban Form: The Neighbourhood Unit in China." *Planning Perspectives* 21, no. 4 (2006): 369–92.

Ma, G. S., et al. "The Prevalence of Body Overweight and Obesity and Its Changes among Chinese People during 1992 to 2002." [In Chinese] *Zhonghua Yu Fang Yi Xue Za Zhi* [Chinese journal of preventive medicine] 39 (2005): 311–15.

MacLeod, Roy. "Scientific Advice for British India: Imperial Perceptions and Administrative Goals, 1898–1923." *Modern Asian Studies* 9, no. 3 (1975): 343–84.

———. "On Visiting the 'Moving Metropolis': Reflections on the Architecture of Imperial Science." In *Scientific Colonialism: A Cross-Cultural Comparison*, ed. Nathan Reingold and Marc Rothenberg, 217–49. Washington, DC: Smithsonian Institution Press, 1987.

MacLeod, Roy, and Milton Lewis, eds. *Disease, Medicine and Empire: Perspectives on Western Medicine and the Experience of European Expansion*. New York: Routledge, 1988.

Magee, Gary B., and Andrew S. Thompson. *Empire and Globalisation: Networks of People, Goods and Capital in the British World, c.1850–1914*. Cambridge: Cambridge University Press, 2010.

Maiden, M. "Putting Leprosy on the Map." *Nature Genetics* 41 (2009): 1264–66.

Manderson, Lenore. *Sickness and the State: Health and Illness in Colonial Malaya, 1870–1940*. Cambridge: Cambridge University Press, 1996.

Marcovich, Anne. "French Colonial Medicine and Colonial Rule: Algeria and Indochina." In *Disease, Medicine and Empire*, ed. Roy MacLeod and Milton Lewis, 103–17. New York and London: Routledge, 1988.

Marks, Robert. *Tigers, Rice, Silk, and Silt: Environment and Economy in Late Imperial South China*. Cambridge: Cambridge University Press, 1998.

Marx, Karl. *Capital: A Critique of Political Economy*. Translated by Ben Fowkes. Harmondsworth: Penguin, 1976.

McFarlane, Colin. "Governing the Contaminated City: Infrastructure and Sanitation in Colonial and Post-Colonial Bombay." *International Journal of Urban and Regional Research* 32, no. 2 (2008): 415–35.

McKeown, Adam. "Global Migration, 1846–1940." *Journal of World History* 15, no. 2 (2004): 155–89.

———. *Melancholy Order: Asian Migration and the Globalization of Borders*. New York: Columbia University Press, 2008.

Meade, Teresa, and Mark Walker, eds. *Science, Medicine and Cultural Imperialism*. New York: St Martin's Press, 1991.

Melosi, Martin V. *The Sanitary City: Environmental Services in Urban America from Colonial Times to the Present*. Pittsburgh, PA: University of Pittsburgh Press, 2008.

Mendelsohn, J. Andrew. "The Microscopist of Modern Life." *Osiris* 18 (Science and the City) (2003): 150–70.

Metcalf, Thomas R. *An Imperial Vision: Indian Architecture and Britain's Raj*. Berkeley and London: University of California Press, 1989.

———. *The New Cambridge History of India. Volume 4, Ideologies of the Raj*. Cambridge: Cambridge University Press, 1995.

———. *Imperial Connections: India in the Indian Ocean Arena, 1860–1920*. Berkeley: University of California Press, 2007.

Metcalfe, Barbara, and Thomas Metcalfe. *A Concise History of India*. Cambridge: Cambridge University Press, 2004.

Meusburger, Peter, David N. Livingstone, and Heike Jöns, eds. *Geographies of Science*. Dordrecht and New York: Springer, 2010.

Miles, Ashley. "Reports by Louis Pasteur and Claude Bernard on the Organization of Scientific Teaching and Research." *Notes and Records of the Royal Society of London* 37, no. 1 (1982): 101–18.

Miner, Norman. *Hong Kong under Imperial Rule: 1912–1941*. Hong Kong: Oxford University Press, 1987.

Mokdad, Ali H., Mary K. Serdula, William H. Dietz, Barbara A. Bowman, James S. Marks, and Jeffrey P. Koplan. "The Spread of the Obesity Epidemic in the United States, 1991–1998." *Journal of the American Medical Association* 282, no. 16 (1999): 1519–22.

Mollaret, Henri H., and Jacqueline Brossollet. *Alexandre Yersin ou le vainqueur de la peste.* Paris: Fayard, 1985.

Monnais (Rousselot), Laurence. *Médecine et colonisation. L'aventure indochinoise, 1860–1939.* Paris: CNRS Editions, 1999.

———."La médicalisation de la mère et de son enfant: l'exemple du Vietnam sous domination française, 1860–1939." *Canadian Bulletin for the History of Medicine/ Bulletin Canadien d'Histoire de la Medecine* 19 (2002): 47–94.

———."Modern Medicine in French Colonial Vietnam: From the Importation of a Model to its Nativisation." In *The Development of Modern Medicine in Non-Western Countries,* ed. Hormoz Ebrahimnejad, 127–59. London: Routledge, 2008.

———. *Médicaments coloniaux. Circulation, distribution et consommation de médicaments au Viêt nam, 1905–40.* Paris: Les Indes Savantes, forthcoming.

Monnais, Laurence, and Harold J. Cook, eds. *Medicine, Health, and Health Care in Southeast Asia: A Modern History.* Singapore: NUS Press, forthcoming.

Morse, Stephen, ed. *Emerging Viruses.* New York: Oxford University Press, 1993.

Morton, Patricia A. *Hybrid Modernities: Architecture and Representation at the 1931 Colonial Exposition, Paris.* Cambridge, MA: MIT Press, 2000.

Moulin, Anne Marie. "Bacteriological Research and Medical Practice in and out of the Pastorian School." In *French Medical Culture in the Nineteenth Century,* ed. Ann La Berge and Mordechai Feingold, 327–49. Amsterdam and Atlanta: Rodopi.

Mulkay, M., and K. Knorr-Cetina, eds. *Science Observed, Perspectives on the Study of Science.* London: Sage, 1983.

Munn, Christopher. *Anglo-China: Chinese People and British Rule in Hong Kong, 1841–1880.* Richmond, Surrey: Curzon, 2001.

Myers, Ramon H., and Mark R. Peattie. *The Japanese Colonial Empire, 1895–1945.* Princeton, NJ: Princeton University Press, 1987.

Nasr, Joe, and Mercedes Volait, eds. *Urbanism Imported or Exported? Native Aspirations and Foreign Plans.* Chichester: Wiley-Academy, 2003.

Naylor, Simon. "Introduction: Historical Geographies of Science—Places, Contexts, Cartographies." *British Journal for the History of Science* 38, no. 1 (2005): 1–12.

Neill, Deborah. J. "Paul Ehrlich's Colonial Connections: Scientific Networks and the Response to the Sleeping Sickness Epidemic, 1900–1914." *Social History of Medicine* 22, no. 1 (2009): 61–77.

———. *Networks in Tropical Medicine: Internationalism, Colonialism, and the Rise of a Medical Specialty, 1890–1930.* Stanford: Stanford University Press, 2012.

Nicholl, Charles. *Somebody Else: Arthur Rimbaud in Africa 1880–91.* London: Vintage, 1998.

Nightingale, Carl. *Segregation: A Global History of Divided Cities.* Chicago: University of Chicago Press, 2012.

Nissim, Robert. *Land Administration and Practice in Hong Kong*. Hong Kong: Hong Kong University Press, 2008.

Njoh, Ambe J. *Planning Power: Town Planning and Social Control in Colonial Africa*. New York: Routledge, 2007.

———. "Urban Planning as a Tool of Power and Social Control in Colonial Africa." *Planning Perspectives* 24, no. 3 (July 2009): 301–17.

Norton-Kyshe, James William. *The History of the Laws and Courts of Hong Kong from the Earliest Period to 1898*. With a new foreword by Sir Ivo Rigby. Hong Kong: Vetch and Lee, 1971.

Otis, Laura. *Membranes: Metaphors of Invasion in Nineteenth-Century Literature, Science, and Politics*. Baltimore, MD: Johns Hopkins University Press, 1999.

Owen, Roger. "The Population Census of 1917 and Its Relationship to Egypt's Three 19th century Statistical Regimes." *Journal of Historical Sociology* 9, no. 4 (1996): 457–72.

Packard, Randall. *The Making of a Tropical Disease: A Short History of Malaria*. Baltimore, MD: Johns Hopkins University, 2007.

Pandya, S. "Regularly Brought-up Medical Men." *Indian Economic and Social History Review* 41, no. 3 (2004): 293–314.

Pant, Rashmi. "The Cognitive Status of Caste in Colonial Ethnography: A Review of Some Literature of the North-West Provinces and Oudh." *Indian Economic and Social History Review* 24, no. 2 (1987): 145–62.

Papin, Philippe. *Des 'villages dans la ville' aux 'villages urbains'. L'espace et les formes du pouvoir à Hà-Nôi de 1805 à 1940*. Unpublished Ph.D. dissertation, Université de Paris 7, 1997.

———. *Histoire de Hanoi*. Paris: Fayard, 2001.

Parthasarathi, Prasannan. "The State of Indian Social History." *Journal of Social History* 37 (2003): 47–54.

Paterson, Edward H. *A Hospital for Hong Kong: The Centenary History of the Alice Ho Miu Ling Nethersole Hospital*. Hong Kong: Alice Ho Miu Ling Nethersole Hospital, 1987.

Pati Biswamoy, and Mark Harrison, eds. *Health, Medicine and Empire: Perspectives on Colonial India*. Hyderabad: Orient Longman 2001.

———. eds. *The Social History of Health and Medicine in Colonial India*. London: Routledge, 2009.

Pickering, Andrew, ed. *Science as Practice and Culture*. Chicago: Chicago University Press, 1992.

Picon, Antoine, and Alessandra Ponte, eds. *Architecture and the Sciences: Exchanging Metaphors*. New York: Princeton Architectural Press, 2003.

Pivar, David J. *Purity and Hygiene: Women, Prostitution, and the 'America Plan,' 1900–1930*. Westport, CT: Greenwood Press, 2002.

Pomfret, David M. "'Raising Eurasia': Age, Gender and Race in Hong Kong and Indochina." *Comparative Studies in Society and History* 51, no. 2 (April 2009): 314–43.

Power, D'Arcy, and P. Wallis. "Sir W. G. Hunter." In *Oxford Dictionary of National Biography*. Oxford: Oxford University Press, 2004.

Prakash, Gyan. *Another Reason: Science and the Imagination of Modern India*. Princeton, NJ: Princeton University Press, 1999.

Prashad, Vijay. "The Technology of Sanitation in Colonial Delhi." *Modern Asian Studies* 35, no. 1 (2001): 113–55.

Preston, Richard. *The Hot Zone*. New York: Doubleday, 1994.

Probert, Henry. *The History of Changi*. Singapore: Changi University Press, 2006 [1965].

Procida, Mary A. *Married to the Empire: Gender Politics and Imperialism in India, 1883–1947*. Manchester: Manchester University Press, 2000.

Pryor, E. G. "The Great Plague of Hong Kong." *Journal of the Royal Asiatic Society* 15 (1975): 61–70.

———. *Housing in Hong Kong*. Oxford and New York: Oxford University Press, 1983.

Rabinow, Paul. *French Modern: Norms and Forms of the Social Environment*. Cambridge, MA: MIT Press, 1989.

———. *Anthropos Today: Reflections on Equipment*. Princeton, NJ: Princeton University Press, 2003.

Rabinow, Paul, and Nikolas S. Rose, eds. *The Essential Foucault: Selections from Essential Works of Foucault, 1954–1984*. New York: New Press, 2003.

Ramanna, Mridula. *Western Medicine and Public Health in Colonial Bombay*. London: Sangam, 2002.

Rambo, A. Terry, et al. *The Challenges of Highland Development in Vietnam*. Honolulu: East-West Center, 1995.

Ray, Rajat. *Urban Roots of Indian Nationalism. Pressure Groups and Conflict of Interests in Calcutta City Politics, 1875–1939*. New Delhi: Vikas, 1979.

Redfield, Peter. "Foucault in the Tropics: Displacing the Panopticon." In *Anthropologies of Modernity*, ed. Jonathan Xavier Inda, 50–79. Malden, MA: Blackwell, 2005.

Rediker, Markus. *The Slave Ship: A Human History*. New York: Penguin, 2008.

Reingold, Nathan, and Marc Rothenberg, eds. *Scientific Colonialism: A Cross-Cultural Comparison*. Washington, DC: Smithsonian Institution Press, 1987.

Reiser, Stanley J. *Medicine and the Reign of Technology*. Cambridge: Cambridge University Press, 1978.

Richardson, Ruth. *The Making of Mr Gray's Anatomy: Bodies, Books, Fortune, Fame*. Oxford: Oxford University Press, 2008.

Robb, Peter, ed. *The Concept of Race in South Asia*. Delhi: Oxford University Press, 1995.

Robertson, Jo. "In Search of *M. Leprae*: Medicine, Public Debate, Politics and the Leprosy Commission to India." In *Economies of Representation, 1790–2000: Colonialism and Commerce*, ed. Leigh Dale and Helen Gilbert, 41–58. Aldershot: Ashgate, 2007.

Rogaski, Ruth. *Hygienic Modernity: Meanings of Health and Disease in Treaty-Port China*. Berkeley: University of California Press, 2004.

Rose, Nikolas S. *Powers of Freedom: Reframing Political Thought*. Cambridge: Cambridge University Press, 1999.

Ross, R. J., and G. J. Telkamp, eds. *Colonial Cities: Essays on Urbanism in a Colonial Context*. New York: Springer, 1985.

Ruscio, Alain. "Du village à l'exposition: les Français à la rencontre des Indochinois." In *Zoos humains: au temps des exhibitions humaines*, ed. Nicolas Bancel, Pascal Blanchard and Sandrine Lemaire, 267–74. Paris: La Découverte, 2004.

Samarendra, Padmanabh. "Classifying Caste. Census Surveys in India in the Late Nineteenth and Early Twentieth Centuries." *South Asia: Journal of South Asian Studies* 26, no. 2 (2003): 141–64.

Saumarez-Smith, Richard. "Rule-by-records and Rule-by-reports. Complementary Aspects of the British Imperial Rule of Law." *Contributions to Indian Sociology*, n.s., 19 (1985): 153–76.

Schiebinger, Londa. *Plants and Empire: Colonial Bioprospecting in the Atlantic World*. Cambridge MA: Harvard University Press, 2004.

Schram, Stuart R., ed. *Mao's Road to Power: Revolutionary Writings 1912–1949*, Vol. 1. Armonk, NY: M.E. Sharpe, 1992.

Sen, Amartya. *Poverty and Famines: An Essay on Entitlement and Deprivation*. Oxford: Clarendon, 1981.

Sharan, Awadhendra. "In the City, Out of Place: Environment and Modernity, Delhi 1860s to 1960s." *Economic and Political Weekly*, November 25, 2006.

Sibley, David. *Geographies of Exclusion: Society and Difference in the West*. London: Routledge, 1995.

Sinn, Elizabeth. *Power and Charity: A Chinese Merchant Elite in Colonial Hong Kong*. Hong Kong: Hong Kong University Press, 2003 [1989].

Smith, Carl. *A Sense of History: Studies in the Social and Urban History of Hong Kong*. Hong Kong: Hong Kong Educational Publishing Co., 1995.

Starling, Arthur, et al., eds., *Plague, SARS and the Story of Medicine in Hong Kong*. Hong Kong: Hong Kong Museum of Medical Sciences Society and Hong Kong University Press, 2006.

Steedman, Carolyn. *Strange Dislocations: Childhood and the Idea of Human Interiority, 1780–1930*. Cambridge, MA: Harvard University Press, 1994.

Stepan, Nancy Leys. *Picturing Tropical Nature*. Chicago: University of Chicago Press, 2001.

Stewart, Jean Cantlie. *The Quality of Mercy: The Lives of Sir James and Lady Cantlie*. London: George Allen & Unwin, 1983.

Stoler, Ann Laura. *Race and the Education of Desire: Foucault's History of Sexuality and the Colonial Order of Things*. Durham, NC: Duke University Press, 1995.

———. *Carnal Knowledge and Imperial Power: Race and the Intimate in Colonial Rule*. Berkeley: University of California Press, 2002.

Sutphen, Mary. "Not What but Where: Bubonic Plague and the Reception of Germ Theories in Hong Kong and Calcutta, 1894–1897." *Journal of the History of Medicine* 52, no. 1 (1997): 81–113.

Swanson, Maynard W. "The Sanitation Syndrome: Bubonic Plague and Urban Native Policy in the Cape Colony, 1900–1909." *Journal of African History* 18, no. 3 (1977): 387–410.

Swislocki, Mark. "Nutritional Governmentality: Food and the Politics of Health in Late Imperial and Republican China." *Radical History Review* 2011, no. 110 (2011): 9–35.

Tagliacozzo, Eric. *Secret Trades, Porous Borders: Smuggling and States along a Southeast Asian Frontier, 1865–1915.* New Haven: Yale University Press, 2005.

Tambe, Ashwini. *Codes of Misconduct: Regulating Prostitution in Late Colonial Bombay.* Minneapolis: University of Minnesota Press, 2009.

Taylor, Charles. "What Is Human Agency?" In *Philosophical Papers.* Vol. 1, *Human Agency and Language.* Cambridge: Cambridge University Press, 1985.

Thomas, Frédéric. "L'invention des 'Hauts Plateaux' en Indochine: conquête coloniale et production de savoirs." *Ethnologie Française* 34, no. 4 (2004): 639–49.

Thomas, Nicholas. *Colonialism's Culture: Anthropology, Travel and Government.* Cambridge: Polity, 1994.

Tinker, Hugh. *A New System of Slavery: The Export of Indian Labour Overseas 1830–1920.* Oxford: Oxford University Press, 1974.

Topley, Marjorie, ed. *Hong Kong: The Interaction of Traditions and Life in the Towns.* Hong Kong: Hong Kong Branch of the Royal Asiatic Society, 1975.

Tsing, Anna Lowenhaupt. *Friction: An Ethnography of Global Connection.* Princeton, NJ: Princeton University Press, 2005.

Upadhyaya, Shaski Bhushan. "Cotton Mill Workers in Bombay, 1875–1918. Conditions of Work and Life." *Economic and Political Weekly* 25 (1990): 87–99.

Vann, Michael G. *White City on the Red River: Race, Culture, and Power in Colonial Hanoi, 1872–1954.* Unpublished Ph.D. dissertation, University of California, Santa Cruz, 1999.

———. "Of Rats, Rice and Race: The Great Hanoi Rat Massacre, an Episode in French Colonial History." *French Colonial History* 4 (May 2003): 191–203.

———. "'All the World's a Stage', Especially in the Colonies: *L'Exposition de Hanoï,* 1902–3." In *Empire and Culture: The French Experience, 1830–1940,* ed. Martin Evans, 181–91. Basingstoke and New York: Palgrave Macmillan, 2004.

———. "Building Colonial Whiteness on the Red River: Race, Power and Urbanism in Paul Doumer's Hanoi, 1897–1902." *Historical Reflections/Réflexions Historiques* 33 (Summer 2007): 277–304.

Vaughan, Megan. "Slavery, Smallpox and Revolution: 1792 in Ile de France (Mauritius)." *Social History of Medicine* 13, no. 3 (2000): 411–28.

Velten, Hannah. *Milk: A Global History.* London: Reaktion, 2010.

Vogelsgang, T.M. "Leprosy in Norway." *Medical History* 9 (1965): 29–35.

Wald, Priscilla. *Constituting Americans: Cultural Anxiety and Narrative Form.* Durham, NC: Duke University Press, 1995.

———. *Contagious: Cultures, Carriers, and the Outbreak Narrative.* Durham, NC: Duke University Press, 2008.

Wang, Longde, Lingzhi Kong, Fan Wu, Yamin Bai, and Robert Burton. "Preventing Chronic Diseases in China." *The Lancet* 366 (November 2005): 1821–24.

Watson, Malcolm, and Mary Sutphen. "Simpson, Sir William John Ritchie." In *Oxford Dictionary of National Biography.* Oxford: Oxford University Press, 2004.

Weindling, Paul, ed. *International Health Organisations and Movements, 1918–39.*
        Cambridge: Cambridge University Press, 1995.
Weindling, Paul. "Scientific Elites and Laboratory Organisation in Fin de Siècle Paris
        and Berlin: The Pasteur Institute and Robert Koch's Institute for Infectious Diseases
        Compared." In *The Laboratory Revolution in Medicine*, ed. Andrew Cunningham
        and Perry Williams, 170–88. Cambridge: Cambridge University Press, 1992.
Weisz, George. "Reform and Conflict in French Medical Education, 1870–1914." In *The
        Organization of Science and Technology in France 1808–1914*, ed. Robert Fox and
        George Weisz, 61–94. Cambridge and New York: Cambridge University Press,
        1980.
Wen, Ku Ya. "Anti-Malaria Policy and Its Consequences in Colonial Taiwan." In *Disease,
        Colonialism, and the State: Malaria in Modern East Asian History*, ed. Ka-Che Yip,
        39–42. Hong Kong: Hong Kong University Press, 2009.
Weng, Xiaoping, and Benjamin Caballero. *Obesity and Its Related Diseases in China:
        The Impact of the Nutrition Transition in Urban and Rural Adults.* Youngstown, NY:
        Cambria Press, 2007.
Wesley-Smith, Peter. *Unequal Treaty, 1898–1997: China, Great Britain, and Hong Kong's
        New Territories.* Rev. ed. Hong Kong and Oxford: Oxford University Press, 1998.
Winseck, Dwayne R., and Robert M. Pike. *Communication and Empire: Media, Markets,
        and Globalization, 1860–1930.* Durham, NC: Duke University Press, 2007.
Worboys, Michael. *Spreading Germs: Disease Theories and Medical Practice in Britain,
        1865–1900.* Cambridge: Cambridge University Press, 2000.
———. "Was There a Bacteriological Revolution in Late Nineteenth-Century
        Medicine?" *Studies in History and Philosophy of Biological and Biomedical Sciences*
        38 (2007): 20–42.
Wright, Gwendolyn. *The Politics of Design in French Colonial Urbanism.* Chicago:
        University of Chicago Press, 1991.
Yeoh, Brenda S. A. *Contesting Space: Power Relations and the Urban Built Environment
        in Colonial Singapore.* Kuala Lumpur: Oxford University Press, 1996.
Yip, Ka-Che, ed. *Disease, Colonialism, and the State: Malaria in Modern East Asian
        History.* Hong Kong: Hong Kong University Press, 2009.
Zinoman, Peter. *The Colonial Bastille: A History of Imprisonment in Vietnam, 1862–
        1940.* Berkeley: University of California Press, 2001.

Index

acclimatization 2, 141
afforestation 4, 5
Agamben, Giorgio 153, 160
Alabaster, C. Grenville 89
Alice Memorial Hospital (Hong Kong)
    127, 128, 134, 137
Ammann, Auguste 135, 136, 261
anatomy 163, 168
Anderson, Warwick 10–11, 111, 217,
    249n11
Annam 7, 83, 90, 93, 95, 131, 142, 195,
    198, 201, 202, 204, 205, 209, 210,
    252n49
anti-plague measures (*see also* bubonic
    plague): in Hong Kong 6, 30–35, 84,
    86, 126–129, 141–142; in India 7,
    61, 72–77
Arbitration Board (Hong Kong) 31, 34
architecture: exportation of European
    models 39, 40, 135, 137; hybridity
    40, 137, 145, 146, 153
Arnold, David 41, 59, 75, 106, 111, 195,
    240n91
Atkinson, John Mitford 83, 84, 90, 249n7
Atkinson, William 46

bacteria: as 'quasi-objects' 3, 4, 228n12;
    cultures of 228n12, 229n34; hybrid-
    ity of 228n12
bacteriology 10, 84, 90, 91, 98, 102, 123,
    139, 140, 146, 147, 182, 217

Bashford, Alison 111, 119
Baudelaire, Charles 143
Beadon, Sir Cecil 114
Beau, Paul 91, 92, 199
Bernard, Claude 138, 139, 184
Bernard, Noël 91, 98, 198, 258n1
biopolitics 105, 106, 110, 111, 112, 119,
    121, 158, 159
bioprospecting 126
Blake, Governor 86, 147
Bombay: 1901 census 7, 41, 61–63,
    69–78, 244n52; epidemic fever
    270n33; housing conditions 245n64;
    leprosy 164, 167–174, 177; plague
    66, 72–77, 108, 115, 119; public
    health initiatives 88
Bombay Improvement Trust 70, 76, 78
Bombay Medical and Physical Society
    271n41, n42
Booth, Charles 5
borders: blurring 57, 126, 140, 141,
    259n16; guarding against disease 88,
    90, 202, 212; hygiene 91, 100, 111;
    colonizer-colonized 2, 18, 19, 35, 84,
    90; crossing 7, 13, 137
Botanical Gardens (Hong Kong) 4
Briggs, Laura 112
British Medical Association (BMA) 164,
    174
British Social Hygiene Council 106, 113,
    118, 119, 121